How to access the supplemental online resource

We are pleased to provide access to an online resource that supplements *ABLE Bodies Balance Training*. This resource offers 15 homework handouts, more than 130 activities, and a certificate of completion, all of which are in PDF format and can be printed out for ease of use. We are certain you will enjoy this unique online feature.

Accessing the online resource is easy! Simply follow these steps:

1. Visit **www.HumanKinetics.com/ABLEBodiesBalanceTraining**.

2. Click the <u>first edition</u> link next to the book cover.

3. Click the Sign In link on the left or top of the page. If you do not have an account with Human Kinetics, you will be prompted to create one.

4. If the online product you purchased does not appear in the Ancillary Items box on the left of the page, click the Enter Key Code option in that box. Enter the key code that is printed at the right, including all hyphens. Click the Submit button to unlock your online product.

5. After you have entered your key code the first time, you will never have to enter it again to access this product. Once unlocked, a link to your product will permanently appear in the menu on the left. For future visits, all you need to do is sign in to the book's website and follow the link that appears in the left menu!

For technical support, send an e-mail to:
support@hkusa.com . . . . U.S. and international customers
info@hkcanada.com . . . . Canadian customers
academic@hkeurope.com . . . . European customers
keycodesupport@hkaustralia.com . . . . Australian customers

 HUMAN KINETICS
The Information Leader in Physical Activity

12–2013

Product: ABLE Bodies Balance Training online resource

SCOTT-9J4L73-OSG

HUMAN KINETICS ONLINE RESOURCE

This unique code allows you access to the online resource

ABLE Bodies Balance Training

Sue Scott, MS

Renewable Fitness

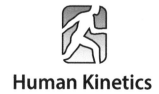

Human Kinetics

Library of Congress Cataloging-in-Publication Data

Scott, Sue, 1952-
  ABLE bodies balance training / Sue Scott.
     p. cm.
  Includes bibliographical references and index.
  ISBN-13: 978-0-7360-6468-2 (soft cover)
  ISBN-10: 0-7360-6468-0 (soft cover)
  1. Physical fitness for older people. 2. Exercise for older people. 3. Equilibrium (Physiology) I. Title.
  GV482.6.S36 2008
  613.7'0446--dc22
                                        2008026527

ISBN-10: 0-7360-6468-0
ISBN-13: 978-0-7360-6468-2

Acquisitions Editor: Judy Patterson Wright, PhD
Developmental Editor: Amanda S. Ewing
Assistant Editors: Lee Alexander and Kyle G. Fritz
Copyeditor: Alisha Jeddeloh
Proofreader: Pam Johnson
Indexer: Joan K. Griffits
Permission Manager: Dalene Reeder
Graphic Designer: Fred Starbird
Graphic Artist: Patrick Sandberg and Kathleen Boudreau-Fuoss
Cover Designer: Keith Blomberg
Photographer (cover and interior): Neil Bernstein
Visual Production Assistant: Joyce Brumfield
Photo Office Assistant: Jason Allen
Art Manager: Kelly Hendren
Associate Art Manager: Alan L. Wilborn
Illustrator: Alan L. Wilborn
Printer: Total Printing Systems

We thank Rose Schnitzer Manor and Terwilliger Plaza in Portland, Oregon, for assistance in providing the locations for the photo shoot for this book.

Printed in the United States of America   10 9 8 7 6 5 4 3 2

The paper in this book is certified under a sustainable forestry program.

Human Kinetics
Web site: www.HumanKinetics.com

United States: Human Kinetics
P.O. Box 5076
Champaign, IL 61825-5076
800-747-4457
e-mail: humank@hkusa.com

Canada: Human Kinetics
475 Devonshire Road Unit 100
Windsor, ON N8Y 2L5
800-465-7301 (in Canada only)
e-mail: info@hkcanada.com

Europe: Human Kinetics
107 Bradford Road
Stanningley
Leeds LS28 6AT, United Kingdom
+44 (0) 113 255 5665
e-mail: hk@hkeurope.com

Australia: Human Kinetics
57A Price Avenue
Lower Mitcham, South Australia 5062
08 8277 1555
email: info@hkaustralia.com

New Zealand: Human Kinetics
P.O. Box 80
Torrens Park, South Australia 5062
0800 222 062
e-mail: info@hknewzealand.com

E3763

To my family, colleagues, clients, and the exercise sciences.

Contents

Part I   All About ABLE Bodies Balance Training *1*

CHAPTER 1   Components of ABLE Bodies Training *3*

There's more to balance training than just balance! This chapter outlines the five components that make up an ABLE Bodies training program: flexibility, posture and core stability, strength for a purpose, balance and mobility, and cardiorespiratory endurance.

CHAPTER 2   Setting Up ABLE Bodies Training Sessions *15*

Now you know the components, but how do you combine them to create a solid training program? This chapter explains how to set up classes, how to select and progress activities, and how to be a more effective instructor.

CHAPTER 3   Ensuring Safety in ABLE Bodies Training *45*

No matter how well you set up your training sessions, they aren't any good without the proper safety guidelines in place. This chapter outlines how to create plans and establish rules, ensure the mental and physical well-being of your participants, and prepare for emergencies.

Activity Finder

vi

(continued)

(continued)

(continued)

ix

(continued)

(continued)

Activity	Page number	Flexibility	Posture and core stability	Strength for a purpose	Balance and mobility	Cardiorespiratory endurance	Beginner	Intermediate	Advanced	Conceptual	Somatosensory	Vision	Vestibular	Gait	Rhythm	Integrated movement	ADL
Walking Sticks	268				✓			✓			✓		✓	✓		✓	
Wall Push-Ups and Wall Push-Offs	224			✓					✓								✓
When Push Comes to Shove	107		✓					✓		✓							
Whooh, Whoohh, Whooohhh!	110		✓				✓			✓							
Words on the Wall in the Hall	68	✓					✓			✓							
You Shoot, You Score!	331				✓				✓			✓		✓	✓	✓	

Preface

So, you want to be an awesome instructor. You want to be confident that the programs you offer will help others live better, more capable lives. *ABLE Bodies Balance Training* is designed for you and any exercise leader or personal trainer working with frail populations.

The *ABLE* in ABLE Bodies is an acronym that stands for Adventures in Better Living through Exercise. This phrase reflects two of my core beliefs. First, I believe that life should be an adventure. Just how adventurous depends on the person, of course, but living enthusiastically and being able to do what you enjoy make life better. Everyone deserves the opportunity to set and work toward goals that have personal meaning. Having purpose and facing challenges are important to quality of life. Everyone values having choice and capability, regardless of age.

My second core belief is from the perspective of an exercise science professional: I believe that physical activity offers incredible tools that we can use to get the results we want. Exercise gives us a stronger, more capable body that allows us to continue doing what we choose and enjoy. Appropriate physical activities can restore, maintain, and improve physical capabilities. Different physical goals require the use of different exercises. Olympic sprinters train for their events by using bursts of speed to create power; cross-country skiers train for endurance using activities that improve their ability to ski at high intensities for long amounts of time. It follows that older adults who want to improve their balance should train using a wide variety of physical activities that engage the principle elements of balance and the tasks of everyday living.

What makes ABLE Bodies a credible program for working with the frail elderly? ABLE Bodies techniques were proven effective in a randomized, controlled trial that used multiple components involved in balance, and meet American College of Sports Medicine (ACSM) guidelines for balance in the frail elderly. In 2003, a grant from the National Blueprint–Active Aging Partnership evaluated the effectiveness of ABLE Bodies techniques. The subjects were 70 years of age or older and living in assisted living or retirement facilities; 38 percent used walkers. Results showed that ABLE Bodies training significantly improved balance, mobility, and activity levels in subjects. A main conclusion was that the multicomponent nature of the program (weaving many types of training together into one program) contributed to its success. This finding is consistent with other research and with current ACSM best practices for working with older adults. Understanding and applying those kinds of ideas is what makes ABLE Bodies training both credible and effective.

I have worked exclusively with the elderly for more than 15 years, and on a daily basis I see the high costs of inactivity and disease. Fear of falling and diminution of balance skills are devastating. They affect quality of life, self-efficacy, physical capabilities, and families and their finances. Previously, little other than strength training was used to bolster balance skills for frail populations. Now there is another tool—*ABLE Bodies Balance Training*.

This book brings together a much broader range of physical activities than has been used previously to improve balance and mobility skills in frail populations. Many activities in this book start simply and become progressively more challenging. This allows for progress to be made, measured, and celebrated. And for older adults who are already fit, the more challenging activities help improve their balance, mobility, and fitness. Because learning is always better when participants enjoy and are engaged in the process of learning, these activities are also designed to be fun and even a little adventurous!

TEXT ORGANIZATION

Before jumping into the activities, it's important to understand how the ABLE Bodies system works. Part I explains the layout of the program and ways to use this book safely so that it best fits your program and population. Chapter 1 looks at the five components of ABLE Bodies training and explains the use and benefits of multicomponent training.

Chapter 2 focuses on how to create programs, set up classes, and progress through activities using the ABLE Bodies activities, and chapter 3 looks at safety concerns when working with frail elders.

Part II provides activities that focus on the five components of ABLE Bodies training: flexibility (chapter 4), posture and core stability (chapter 5), strength for a purpose (chapter 6), balance and mobility (chapter 7), and cardiorespiratory endurance (chapter 8). The activities in these five chapters are outlined so that you know exactly how to prepare for and teach each activity. Every activity includes some or all of the following elements:

▶ **Benefits**—Lists what participants will gain by completing the activity.

▶ **Set It Up**—Describes work you need to do before the activity, such as preparing equipment or practicing the activity a few times so that you're familiar with the steps.

▶ **How to Do It**—Provides step-by-step instructions for exactly how to execute the activity, including the beginning positions, specific movements, and sample phrasing you can use to encourage participants. Photographs illustrate various movements of the activities.

▶ **Take It Further**—Provides ideas for making the activity progressively more difficult.

▶ **Give It More Balance**—Provides ideas for increasing the balance challenge of the activity.

▶ **Keep It Safe**—Offers reminders and tips to ensure that each activity is done safely.

▶ **Live It**—Provides quick reminders of why the activity is helpful. Stressing these reminders with participants will help them live the lesson of the activity outside of class.

As discussed in chapter 2, activities from each of these five areas can be combined to create a solid program for improving balance. The book can be used as if it were a big box of tools with sections for various or specific balance maladies. You can choose to use the tools you like where needed in your class or with your private clients. However, if you prefer more guidance and would like to start with a prepared lesson plan, then appendix A will be particularly useful. Appendix A provides 16 progressive lessons that you can follow when you teach your first courses. These 16 lessons give an idea of how you can combine activities to create effective classes. After a few times through, you will be able to make this program your own, using what works for you and your students.

You can use the Activity Finder provided at the beginning of this book to quickly find a particular activity. The Activity Finder has four sections, shown as groups of shaded or non-shaded columns. Each section of the activity finder lists in the top row categories that will allow you to locate an activity in several different ways. You can find an activity by its page number, the ABLE Bodies training component that it focuses on, its intensity level, or the specific need it addresses. The second section of the Activity Finder lists the components as they appear as chapters in the book and shows in which component you'll find an activity. The next section shows the intensity level of each activity, which increases as the activity works multiple muscle groups or combines different tasks. The last section of the Activity Finder shows which specific needs are addressed by each activity, such as conceptual, somatosenory, vision, vestibular, gait, rhythm, integrated movements, or activities of daily living. Using the Activity Finder should make it easier to locate activities that will fulfill the specific needs of your training sessions.

ONLINE RESOURCE

A companion online resource provides many items in PDF format, making it easier for you to print out items. Every activity in the book is available, and you can print them out, making it easier to structure and plan your classes. The online resource also features 15 homework handouts that you can give to your participants so that they can practice different activities at home. A certificate of completion is also available for you. You can print and fill out the certificate as a "Congratulations, you did it!" reward for your participants. The online resource is available at www.HumanKinetics.com/ABLE BodiesBalanceTraining.

ABLE Bodies Balance Training will change your view of frail adults and what you can do in your classes. I sincerely hope this book will be a favorite resource for you that will inspire you to do more balance activities with your clients. Preventing, deterring, or reversing declines in health and function with appropriate physical activities is one of the most important contributions an exercise leader can make in the lives of others. Take this journey with me and change a few lives for the better. Able, capable living is what we all want. Soon you, too, will be ready, willing, and ABLE!

Acknowledgments

Connections to others are truly what I think makes the world hum and work. We all hold hands with many people on any great project. This may be my book, but my journey to its completion was shared with so many others from start to finish. Family, mentors, colleagues, bosses, staff, clients, and residents all made this book sing for me.

This is my first book. It is such an honor; but there are many exceptional people to acknowledge and thank whose contributions made this book possible.

This project truly began with Rae Rosenberg, an amazing community advocate and friend who saw potential in me and said, "I'll help."

I am grateful to Fay Horak for the amazing opportunity to work with her in balance research and for her expertise and time in reviewing parts of the text.

Thank you to all of my wonderful clients and class participants. You've taught me what I've written here.

Thank you Rose Schnizter Manor and all of your great staff. You guys are incredible. Thank you Terwilliger Plaza whose leadership and support changed my life.

Human Kinetics. How lucky was I to have found them. They are kind and respectful in dealing with me as an author and a person. They are talented, flexible, team-oriented, productive. All those whom I've met and the many I e-mail seem to be the nicest of people that anyone would enjoy working with. Thank you especially Judy Wright, Amanda Ewing, Neil Bernstein, and Rainer Martens, who first found me in Nashville.

Gary Brodowicz, my former professor, thank you for your mentoring, guidance, kind words, and encouragement. You support helped keep me motivated and moving forward.

Wojtek Chodzko-Zajko, thank you for your leadership, stewardship, and National Blueprint Mini-Grant in 2003. You gave me the chance to step up and an opportunity to make a difference.

And my family. A family helps in so many ways. My husband has been amazing; he listens, he cajoles, he supports, he does the heavy lifting, and he can always make me laugh. He often waited up for me late at night while I wrote. My children, Ashley and Jordan, who have inspired me from Day One; and whose lives I look so forward to seeing unfold. My daughter, a recent graduate in exercise science, often works beside me, now making her own contributions to this great field of ours. I give my family many kudos for allowing my computer to move to the kitchen table; so my work could stay in the center of my family. In my extended family there are many teachers; some without degrees; I feel I come from all of them. I know this book will make them proud.

I am grateful to God for making me just who I am. Talented in my own special way and with a passion to make a difference. I love my life and I am grateful for all I have.

It's been quite a journey; shared by many. I hope this work will continue to bless those who find it useful; and inspire others to believe even more in the potential of exercise.

And now you and I are connected as we share this path. Your journey will continue from here. I've so enjoyed this work and believe in its potential; I hope my next journey allows me to do more training and teaching. If you are interested in having me help train you or your staff, please contact me. I hope my work will help your journey be that much better, and that you will make wonderful differences in the lives of those you touch and work with. May your journey be grand, rewarding, and happy.

All About ABLE Bodies Balance Training

ABLE Bodies is a program with many components and options. This manual uses physical activities as if they were tools in a toolbox. I hope you will take the time to learn what this box of tools is all about—you will be more effective if you read part I before using the activities in part II.

Part I of *ABLE Bodies Balance Training* explains the layout of the program and suggests ways to use this book so that it best fits your program and your participants. Chapter 1, Components of ABLE Bodies Training, explains multicomponent training and why these kinds of programs are more effective than single-mode programs that use only strength or flexibility to improve balance. The major ABLE Bodies components are described and explained in detail. Included are flexibility, posture and core stability, strength for a purpose, cardiorespiratory endurance, and, of course, balance and mobility training.

Balance and mobility training is discussed in the greatest detail. This is partly because there are so many parts to balance. There are three sensory systems (somatosensory, vestibular, and visual); a central or integrative system; and a motor system that carries out the actions you want to do. In addition, there are reflex systems that help you stay balanced and upright. Engaging all of these systems in a progressive, ordered manner will offer you ways to improve the balance of others.

Chapter 2, Setting Up ABLE Bodies Training Sessions, focuses on the nitty-gritty work of creating balance programs with ABLE Bodies activities. Do you test or not test? Screen or not screen? What class structure is best? How do you select activities and then how do you progress them? The chapter concludes with some suggestions that any instructor can use to become more effective. It includes suggestions for being more professional, entertaining, interactive, and engaging.

Chapter 3, Ensuring Safety in ABLE Bodies Training, looks at safety concerns for working with frail elders. It begins with always having a written plan and certain safety rules. The physical safety of participants is your primary concern. Physical safety includes watching for signs and symptoms of trouble (e.g., dizziness, nausea), preventing falls, taking turns, and having a fall policy. In most classes, participants will have a variety of chronic health issues. Chapter 3 also discusses emotional safety. Ensure emotional comfort by showing respect for participants' decisions, making sure they are comfortable with the challenges, minding your manners, guarding their privacy, and explaining the activities in ways they understand. Don't talk down to them; watch their eyes and talk to them as equals. This will go a long way toward earning their trust and respect. Chapter 3 offers guidelines for dealing with the most common challenges, such as osteoporosis, diabetes, and so on.

Taken together, these three chapters will enable you to understand the program so that you can implement it effectively and safely. Dig into part I, and please take the time to learn it well.

1

Components of ABLE Bodies Training

Exercise is powerful medicine that can change lives. An effective exercise prescription can improve strength, endurance, balance, function, and quality of life. Exercise science can prescribe exercises to rehabilitate a hip, a knee, or a heart; train a sprinter to be faster; or train a weightlifter to be stronger. Whether you want speed, strength, agility, or simply less back pain, there are established protocols for achieving those goals. Today new exercise protocols are being developed, tested, and implemented to improve the balance of frail adults. Evidence-based, multicomponent balance training such as ABLE Bodies training can play a significant role in that improvement.

In this chapter, we'll take a closer look at each component of ABLE Bodies training and examine how its multimodal approach can improve balance. *Multimodal* simply means weaving many types of training together into one comprehensive program. Achieving and maintaining balance involves many systems working together. The central nervous system must continually interpret, monitor, and coordinate feedback

from muscles, senses, reflexes, motor skills, and our knowledge of the world and then respond to that ever-changing information by using the motor system to achieve goals. This dynamic interconnectedness between systems explains why multicomponent programs work better than training for just one component. ABLE Bodies programming is effective in large part because it offers a multimodal approach to balance.

FIVE COMPONENTS

ABLE Bodies balance training centers on the five components that have the greatest potential for instructors, trainers, and therapists to use in their everyday work with the elderly:

▶ Flexibility
▶ Posture and core stability
▶ Strength for a purpose
▶ Balance and mobility
▶ Cardiorespiratory endurance

Think of these five components as the main compartments in your balance training toolbox. Each compartment

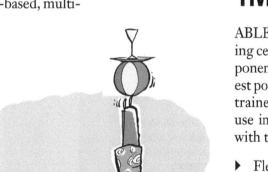

I THINK MY WORK HERE IS DONE.

www.CartoonStock.com

3

contains tools (physical activities) designed to improve balance and mobility in an older or frail adult. The section of the toolbox marked balance and mobility will actually have several subcompartments; the activities are divided into their related systems for balance and mobility, with a few side components for incidental tools to consider as needed. You can use activities from just one compartment to suit a specific need, but generally you will want to use combinations of tools from various compartments to create comprehensive, multimodal programs.

Balance difficulties, also called *postural instability*, usually have multiple causes in older adults. Not all of them can be fixed or positively altered with activities—but many can! For those many possibilities, a multimodal program makes sense and promises to be effective (Day et al., 2002; Lord et al., 2003; Mazzeo et al., 1998; Rose, 2003). Let's take a closer look at the five components of the ABLE Bodies training program.

Flexibility

Wrap an elastic bandage around one knee or an ankle to restrict movement and then try to walk up a flight of stairs or get in a car. It's not so easy. You've got to hike up your whole leg for each stair and you may almost fall over from the increased

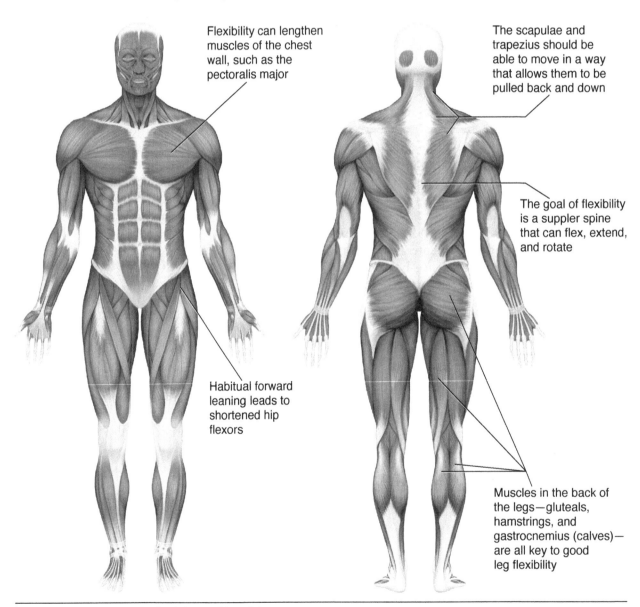

Flexibility can lengthen muscles of the chest wall, such as the pectoralis major

The scapulae and trapezius should be able to move in a way that allows them to be pulled back and down

The goal of flexibility is a suppler spine that can flex, extend, and rotate

Habitual forward leaning leads to shortened hip flexors

Muscles in the back of the legs—gluteals, hamstrings, and gastrocnemius (calves)—are all key to good leg flexibility

Figure 1.1   Key muscles for flexibility in older adults.

lean. Then pretend you're 90 years old. Your back feels stiff and sore; it hurts to stand up at all. Your chest muscles are tight and shortened because your shoulders have slumped forward for many years. You mostly look down. Use this hunched position while trying to take a deep breath or navigate a crowded room. Did you feel limited? Did pulling up a stiff knee to climb a stair change your balance? How about your perspective on flexibility?

Stiff joints and tight muscles often limit function, inhibiting both posture and movement. (See figure 1.1 for muscles important to flexibility). For example, if your back and shoulders are tight and hunched forward, standing tall may not be possible or may be painful. The resultant forward-leaning posture affects where you feel your balance over your feet. Lean far enough forward and you'd need a walker, too. A forward-leaning posture may also affect stride. It is much easier to take a step when you're standing tall than when you're leaning forward—try it and see for yourself. Spinal, shoulder, and hip flexibility may lessen these effects, thereby improving balance and function. By alleviating tightness and renewing functional range of motion, flexibility can improve with gentle exercises, such as walking, dancing, tai chi, and stretching. Participants can attain upright posture and move more efficiently with improved functional range of motion.

Flexibility training is also beneficial for building body awareness. The most effective stretches also focus on breathing and awareness. Ask your participants to relax, breathe, and pay attention to how and where they feel a stretch. Stretching is easy; almost anyone can stretch at least a little. Stretching gets people in the mood for exercise and it feels good. A good stretch with exercise is like a good wine with dinner—relaxing and inspiring! Your participants will feel and move better after a good stretch that focuses on their needs. For all of these reasons, appropriate flexibility is a cornerstone of ABLE Bodies training and a key component in your toolbox.

Flexibility is one if the easiest and best places to start your program. This is partly because anyone can do at least some stretching and feel better and gain benefits for having done it. Increasing range of motion will bring about important improvements in movement and posture. In ABLE Bodies training, participants learn a gentle whole-body stretch in an easy-to-remember routine. They are coached

to use breathing, awareness, and relaxation to further enhance the quality of their stretches. Two of my favorite flexibility activities are Venus de Milo Arms and Supple Spine. You can find these activities and many more in chapter 4.

Posture and Core Stability

Structure dictates function. Posture is the structure of the human body, and that structure has a direct relationship to balance. If you lean forward, your center of gravity moves forward toward your feet. When you stand tall, your weight stays centered over the feet. Positioning and posture affect how you balance and move. In frail adults, a forward-leaning, hyperflexed posture makes them more vulnerable to falling and often precipitates the need for a walker.

Posture even plays a role in mood and confidence. Bodies are integral to self-expression and emotion. Proud, courageous, mousy, sad—these emotions have body patterns that everyone recognizes. Filling the lungs and standing tall leads to feelings of confidence and capability, and building confidence in participants is an important goal. Try comparing fearful versus confident postures in the Feel-Good Posture activity in chapter 5.

Creating activities that help participants use, appreciate, and understand posture is a core value in ABLE Bodies training. Are participants Eiffel towers or leaning towers? How can they successfully change their posture during gait or other challenging situations? When teaching, frequently prompt awareness for posture with cues such as abs braced, ribs lifted, and shoulder blades back and down. Chapter 5 offers many simple tools to enhance posture and build core strength. Good posture is good form for strength training, movement skills, and balance. See figure 1.2 for key muscles in posture and core stability.

Related to good posture is core stability. Pretend for a moment you are 10 years old. You and your 8-year-old brother are planning to punch each other in the abdomen as hard as you can, just to see if it hurts. When it's your turn to be hit, you brace your core to protect against the oncoming punch. That bracing is core stability. Core muscles can also be described as the muscles that cinch in the waistline and draw in the rib cage. Core stability, paired with good posture, is a main component of ABLE Bodies. Core stability helps steady the body against everyday balance disturbances, including head turns, arm swings, or a jostling crowd. A combination of good posture and core stability is a powerful combination for better balance. It greatly improves stability in stance or movement. ABLE Bodies activities for posture and core stability target muscles of the abdominal wall, the shoulder girdle, and the back extensors. Check out When Push Comes to Shove in chapter 5 for a fun, social interactive core-stability activity. This ABLE Bodies activity is one of my participants' favorites for learning why they need a stable core.

Strength for a Purpose

Among other significant accomplishments, strength training is widely recognized as an effective way to improve balance and function in older adults. Strength training reduces muscle weakness and sarcopenia and increases physical activity (Mazzeo et al., 1998; Shumway-Cook and Woollacott, 2001). The American College of Sports Medicine (ACSM) further recommends that for the frail adult, strength training should precede cardiorespiratory training (Mazzeo et al., 1998). The reasoning is that leg strength may need to be developed before a walking program

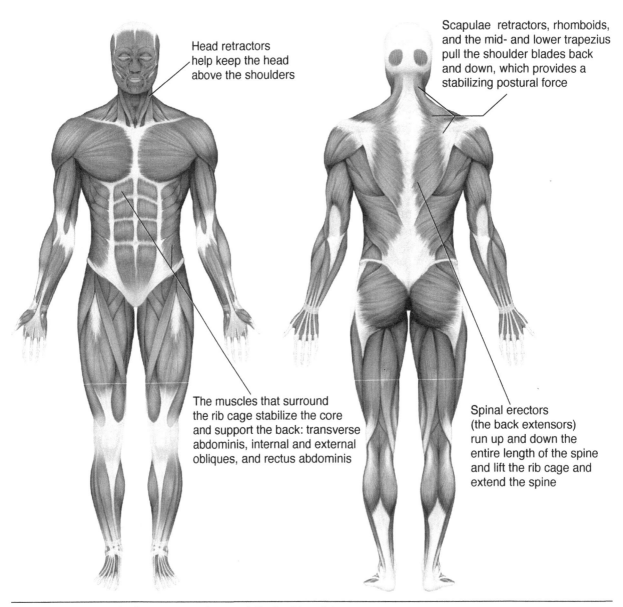

Head retractors help keep the head above the shoulders

Scapulae retractors, rhomboids, and the mid- and lower trapezius pull the shoulder blades back and down, which provides a stabilizing postural force

The muscles that surround the rib cage stabilize the core and support the back: transverse abdominis, internal and external obliques, and rectus abdominis

Spinal erectors (the back extensors) run up and down the entire length of the spine and lift the rib cage and extend the spine

Figure 1.2   Key muscles for posture and core stability in older adults.

can be considered safe. ABLE Bodies training also recommends strength training before balance training for frail adults with balance difficulties.

ABLE Bodies training pursues particular goals in selecting strength training activities—the focus is on balance and function. The strength exercises in ABLE Bodies target muscles used for balance by using them in movement patterns that mimic patterns found in daily activities. Our target muscles include muscles in the legs, especially the extensors, as well as muscles involved in posture and the triceps, which older adults often need to help push themselves up from a chair (see figure 1.3).

The patterns of many ABLE Bodies strength exercises use functional movement patterns. Flag Salutes (chapter 6) uses an arm movement almost identical to that of when a person gets up from a chair. The triceps are get-up-and-go muscles. If participants can get out of their chair, they can go places. As another example, the program could have included squats more predominantly in the strength section, but because one of the key functional movement patterns for this population involves chair stands, we instead focus on chair stands to build leg strength. Teeter-Totter Chair Stands (chapter 6) is a strength activity that also helps maintain mobility by making getting up

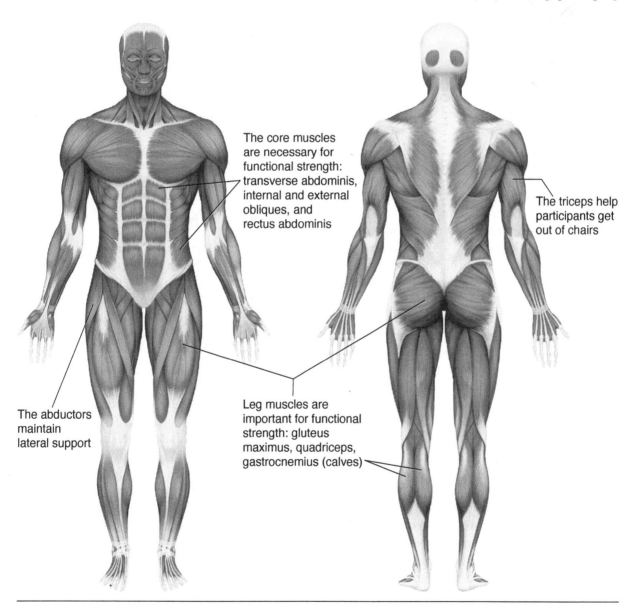

The core muscles are necessary for functional strength: transverse abdominis, internal and external obliques, and rectus abdominis

The triceps help participants get out of chairs

The abductors maintain lateral support

Leg muscles are important for functional strength: gluteus maximus, quadriceps, gastrocnemius (calves)

Figure 1.3   Key muscles in strength for a purpose for older adults.

from a chair a lot easier. It also teaches concepts of momentum and leverage. ABLE Bodies strength training uses chair stands as both a functional movement skill and as a strength-building activity. It's strength for a purpose—a great way to preserve active, independent living!

In ABLE Bodies training, activities to improve flexibility and posture precede strength training. Because these components are gentler, easier, and feel good, they have the potential to build self-confidence. Enjoying exercise activity, building balance confidence, and getting participants tuned into their own bodies is as important as any other components of fitness. Early on, it's important for participants to think, "If I can do these things, then I might be ready for . . . . " Confidence and body awareness is built gradually through linked successes in the ABLE Bodies training program starting with the simpleness of a good stretch and building from there. Hence, strength follows flexibility and posture in ABLE training. The harder stuff can come later.

Cardiorespiratory Endurance

Moderate physical activity accumulated in two or three short bouts of 10-minute durations can be as effective for frail elders as 20- to 30-minute continuous sessions (Wood et al., 2001). Among the least fit participants, even the smallest amounts of regular aerobic exercise can make positive differences (Takeshima et al., 2007). Anything your participants do on a regular basis that is more than they normally do will increase their stamina. Among the least fit participants, even the smallest amounts of regular aerobic exercise can make positive differences. The amount of gain depends on the effort, but even low levels of intensity are beneficial for older adults (Mazzeo et al., 1998; Nelson et al., 2007).

Cardiorespiratory and muscular endurance can put the spring back in an older person's step. Cardiorespiratory training is to be added gradually. The ACSM position stand for working with the frail elderly says improved strength and balance may be necessary before introducing aerobic conditioning, because stamina may well require both (Mazzeo et al., 1998). A myriad of conditions is common among the frail elderly that preclude them from the usual recommendation of walking.

Several gait disorders, arthritis, dementia, orthopedic problems, cardiovascular disorders, and visual impairment are examples cited. Begin endurance gradually, when balance and exercise tolerance are both apparent, and only then as well tolerated by your participants. Be patient and conservative; over time their stamina will improve and make a difference. Endurance may be the last piece of the puzzle to put in place to enable frail adults to stay involved in their everyday activities, hobbies, and adventures.

In ABLE Bodies training, endurance can begin by simply linking seated exercises together in a continuous manner for 3 to 5 or 10 minutes. Or, you might encourage participants to do Walk-Abouts (see chapter 8), where they meet and greet each other a little ahead of class and then simply walk about the room (with good upright posture and stable cores, of course). There are trips you can take with them to the Olympics or Africa (see chapter 8). Your goal above all is to keep participants active and connected to their communities and the things they love to do. Endurance plays a key role, but please remember that it should follow and build gradually from other components.

Balance and Mobility

Chapter 7 explains the balance and mobility tools; it is by far the largest section of the ABLE Bodies toolbox and probably the most fun and unique. Expanding balance training options for the frail elderly, especially for specific balance components, is a primary purpose of ABLE Bodies training.

In chapter 7, the components of balance are divided into several smaller categories, including the three sensory systems for balance, as well as areas of motor coordination such as transitions (weight shifts, anticipatory balance), sequential coordination (gaits and activities of daily living [ADL]), and integration of balance systems. These activities facilitate balance awareness and kinesis, use of visual and vestibular input, coordination for everyday skills, and overall balance confidence in ways that are fun, challenging, and engaging.

You will likely find that balance training is what your participants are most excited to learn. Improved balance will highly motivate your participants. However, you must remind them

Components of Balance

- **Somatosensory or proprioceptive activities:** These activities help participants relate to their position in space by engaging the somatosensory system. Somatosensory comes from two words: *soma* (body) and *sensory* (sensory receptors). Soma receptors are sensitive to pressure (including center of gravity pressure), limb position, surface characteristics, temperature, and changes in position. This proprioceptive system gauges balance and how the center of gravity is situated.

- **Visual activities:** These activities enhance the ways participants use visual information for balance. Some activities expand how vision is used; visual targeting is an example. Activities that reduce visual input cause the participant to rely more on their other balance systems.

- **Vestibular activities:** The inner ear's balance system relays gravity and motion information to the brain. No fitness activity can repair inner-ear function, but some can make living with related problems easier. Vestibular training activities improve how the inner ear performs relative to balance.

- **Gait activities:** These activities address components of gait. Some activities develop just one aspect of gait, and others put several sequential gait movements together.

- **Rhythmic activities:** Under the influence of rhythm, whole movement patterns fall easily into place. Rhythmic activities improve anticipation of and preparation for movement. Rhythm can help participants develop a cadence to their gait and know when to put which foot where.

- **Integrated movement activities:** Every time you accomplish a physical goal, you have integrated more than one system in a coordinated manner. Integrated movement requires coordination of more than one system of balance and sequential movements of muscle groups.

- **Activities of daily living (ADL):** Balance training should underpin everyday balance situations. This category includes activities that teach participants how to make the tasks more efficient, as well as activities that practice everyday skills either in part or as a whole function.

that they're on a journey. Their first steps are to improve posture and alignment and increase core strength. Then they can develop the strength necessary for tasks in balance control.

With posture, core stability, and strength as a background, let's get started with balance and mobility training. How does the body achieve and maintain balance? What are the three main sensory systems (proprioception, vestibular, and vision) that help orient the body? And how do these systems interact with the overlying system that helps integrate the three systems for postural orientation and equilibrium?

We are truly amazing creations! Our movements are mostly goal driven by higher systems and each functional goal requires the brain to automatically anticipate the movement with weight shifts and other postural preparations throughout the body. This kind of anticipatory processing goes on for every movement we make. It is complicated, impressive, and partly automatic—at least until we begin having trouble with one or more systems. Then we need to rely more heavily on the remaining systems and pay more attention to compensate.

Generally a trainer or instructor will be more successful with balance training if they can identify the system that is compromised and then use their activity tools to help the participant compensate for these deficits. However, if pre-testing is not feasible, the best way to approach balance training for untested participants, who may have multiple balance deficits, is to use a broad spectrum of modes.

Think of the balance components discussed in this chapter as belonging to one of three systems: (1) a peripheral sensory system that receives and transforms incoming information; (2) a central system that evaluates, integrates, and responds to that information; and (3) a neuromuscular or motor system that carries out selected goals. The peripheral sensory systems important for balance include the proprioceptive, vestibular, and visual systems. The central, integrative system includes parts of the brain responsible for sensory integration, interpretation of sensory information, and selection of appropriate motor plans. The motor system consists of the brain areas responsible for selecting the patterns of muscle activation that generate joint forces to control limb movements. Continuous interplay among the sensory, integrative, and motor systems maintains dynamic equilibrium. Let's take a closer look at these systems.

Sensory Systems

The three sensory systems—proprioceptive, vestibular, and visual—provide sensory information to the brain about where the body is in space. Specifically, the proprioceptive systems contribute information about body segment position with respect to each other and the surfaces the body is in contact with. The vestibular system provide information about head motion and position in space. Finally, the visual system contributes information about the relationships between objects in our field of vision and ourselves.

▶ **Proprioceptive system.** This system (also called the *somatosensory system*) helps you perceive your body position, your movements, and the surfaces you contact. Sensory receptors throughout the muscles, joints, and skin are mechanical structures responsive to pressure, touch, stretch, force, temperature, and position. The proprioceptive system is an important sensory system for balance control. Where do you feel something touching your body? What type of surface are you standing on? Is your balance point over your toes or your heels? Is your foot here or there? You know the answers to these kinds of questions because your body communicates sensory information to your brain via these soma (body) receptors. ABLE Bodies training for the somatosensory system involves sensation cues, asking participants to pay attention to information they feel from their bodies. Frequently ask them sensory-oriented questions, such as how or where they feel an activity in their body; whether they can tell if the ground is slanted or flat, soft or firm. Ask if they are more aware of the floor surface when the lights are low or whether pressure from their center of gravity is over their toes or heels when standing. Those kinds of questions get participants to tune into their somatosensory system.

▶ **Vestibular system.** The vestibular system refers to the inner ear system for balance. Vestibular senses use information about how the head tilts and rotates to relay gravity and motion information to the brain. The vestibular system includes a sensor for gravity and three fluid-filled semicircular canals oriented in three directions in each inner ear. These fluids move sensors in response to gravity and head acceleration whenever you tilt or turn your head. The system keeps track of how the head is oriented to the earth and how it is moving. For people with abnormal vestibular function, something as simple as a head turn can be a nauseating challenge. Training vestibular function may include practicing slow head turns while maintaining gaze on a stable object, or dimming lights (reducing visual input), or using balance pads (reducing somatic input). These activities increase use of vestibular information for balance. When both visual and proprioceptive inputs are reduced, the brain depends more on vestibular inputs. In other words, when standing on a balance pad in a dim room, both somatic and visual input are reduced and so participants must rely on input from their vestibular system to maintain balance.

▶ **Visual system.** Your eyes gather most of the information about the world around you. Visual input provides a wealth of information about relationships among objects in your view. As you sway back and forth, visual motion across your eyes tells the brain that you are moving with respect to the surroundings. Everyone sets visual targets to help orient them to the world. When learning to drive, for example, student drivers set their eyes on the road ahead. By using this visual target, the car stays on track. When you walk from one place to another, you quickly see obstacles in your path and plan avoidance strategies. The continuous interplay among the sensory, central, and motor systems allows you to avoid obstacles smoothly. You can improve participants' gait and balance by helping them use their visual system to set their path. Cue participants to set and maintain visual targets when crossing a room or negotiating a difficult path. Tell them to look ahead at a goal or to keep their eyes at the horizon. Visual targets are a powerful training tool for improving balance.

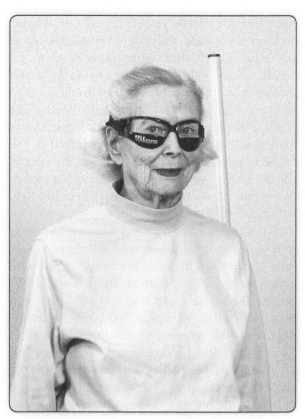

Heads-up glasses may look silly, but they are effective and challenging for most participants. Heads-up glasses reduce a participant's field of vision; looking down while wearing the glasses is difficult. Participants tend to do a much better job of looking ahead when wearing the glasses.

to you, it means that balance is such a tough task that they must concentrate on it fully to keep walking.

To improve automatic balance, ABLE Bodies tools challenge this system with the use of dual tasks, which are basically distractions designed to put motor tasks on autopilot. Distractions make the automatic balance system start working (Rose, 2003). You can probably walk and talk and chew gum, but this kind of multitasking is much more difficult for frail seniors. However, adding some simple distractions while practicing mobility tasks will help participants manage everyday tasks better. For example, counting backward, singing a song, reading wall signs, or tossing a ball from hand to hand while walking are all dual tasks that distract participants from the work of maintaining balance. Another distracting task might be adding competition to an activity. The idea of automatic training is to distract the mind from the task and coax the body into autopilot mode. Dual tasks are fun, odd, and sometimes a bit annoying for participants at first. But keep trying to find ideas that work for your participants and keep their attention. They will laugh at each other and themselves, but they will be learning and pushing their automatic system, and soon they'll want to try it again.

Central Integrative System

The central, integrative balance system, which includes the cortex, basal ganglia, cerebellum, and brain stem, is mostly automatic. Without your conscious awareness, it integrates and interprets incoming sensory information about where you are located in space relative to other objects and initiates an appropriate response using the motor system in order to accomplish goals. A functioning automatic balance and mobility system allows you to talk, read, or otherwise attend to the environment while walking and even while avoiding obstacles. As another example of automatic postural control, when you reach for an object, the body has already prepared the legs and trunk for the weight shift forward, even before the arm begins to move. Rose (2003) suggests using a simple test of the automatic system—the Walkie-Talkie Test. Walk beside participants and initiate a conversation. If they must stop walking in order to talk

Motor System

Balance and mobility require strength, endurance, and coordination of many muscles throughout the body. Getting up from a chair, for example, takes leg and torso strength, but the muscles involved must all work in a sequential pattern to be effective. For everyday mobility tasks, participants must generate a sequential movement pattern, or a rhythmic pattern, that involves a goal, a gait pattern, and a transition from one posture to another. In addition, proper coordination of the motor system involves anticipating, initiating, or completing movement. Practicing all of these parts, in part or whole, can help our participants improve their motor control.

ABLE Bodies training addresses the motor system's function for coordination and agility in a variety of ways. Some activities focus on gait or activities of daily living. Others practice difficult movements, either in parts (Step and Stop) or as a whole pattern (Teeter-Totter Chair Stands). Adding sensory awareness is another tool that can help train coordination and motor skills. Completing weight shifts, for example, is part somatic and part coordination. Activities that use rhythm envelop many systems and can further improve performance. Providing a variety of challenges similar to everyday tasks and obstacles will make work with your clients more functional and effective. Check out Traffic School, Clock Stepping, Agility Grids, or other motor coordination activities in chapter 7 for some new ideas in agility training.

Other Contributors to Balance

Achieving and maintaining balance is complicated. The list detailed thus far is fairly comprehensive, but there are other components to consider, too. You also use past experience, learned skills, reflexes, cognition, and even sound to assist in maintaining balance. These components help us anticipate and select responses that keep us balanced and mobile. The best kinds of balance training will also integrate these components making the training more specific to real life.

Past experiences are profound teachers of many lessons. Feedback from past experiences can affect your choices and self-confidence. Prior experience helps you learn skills that make you more confident and efficient as you apply these new skills to the next experience. The skills and experiences that participants have learned previously will influence their approach to your balance challenges for them.

Built-in reflexes and automatic responses help with balance as well. Automatic balance responses are faster than voluntary responses but take longer than simple reflexes. These balance responses help you stay upright when your head tilts or you lean too far in any direction. Reflexes help keep the head over the shoulders. They prevent you from falling when you step on a sharp object, and they cause you to quickly pull your hand away from a hot stove.

The brain also processes information for balance and mobility from what you hear. You learn about your movement and the environment from speed noises or sounds things make when you touch them. Swooshing, stretching, whirling, clothes touching (such as pant legs), feet touching ground—these are all sounds that give distance perception. You can anticipate the surfaces you are about to walk on based on the sound of it beneath your feet and adjust your strategies for safe walking. Perhaps the most powerful use of sound, though, is rhythm and music. Music can add rhythm to walking and movements, and it is often easier to dance than to move without music. In his book *Musicophilia* (2007), Oliver Sacks, a clinical neurologist, shares evidence that the motor system is linked to the capacity to perceive music, and that the area in the brain that "perceives, processes and responds to music occupies more terrain in our brains than language" (Dunn, 2007).

Enjoyable musical rhythms improve coordination and sequential movement, reduce perceived rate of exertion, increase psychological arousal, and make time fly (Harmon and Kravitz, 2007; Sacks, 2007). Music can help you anticipate each next move with your whole body, building amazing mind–body connections (Shumway-Cook and Woollacott, 2001; Wagenaar, Holt, Dubo, and Ho, 2003). ABLE Bodies' Rhythm and Moves in chapter 7 will help you begin using rhythms. For example, sidestepping is just something bland for the legs to do, until participants begin sidestepping to a beautifully lilting waltz such as Percy Faith's "Theme From *A Summer Place*." Once participants begin to feel the music, you'll see side steps done with the whole body. It's an amazing transformation! Trunks, arms, legs, and heads all move in a rhythm that seems as melodic as the tune. Participants move more surely, with greater skill. For best results, use participants' favorite music and you'll also be adding a pleasant waltz down memory lane. Music can easily be added to activities such as stretching and stepping. Music has its own powerful way of telling the body how to move.

COGNITIVE AND CONCEPTUAL COMPONENTS OF ABLE BODIES

Before moving on, I wanted to discuss one more significant aspect of balance training: cognitive and conceptual learning. Cognitive and conceptual learning helps participants make important mind–body connections. I like to say, teach their minds and their bodies will more willingly follow.

Curiosity and the desire to learn are universal qualities that keep people connected to the world around them. Over the years while teaching and developing *ABLE Bodies Balance Training*, I've noticed that participants love learning new information and hearing the theories behind the activities. In addition, their increased understanding added to what they learned and affected their balance confidence. In other words, the intellectual learning seemed to add another layer to the skills they were developing.

When learning both physically and cognitively, what participants learn with their body is reinforced with their mind and vice versa. Reinforcing physical learning with cognitive learning is important to building balance confidence and it greatly improves the chances they will incorporate these ideas into everyday life. Conceptual learning strategies used in ABLE Bodies training anticipate this kind of mind–body learning. This interactive way of learning enhances cognitive learning and reinforces a healthy mind–body connection. It is an awesome tool.

Conceptual activities are one way to begin with cognitive learning. Conceptual activities provide a unique way of framing knowledge or putting it into a simpler form with a few words. ABLE Bodies conceptual activities are interactive, big-picture ways to tell a story about posture, core stability, or balance. Concepts may introduce the big picture before the smaller details are discussed, or they may offer just parts of the story. The goal is to tell an unforgettable story that makes the big picture clear. Venus de Milo Arms is an interactive way to help participants understand the functional potential of flexibility. Posture Affects Function and Balance will drive home how good alignment affects breathing and every step they take. Torso as a Cylinder teaches that core stability is practical and good posture is renewable. Some activities provide insight regarding visual learning (Eyes on the Prize), and others encourage learning from internal sensations (Coming to Your Senses).

Discussing activities, spurring questions, and coaxing answers from participants will also help them learn using reason and logical understanding. These discussions allow participants to convince themselves that what they are learning is good, right, and possible. Another powerful interactive cognitive tool is asking participants to make a plan before trying an activity. Give them choices for how they'll approach a balance challenge. For instance, for the Alligator Pit or Lazy River (chapter 7), have them select a route and devise a plan they think will work for them. Ask them what skills they have that will help them do the challenge better. This will get participants to recall and use information they have learned previously.

Cognition is a powerful tool we should all use. These cognitive experiences become more layers of learning that enhance understanding of balance and increase balance confidence. Good conceptual and cognitive activities together build toward giving participants that wonderful light-bulb sensation of "Aha! I get it!" I am confident that using these strategies will help you be a better teacher.

Another benefit of cognitive strategies is that they can give your lessons more staying power. A good message should stick with a person if it is going to make a long-term difference (Gladwell, 2002). Conceptual activities reinforce intellectual learning and are great aids when you introduce new material or want to prompt a particular behavior. I think it's best to use these tools like salt and pepper—sprinkled here and there as needed when served. For this reason, there isn't a specific chapter devoted to cognitive and conceptual learning; rather, these important ideas are dispersed throughout the book.

MULTICOMPONENT TRAINING

Whew! By now you've probably found that there is much more to balance and mobility training than you'd imagined. You may even have already concluded that mixing all five elements and a bunch of smaller ones together would make for the best balance training. You'd be right, and many researchers would agree with you. Following is some of the research that helped create the ABLE Bodies Multicomponent program (American Geriatrics Society, British Geriatrics Society, and American Academy of Orthopedic Surgeons, 2001; Berg and Kairy, 2002; Campbell, Robertson, Gardner, Norton, and Buchner, 1999).

Multicomponent exercise programming has been shown to improve function and decrease falls among adults aged 65 and older (Barnett, Smith, Lord, Williams, and Baumand, 2003; Berg and Kairy, 2002; Campbell et al., 1999; Day et al.,

2002; Province et al., 1995; Rose, 2003). Research suggests that group exercise and balance programs incorporating multimodal techniques should be evaluated for implementation in assisted living facilities and retirement communities where group cohesion is easily achieved (American Geriatrics Society, British Geriatrics Society, and American Academy of Orthopedic Surgeons, 2001; Berg and Kairy, 2002; Campbell et al., 1999). Group programs using existing facilities and inexpensive equipment are more sustainable and less expensive than off-site or individually tailored programs (Eng et al., 2003; Lord et al., 2003) and can increase strength and balance and decrease falls among older adults (Day et al., 2002; Eng et al., 2003).

As discussed previously, the technique of weaving together the components of balance is called *multimodal*, or *multiple component, training*. Balance, as you have seen, is not simple. It requires the integration, monitoring, facilitation, and synchronicity of many components. If training for balance is to be specific, these components should be used in integrated ways.

The principle of specificity for effective exercise further says that training should be specific to the goal as a whole or to parts of the goal (Horak, Mirka, and Shupert, 1989; Rose, 2003; Rose and Clark, 2000). In other words, it is acceptable to work on the parts of a goal individually if necessary. For example, if a participant is having difficulty with just one component, such as strength, you can work on just that one part and you will improve its contribution to balance. This is especially true if the training mimics the role of strength in the larger picture of balance and mobility.

Multimodal training is a fairly new method for working with the frail elderly, and to some extent is still being developed. You may remember that a complete exercise prescription needs a specific mode, intensity, frequency, and duration. For balance, however, we know only parts of this recipe. The exercise science literature supports functionally based multimodal training as the best mode. We know too that intensity should be based on the overload principle and that activities need to challenge the targeted balance system and the person to be effective. But we don't yet know what frequency or duration works best. More research will help better define those variables.

Balance is multifaceted, and therefore so should be balance training. ABLE Bodies participants are encouraged to be aware of and use good posture and to build functional strength. They are challenged to move a little differently and to sharpen their visual and kinesthetic skills. They're coaxed to breathe deeply and feel movement and their balance. Sometimes training may include reducing the input of one system to make the others work harder. Movement patterns are based on activities of daily living. And cognitive activities include concepts, common sense, discussions, planning, rhythm, and other ways to connect mind and body and increase self-confidence.

Any of the ABLE Bodies tools are strategies or activities useful for balance training. You can focus on components separately to achieve improvements in weak links, or you can offer a broad range of components for real-life practice. Choose what tools will work best for your application. Create your own emphasis to meet the needs of your participants.

It was not so long ago when, upon discovering deteriorating balance in a patient, a physician would prescribe only strength training. But now we have new tools; and we've come a long way. These new ideas have proven to be effective at improving balance deficits in fit and frail seniors. We have discovered that it makes sense to incorporate many other components alongside purposeful strength training. This ABLE Bodies toolbox is chock full of appropriate, everyday kinds of physical activities that will become your tools for change. Tools that are fun, engaging, and effective. How cool is that?

TAKE-HOME MESSAGE

The ABLE Bodies toolbox is *not* like a box of chocolates. You *do* know what you're getting here. The primary ABLE Bodies components—flexibility, posture and core stability, strength for a purpose, balance and mobility, and cardiorespiratory endurance—are organized into separate compartments of the toolbox. There is a chapter for each in this book. The smaller components are sprinkled throughout. Taken as a whole, this toolbox contains tools of our trade—physical activities that will help your participants improve and maintain their balance, independence, confidence, and zest for life!

2

Setting Up ABLE Bodies Training Sessions

Balance normally happens while you're busy doing other things. You see something you want and you reach for it. There's no need to consciously shift your weight backward and brace your trunk before lifting your arm up and forward just the right number of inches to grasp a desired object. You just do it! Balance it seems is complicated, multifaceted, and mostly automatic. However, time catches up with all our bodies. Balance systems begin to struggle or even fail, strength diminishes, and joints freeze up. Suddenly balance is not so certain. Call in the balance mechanic—but wait, that's you! If the thought of you working on somebody else's balance difficulties is leaving you feeling like a deer in the headlights, then this chapter is for you.

Good balance training, especially for groups where individual needs vary, should be comprehensive and include as many elements for balance as possible. Include activities for flexibility, posture, and strength, as well as traditional balance components and everyday skills (see chapter 1 for a discussion on multicomponent training). Chapter 2 will help you learn how to pick appropriate activities from the ABLE Bodies toolbox that will address multiple components of balance and will raise your confidence in working with the elderly. In turn, your skills and adaptations will inspire your participants' confidence in you.

Chapter 2 is about creating an organized approach to multicomponent balance training. Whether you are an inexperienced activity leader, a seasoned personal trainer, or a physical therapist,

this chapter has ideas that will help you teach better balance. After reading this chapter you will know how to

▶ set up balance training adapted for your group classes or individuals,

▶ progress and pace activities, and

▶ make your teaching style more effective, engaging, and entertaining.

More specifically, this chapter will answer questions about how to set up balance classes to suit both your own and your participants' skill level. It will answer questions such as, Should you test your clients or not test them? How will you set up your sessions? Should you consider seated, standing, or circuit work? What about changes for small groups or for large groups? Would a short series of classes work best, or should you spread ideas over the year? Can you use portions of the program and still be effective? You'll discover how having a clear structure for your selections will help your classroom function better.

Once you've decided on a structure for your class, you'll want some guidelines for progressing activities. Exercise progression is an art. This chapter will provide useful guidelines for progression and pacing and for learning how to listen to a body. What are safe ways to progress and pace various activities? How long should you stick with introductory activities for posture and flexibility before moving on to strength and balance? What are the signs that an activity is too hard for participants? How many repetitions do you use for strength? What is the best level of intensity for a participant? When should participants take turns? When do you push and when do you pull back?

The chapter concludes with suggestions for making your teaching style more effective and creating a message that has longer staying power. Malcolm Gladwell calls it making your message "stickier" (Gladwell, 2000); you want your participants to remember what they've learned for a long time and to link it to what they already know and enjoy. Look for ways to fill your classes with laughter and learning, discussions of concepts, and confidence-building events to elicit greater efforts. These ideas will add "stickiness" to your classes and make them more fun, engaging, and effective. Together with your flair and talent, chapter 2 can make these ABLE Bodies activities come to life in your classroom. I hope you will take ownership of these materials and activities, adapt them to suit, and make them truly yours.

If you watch your class carefully, over time you'll develop a sense of what to choose each day and when to add new materials. It comes with the territory of a perceptive instructor. Your confidence will grow, and in turn the participants will feel more confident and relaxed with you. Your adaptations will make the biggest difference in how ABLE Bodies training works.

Use ABLE Bodies tools in ways that work for your own style and skill and for those of your participants. You and they will take this journey together as you discover and enjoy both your capabilities and theirs. Be intuitive about your choices and trust your perceptions of what you feel is best for your situation. Always err on the side of caution. This toolbox and its contents are in your hands now—the final design is yours. With time and practice, you will become the tool master for your group. Let's get started!.

SETTING UP A BALANCE TRAINING CLASS

So many activities, so little time—where do you start? I always say, "At the beginning."

Many of this book's readers are not physical therapists or doctors and cannot diagnose medical conditions. However, it is still every instructor's responsibility to find an appropriate starting point for their group or client. Starting points should be based on capabilities you can reasonably discern, observe, or measure based on your training and the information you are given. Assessing participants will help you spot exercise limitations, identify risk factors, and select appropriate activities. Typically, some type of assessment is the first step in setting up a balance class.

Instructors can either profile (observe abilities) or test (do actual fitness assessments) participants. This section will give examples of both, and you will see that assessments need not be complicated or difficult. Once you have a starting point based on the group's abilities and needs, you will want to select a class structure that works well for the group. This next section will give suggestions for structuring your classes.

Profiling Participants

Profiling suggests that you get to know participants' abilities using your eyes, ears, and common sense rather than formal testing. You make observations and use available written information or other communications, and you initiate discussions with the parties concerned, including your participants. Putting together this kind of information is a valid way to get a comprehensive feel for your participants and their abilities and needs. Here are some questions to ask and areas to look at that will help profile participants and guide your training decisions.

Learn From Previously Available Information

▶ Are there any recent written evaluations, suggestions, or lists of exercises from their doctor, physical therapist, or occupational therapist? This is more likely if you are preparing to work with an individual as opposed to a group. But even for groups, check for prior testing. The test results can give you insight into where to begin.

▶ What are their ages?

▶ What are the typical medical conditions in your group?

▶ How have previous classes been structured? Seated only? Seated and standing? Up and active?

▶ Do you already have a sense for their needs based on previous discussions or visits?

Observe How Participants Function

The answers to these questions have to do with abilities, strengths, and limitations you can observe. Be your own video camera and mentally record what you see, hear, and learn (or use a real video camera). Make written notes too. What you see is what you will get. If participants move in frail ways, you can assume they are frail, so you'll be starting with easy, seated activities. If participants appear more robust and are comfortable on their feet, you may be able to structure more of the class for standing participants. If you are unsure where to start, assume frail and build from there. Here are some observations that will help your zero in on their abilities.

▶ How many participants use walkers or canes?

▶ Can they walk and talk at the same time, or do they need to stop and talk?

▶ Flexibility—Can they turn their head independently of their body, or does their body follow when they turn their head and they deviate from a straight path? When participants are seated, observe how many can lift their hands over their head without pain.

▶ Posture—Can they stand upright? Is their posture symmetrical or asymmetrical? Do they have flexed knees? Bowed backs? Forward heads? Are they leaning so far forward that they need a walker?

▶ What are their strength and endurance abilities? How many can get out of a chair easily? Of those who do get up, do any wobble upon standing? What percent need to use their arms to get up? Do some participants need to rest frequently? Do they move slowly?

▶ Agility—How well do they walk? Do they walk confidently, or with shuffling, slow gaits? Can they change direction smoothly? Can they slow down and speed up on demand? Can they maneuver comfortably around obstacles?

Interview Participants

Interviews give you more and varied information you can use in setting up the class. They will help you better meet participants' expectations and build confidence between you and them.

▶ What kinds of everyday activities are difficult for them? Do they do housework? Dress themselves? Can they walk across a street before the crossing signal changes? Can they step up and down curbs? Climb stairs?

▶ On a scale of 1 to 10, how would they rate their balance confidence?

▶ Have they been exercising regularly? For how long and how hard?

▶ What kind of exercise have they been doing? Do they like the activity?

▶ How far can they walk without resting?

▶ What kind of help would they like from you? This is a very important question. Be sure to ask it early on.

After these questions are answered, ask yourself what types of class structures and goals seem reasonable. Do not plan class for the most able participants; rather, tailor class content to suit the frailer participants in your group. If several participants have trouble with instructions or are very frail, or if your class is large, then you must keep activities simple and seated. Another option is to divide the class into two groups, but name both of them something respectful and hopefully inspiring or fun. Nobody wants to be in a group called Frail and Old. I've used names such as Sitting Pretty (seated class) and Arm's Length Balance (some standing but near chairs), and Ready, Willing, and Able I & II (both have ABLE elements, but I is much easier and seated).

Testing Participants

To test or not to test? That is always a tough question. Is it reasonable for you to run formal tests beforehand? Testing takes a lot of time, qualifications, and experience. Are you qualified and able to do these tests? Which tests are appropriate and which are you competent at using? Can you interpret the results meaningfully and offer training ideas to help improve identified deficits? If your answer to most of these questions is no or you aren't sure, then do not test; profiling participants is a better option for you than formal testing. Compiling observations, interviews, and other information is a very helpful way to gauge abilities. Remember the goal is merely to know where to start safely.

Individual or Small-Group Testing

For individual clients or small groups it's almost always reasonable to do some assessments before commencing training. One of the greatest reasons for testing is to allow you to measure and then later celebrate results. Normally when you work with a client, it is ethical that you set goals and agree on ways these goals will be measured. Testing is a great way to measure results over time. Clients who make progress will have tangible, measurable results that buoy their confidence and validate your training.

There are lots of great tests that are valid and ready for use. The *Senior Fitness Test Manual* (Rikli and Jones, 2001) has several tests that can be easily used for groups or individuals. The tests are easy to do and are well validated with norms presented. I most frequently use the flexibility, strength, endurance, and Get Up and Go tests. Debra Rose's *FallProof* (2003) offers tests that are more balance-oriented, including the Fullerton Advanced Balance (FAB) scale; Rose also presents a very solid and useful explanation for how to use a modified Clinical Test of Sensory Integration of Balance (CTSIB). Rose's tests are more complex and time consuming than those in the Rikli and Jones manual; they require more subject supervision and the tester should be experienced, trained, and knowledgeable. As an instructor, you should use only what your training merits and what you feel comfortable doing.

If you do decide to test, keep things simple. Pick only a few tests you understand and feel comfortable using. Pick tests that can be done safely with your class size and that measure something you think your training will affect. My recommendation is to choose one test for each balance training component: the modified sit and reach for lower-body flexibility (Rikli and Jones, 2001); chair stands for leg strength (Rikli and Jones, 2001); Get up and Go test for agility, strength, and balance (Rikli and Jones, 2001); and the modified CTSIB for general information on sensory integration (Rose, 2003). Rikli and Jones' Scratch Test for upper-body flexibility also gives insight on posture (Rikli and Jones, 2001). There are other tests you can use depending on your situation and training. Alongside any good

set of tests, remember to use the profiling information discussed previously. The answers from these assessments should mirror or confirm what you see in the profiles. Once you have finished the assessments or profiles, this becomes your baseline and starting point. Plan your sessions according to what is revealed. Then plan to retest in 3 to 6 months in order to measure (and hopefully celebrate) progress.

Large or Open-Class Testing

If you are teaching a large class or a class with constant open access in which members come and go or change frequently, then individual testing would be impractical and cumbersome. Instead, you may want to periodically conduct self-monitoring, or group types of tests. That is, select a few your participants can do easily as a group. Every few months have your class repeat the two or three tests. Participants can keep track of their own progress or perhaps you can keep a roll-call type of sheet for them. Remind them of their progress or milestones and the work it took on their part to achieve it. You can help them set reasonable goals. Periodically ask them to share their progress or any concerns they have. Sharing even the little things will buoy the group as a whole and build connections based on these common experiences. One simple test to try with your larger groups might be Teeter-Totter Chair Stands in 30 seconds (Rikli and Jones, 2001) or, with good balance support provided (such as a chair placed behind each participant or a railing placed in front), you might consider Stand on One Leg (Rose, 2003) or the 2-Minute Step Test (Rikli and Jones, 2001).

Developing Class Structure

Once you know the general abilities of your participants, you can figure out how to best structure your class. For the purposes of this book and particularly this section, I assume the clients are frail and that most participants should be closely supervised (i.e., you are standing by them if they are standing more than an arm's length away from a sturdy chair or handrail). To begin deciding on an appropriate structure for such participants, here are some questions to ask yourself:

- How large is the class?
- What type of class will you teach? Based on your earlier assessment, will activities be mostly seated or mostly standing?
- What can you use for balance supports? Do your chairs have arm rests? Are there railings on the walls? Are there extra walkers?
- How frequently will you work with your class? More frequency means more progression.
- Will the class be short term or long term?
- What kinds of activities do you anticipate doing frequently?
- What equipment do you have? Bands, balloons or Slo Mo balls, light weights, balance discs, balance pads, balls, agility dots, or poles? Will equipment be shared, or is there enough for everyone?
- Will you be able to use music?
- How many minutes long should the class be for this group or individual?

Group Ability and Class Length

Group ability will always play a role in the mix of tools you use and in how you set up a class. In assisted living facilities, 75 to 95 percent of the work might be seated, and the classes should be kept short, around 30 to 45 minutes. In retirement facilities, groups can likely spend more time standing and moving in slightly longer classes. These participants should be able to do about half the class or more on their feet, and classes of 45 to 60 minutes are appropriate.

Class Size

Class size will also always play a key role in how you are able to structure your class. Size will affect activity selection, participant safety, equipment, space requirements, and testing. Activities need to be safe with less supervision (keep them close to their chairs or have them take turns doing activities). Balloons or Slo Mo-type balls and bands are plenty of equipment to manage and are affordable for large classes. Equipment gets expensive and can quickly use up a nominal budget. For these large groups, you might consider having occasional Game Days or Balance Challenge days (such as River Fun) when more

equipment is brought in for participants to take turns using. Or have partnered activity days when participants provide each others balance support when away from chairs.

Individual Clients or Very Small Classes

Solo or very small classes provide participants with more individual attention, greater focus on specific needs, and the opportunity to progress faster because more activities can be experienced safely. For example, by the time a large group takes turns crossing the Alligator Pit (see River Fun), class time is almost over. Small groups and individual participants can do many more activities in the same session length. Small classes can also do more challenging work sooner because you can provide so much more supervision. Testing is more feasible, too. You should plan according to these kinds of parameters. Equipment also influences class structure. Equipment is more affordable when less is needed and it is easier to

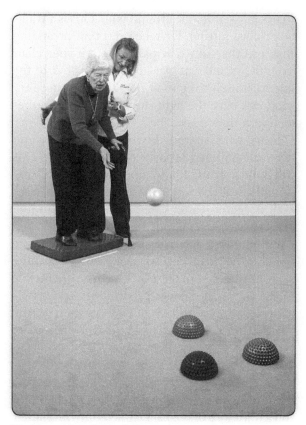

Working with individual clients gives you the opportunity to interact one-on-one, which can create a more meaningful experience for both you and your client. More activities as well as more challenging activities can easily be accommodated under your close supervision.

manage during sessions. Additional equipment such as balance discs, mats, and beams may be more affordable and worth considering.

Almost any class structure will work for small groups. Plan to offer a variety of the five ABLE Bodies components activities in each class setting. Most of the balance activities in chapter 7 were written for groups smaller than 10, so look there for many and varied balance activities to easily do with small groups. On some days, consider setting up work stations, one for each kind of challenge, circuit class style. Plant yourself by the toughest stations to ensure balance safety for participants. You might also choose to provide class themes with extra focus on the group's needs, as identified by your assessment testing.

Large Classes

Large classes (10 or more frail participants in one class) require special planning and adaptations, especially for the balance activities. For large classes that meet several days each week, set up chairs in a semicircle around you. This is a traditional class setting. Do take extra time arranging chairs so that all participants can see your chair from theirs and can spread their arms out to the side without hitting their neighbors. If there are windows, have the light shine toward you rather than into their eyes.

Start with seated flexibility, posture, and strength-building activities on most days. This will build a strong foundation for balance. Occasionally, test the waters with standing exercises such as Teeter-Totter Chair Stands and Standing Heel Raises. After about 3 months, begin to add a few standing activities more regularly. Once the class begins to do standing work, continue to show seated versions for those who are unable to stand. When standing, always keep participants beside, behind, or in front of their sturdy chairs, that is to say, within an arm's length of support.

From there, decide what other balance activities will work for your large class. Begin to peruse the intermediate strength exercises in chapter 6 and a few more of the balance activities in chapter 7. If you have a large, mostly frail audience, you will be limited regarding any standing and balance activities; unless you can arrange for extra staff, some activities cannot be done for large groups in a timely, effective, and safe way. However, seated groups and seated/standing-by-their-chair groups, will still enjoy and benefit greatly from many ABLE Bodies core strength, posture, flexibility, and balance activities. It will not be difficult to derive an effective multicomponent program for your large groups.

Ongoing Classes

Big or small, ongoing classes can be a challenge to keep interesting and effective week after week. Your core group of participants will become people you know well and enjoy spending time with. Camaraderie will boost and maintain attendance, so be sure to have fun and enjoy your group. Basics in strength and flexibility need to be a regular part of these classes, but you have the option of varying what you offer daily, weekly, or even seasonally. These kinds of changes keep your classes fresh and interesting. I've taught a large class of 25 to 30 mostly frail assisted living residents for more than 10 years. Our work is mostly done seated; standing work is done beside sturdy chairs, with a seated variation always shown. Sometimes, though, even I have become a little bored, so to keep it interesting and varied, I began offering daily themes that emphasize different aspects of balance on different days.

- Back at It Mondays—Spend extra time on back and core strength.
- Take It Easy Tuesdays—Work on small muscle groups, single muscle groups, easier exercises, and those 90 percent seated.
- Two for Tuesdays—Do double sets of each exercise.
- Whole-Body Wednesdays—Work on multiple muscle groups, integrating upper and lower body whenever possible. About 40 percent of the class is done standing.
- Tai Chi Thursdays—A few tai chi moves are included alongside other exercises.
- Rhythm and Moves Fridays—Music is played, and sometimes moves are choreographed to the music. About 40 percent of the class is done standing.

- Sport-Themed Fridays—Pick exercises that mimic kayaking, bowling, or skiing.
- Balance Challenge Fridays—always one of their favorites, because the toys are out, I think. But I do these *only* if I can get extra help from facility staff, family come to visit, or a local community service group such as Scouts or high school students.

I always begin with flexibility, and I always include some functional strength work. But beyond those basics, I add variety so that the program is still comprehensive, multicomponent, and fresh.

Circuit Classes

In a circuit class, the instructor sets up various stations with various activities. You might set up a few stations for stretching, another for a warm-up walk, and another as a simple obstacle course. Other stations could be strength activities and others could be simple balance activities. Always place yourself at the most difficult balance station so that you can hold their hands, give them encouragement and verbal cues, and monitor for participant safety. A large-group instructor may find that circuit classes can work well if the activities are kept simple and safe. At the very least, circuits are a fun idea that can add variety to your classes.

Short-Term Classes

You may be offered a job based on a short-term commitment. Perhaps after reading this book, you'll offer your services for a set number of classes to introduce yourself and your skills to a community. You might consider using the 16 sample session plans that have been assembled in appendix A. The plans are 16 sessions meant to be spread out over 4 to 6 months or even longer for larger groups; and can be taught in more than one way. You could pace your participants through the many activities based on your observations and assessments. You choose which activities and what progressions or digressions to use. You could teach 16 progressive classes that are 45 minutes to 1 hour each by following the outline in appendix A. If you do a short-term class, it makes good sense to do pre- and post-testing with your group

to show participant improvement. The appendix A section of preplanned classes is one of the best places for new balance instructors to begin using this book. You get a wide sampling of the activities across the 16 sessions, and I've already done the work of choosing, ordering, layering, linking, and suggesting progressions and digressions for the 16 lessons. You'll still need to apply your own discretions and special touches but appendix A can be an easy, mentored way to jump in and get your feet wet with ABLE Bodies training. At the least, it could be a template you use to create your own great work.

Individual Parts of the Program

Will using just some of the tools provide benefits? Yes, without a doubt! Any one part can stand alone and make a difference in the lives of those you work with. That is one of the great strengths of how ABLE Bodies is organized in this book. Activities are laid out by section from easy to difficult. And different sections work on different specific components of balance. For example, if your group or individual client is very frail and limited, you may choose to use only the flexibility activities. Flexibility can improve range of motion, which can affect posture, function, and many everyday activities. Perhaps your group can only do seated activities. Participants would still benefit from the many seated activities that bolster posture, core stability, kinesis, and strength. Perhaps your clients have lost sensation in their feet from diabetes or neuropathy. Using somatosensory activities (balance pads and hedgehogs) would not be reasonable or beneficial because they are already living life on a balance pad, but most other activities would benefit them as much as anyone else.

Studies of systems have given us the oft-quoted adage that the whole is greater than the sum of its parts. ABLE Bodies training tools can be effective individually and collectively. Use the tools that work best for you and your group. You can work on what is needed and trust that those activities will contribute to the whole of your participants' needs. Or you can offer a comprehensive program for many that will offer something for everyone.

ORDERING AND SELECTING ACTIVITIES

Keep these guidelines in mind when selecting and ordering ABLE Bodies activities.

▶ **Start simple and see what works.** Introduce one component at a time, beginning with flexibility, or introduce a component first with a conceptual activity. It is always doable to start with conceptual and seated activities. If these go well, keep going back to the toolbox for more ideas. Gradually begin to assemble other components and activities into your multicomponent balance training program. Soon you will be creating your own remarkable program.

▶ **Have a clear and specific purpose for each activity.** Any activity you choose should have a clear reason for its selection. Use program goals to choose activities. Generally you'll choose the activity because it meets a specific need of participants or because you're looking to make your program multicomponent. Meeting particular needs likely means you've done some pre-testing. If you do this for a whole group, look at the results to identify common difficulties—usually it is easy to find at least a few. Once you've identified a few common deficits, go to the relevant section of the ABLE Bodies toolbox and pick activities that address those difficulties. For example, if the group is low on strength and transitional skills, choose activities from the strength and mobility sections. If tests showed balance difficulties when standing on balance pads, look for vestibular or visual activities. You may find that strength training activities will help your participants who showed trouble with tandem stances (using narrow bases of support), and then you can introduce visual targeting activities and also strength training for the hip abductors. If poor flexibility was found in testing, go to sections of the toolbox that contain stretches. Focus on specific joints that are tight. In other words, you can look to fix what's broken, or you can take a more comprehensive approach. Either way, pick activities for a reason.

▶ **Use conceptual activities.** Conceptual activities draw a big picture of the idea you want to get across. Concepts aren't like strength training; you won't be working a muscle group two to three times each week for 16 weeks. Conceptual activities get the work done in just one "A Ha!" moment. Usually conceptual activities are not physically difficult. Concepts feel more like recess, a fun break in the usual curriculum. It's a time when participants will learn something memorable that they will think back on later. You will remind them of these concepts occasionally during other training and they will recall them easily because they were so fun and interesting. To keep concepts fresh, use them just once in a while. Use them in the beginning, with new groups, or to illustrate an important principle. Intermittent or occasional use of conceptual activities is best. Think of these activities as salt and pepper—they're a nice finishing touch to what you serve.

▶ **Prepare a variety of activities.** For large groups especially, a variety of challenges makes sense. Select activities from each category as is appropriate for the needs and abilities of your group. Hitting a little of every main category or element will offer something for everyone. There are several important categories in which to challenge participants. As flexibility, posture, and strength improve, continue to add more varied and complex activities from the balance and mobility section of your toolbox. For a broad application of balance components, use a wide range of activities.

▶ **Practice, practice, practice.** Once you discover what activities might work, practice them until you feel fully confident using them. Please don't read through these activities and then take them to class. Practice first by yourself. Rehearse the activity mentally, pretending you are in class. Try to imagine any problems you might encounter or who might have a problem with the activity. Write down what props you'll need so you will remember them for class. If the activity is long and a bit complicated, like Supple Spine, think of the main points or write them down; most likely, the subpoints will follow naturally. Work on any weak points and practice parts you might forget until you have the whole activity down. Next practice with a colleague or friend. Then, try them with your participants.

Order of ABLE Bodies Components

So far in preparing to teach, you have assessed the general abilities of your class or participant, and you have decided on a structure you believe will work best. Your next job is to begin assembling activities from the five ABLE Bodies training components into classes you can teach successfully, comfortably, and safely.

You may remember that the ABLE Bodies toolbox is divided into five compartments, one for each of the main components of ABLE Bodies balance training: flexibility, posture, strength, balance, and endurance. Each compartment holds activities addressing its components. A comprehensive approach suggests you should regularly select activities from each category of activities. I recommend a particular way to progress through the components, especially for frailer participants. Begin with an emphasis on flexibility; it feels good and they begin listening to their own bodies. You can cue them to notice where they feel a stretch and learn what a comfortable tightness is for them. It's a great beginning to kinesthetic learning. Next add just a few activities from the other components; tall sitting exercises are a good start from chapter 5. Work in more posture and core activities, and then begin using more strength

and balance, and finally consider an emphasis on endurance, perhaps as long as 6 to 8 months later. This order is in line with ACSM recommendations for frail adults (Mazzeo et al., 1998) and is the same order in which the book is arranged:

▸ Flexibility
▸ Posture and core stability
▸ Strength for a purpose
▸ Balance and mobility
▸ Cardiorespiratory endurance

Selecting Flexibility Activities

A good whole-body stretch feels good and relaxes us. It directs the focus inward to the body and improves range of motion, which can improve posture and function. Table 2.1 shows key areas for older adults to stretch in order to improve posture and mobility. It gives a few suggestions for activity selections as well. They are my personal favorites, the feel-good stretches. See how they work for you.

TABLE 2.1 Key Areas to Stretch for Older Adults

Target Area	Suggested Stretch
Chest and shoulders	Shoulder Rolls (seated or standing)* Sunbursts (seated or standing)* Lariat Arms (seated or standing)*
Hip flexors	Proud Mary* Farmer's Stretch Lunge Stretch
Hamstrings and gluteals	Gentlemen's Bow (seated or standing) Knee Hugs*
Hip abductors, ribs, and shoulders	(Parentheticals)* Cross Overs* Carry the Baby
Hip abductors	Pull-Aparts*
Spine and Ribs	Supple Spine, Inside-Out Arms* Sunbursts* Wrist Pulls* Head Turns* Head Tilts* Chin Dips*
Calves, feet, and ankles	Ankle: Circles, point, and flex Toes: Wriggle, scrunch, and spread

* = Stretches are under the Seated Whole-Body Stretch activity.

Just about anybody can do and enjoy stretching of some kind; so it's a good place to begin your class. Stretching is an appropriate warm-up that prepares the body for other activities. You can repeat the mechanics of most any stretch slowly, several times, for a relaxing dynamic effect; then hold end positions for a lovely static stretch. To understand what I mean, stop a moment and roll your shoulders around and back several times. Find and hold the tight spots for a long static stretch. Then add head turns and tilts and some deep breaths. Feel better? Could you feel yourself listening to your body? Dynamic and static stretches, listening to your body, and deep relaxing breaths work well together. Bring that message to your groups and clients. For a frail group, a seated flexibility routine may be most appropriate; try the Seated Whole-Body Stretch with gentle, continuous moves and deep breathing. For a more able group, see if you can get them warmed up with a short WalkAbout before your class begins and then do some of the standing stretches.

Keep the flexibility routine simple and easily learnable. It would be great for participants to learn the routine well enough to do it on their own. I like to start with the feet and work up; I pretty much do the same routine each time. The familiar routine gives us time to chat and catch up a bit. Don't forget to occasionally include some of our great conceptual flexibility activities, such as Venus de Milo Arms or Look and See flexibility. It is also important to remind them frequently that nothing should hurt and they should only do what they are comfortable doing. Stretching should feel great!

Selecting Posture and Core Stability Activities

Working on posture is another activity almost anyone can do. "Abs in, ribs lifted, shoulder blades back and down, core braced" is the mantra for posture in ABLE Bodies; and it is one of the most frequent cues participants will hear from you. To sit or stand tall they need to draw their abdominals in and up, moderately, and then lift their ribs away from their hips, bringing shoulders over hips. Next they draw shoulder blades back and down. Then they are ready to brace that posture. Because form is central to all exercises in ABLE Bodies training, tall posture and core stability are parts of almost every activity. Several conceptual activities address core stability, including When Push Comes to Shove and Torso as a Cylinder. Place these activities in your program wherever needed. More instructions for selecting other core strength exercises are included in the following section on strength for a purpose, but in general, select two to four posture and core building exercises for 2 to 3 days of each week.

Selecting Strength for a Purpose Activities

For older adults the ACSM recommends 8 to 10 strength exercises for a wide range of muscles done on at least 2 nonconsecutive days each week, done in sets of 10 to 15 repetitions requiring moderate to high effort (Nelson et al., 2007). For the frail and very old adult the ACSM Position Stand for strength training frequency is 2 to 3 nonconsecutive days per week (Mazzeo et al., 1998). The conservative ends of these ACSM recommendations were used to build a strength training template for ABLE Bodies strength training. The progressive ABLE Bodies strength exercises in this book are presented in order of difficulty, beginner to advanced. Proper form is emphasized, especially core-stable good posture as a beginning position. Participants should be able to feel the targeted muscles as they do the repetitions. Guide participants through appropriate repetitions. You may notice that some of our repetitions begin at fewer than 10 repetitions. For some of the more difficult strength activities, such as Teeter-Totter Chair Stands, our text starts with only 4 repetitions (I use a minimum of 4 repetitions as an arbitrary gauge of effort; if they cannot do 4, I look for an easier strength exercise). The correct number to begin at has to do with the relative fitness and tolerance of the individual. Start with the number of repetitions that are well tolerated, done with moderate effort and in good form. Progress from there toward the ACSM range of 10-15 repetitions.

Table 2.2 shows the key muscle groups for balance and mobility, the rationale for choosing them, and the ABLE Bodies' recommended number of choices.

TABLE 2.2   Key Muscle Groups to Strengthen for Older Adults

Target Muscle Group	Emphasis	Rationale
Torso and core	2-3 choices	The torso and core muscles assist in posture and core stability
Legs	3-5 choices	There are many muscle groups in the legs that contribute to balance and daily activities.
Back and biceps	1-2 choices	Back muscles are important postural and anti-gravity (extensor) muscles. Strengthening back and arm muscles provides strength for everyday activities, such as carrying groceries.
Triceps and chest	1-2 choices	Triceps help participants push themselves out of a chair.

These four categories were selected for their contributions to balance, mobility, and everyday activities. For more optimal balance results, I recommend doubling up on strength exercises for posture, core stability, and legs. Doubling up in one category is similar to doing two sets of an exercise.

To summarize, for 2 to 3 classes per week, choose a total of 8 to 10 strength exercises from these target muscle groups, selecting at least one from each category.

Torso

Select two to three strength exercises for posture and core stability in each ABLE Bodies strength training session. The torso, or core, is the centerpiece of human anatomy. Core and postural muscles include abdominals (transverse is especially important for core support), obliques, back extensors, and scapular retractors. These muscles surround the torso on all sides, providing strength and stability. Increased core strength improves function, stability, and posture. It lessens the likelihood that the torso will be jarred by everyday kinds of perturbations including limb motion, jostling crowds, and transitions. In addition, stable, strong braced torsos reduce many kinds of back pain (McGill, 2007). In chapter 5, you will find descriptions of ABLE Bodies posture and core exercises to strengthen muscles that surround the torso.

Legs

Pick three to five ABLE Bodies strength exercises for legs. There are many leg muscle groups that merit consistent strength training; they are subdivided into six groups for discussion. I have listed them in order of priority.

▶ Quadriceps help strengthen and extend the knee, enabling participants to stand up from a chair. Hip flexors lift the knee, which contributes to step height and length, two vital parameters of gait. A caveat regarding hip flexors: Very often in older adults overly tight hip flexors contribute to forward leaning posture. A balance between strength and length is needed. Special attention to stretching hip flexors should be part of a good program; try the Farmer's Stretch in chapter 4.

▶ Hamstrings, gluteals, and other hip extensors provide for upright posture when standing or walking. They help us get up and go.

▶ The gastrocnemius and soleus (calf muscles) controls sway during standing activities, and their strength and function provide extra oomph during the push-off phase of walking.

▶ Abductors (outer thigh muscles) are important in preventing falls to the side. Strong abductors provide greater lateral stability and reduce the risk of falls to the side. Falls to the side, more commonly than others, result in hip fractures, which can be devastating.

▶ Adductors (inner thigh muscles) also help stabilize side-to-side movement. They are especially important during the single-leg support phase of walking and also provide proper knee and hip alignment.

- The tibialis anterior (shin muscle) helps control backward sway when standing. Shin muscles and calf muscles work synergistically to control sway. Shin muscles are responsible for flexing the foot between steps, allowing the foot to clear the ground and not drag or catch. Shuffling gaits or catching the tip of your own foot, could easily result in a trip and fall.

Back and Biceps

Pick one to two ABLE Bodies back strength exercises for each class. These exercises are in addition to those chosen for posture and core stability from chapter 5. Back and torso work together, all day long. Increased strength in an individual's back and arms will make many everyday activities easier: Lifting, carrying, pulling doors open, recovering balance, and leaning forward are a few examples. Another benefit of a stronger back and torso may be better management of common types of back pain. Coupling biceps and back training is functionally the best option for older participants because the biceps are often naturally recruited by most back exercises.

- The trapezius is the trapezoid-shaped muscle that covers the top and middle portion of the back. This muscle and synergetic other ones, including the scapulae retractors, provide upright posture, upright sitting and standing, and head position. They're also important for stabilizing shoulder function.

- The latissimus dorsi is a wide, V-shaped muscle covering the lower and middle back. They also contribute to upright posture and play an instrumental role in many arm and shoulder movements. Their strength can enhance low back function and health.

- The biceps are the muscles on the front of the upper arm. If you remember what spinach did for Popeye, you know biceps. Biceps assist in pulling and lifting. ABLE Bodies training suggests biceps be strengthened while doing certain back exercises, such as rowing. This will keep the priority on back and posture muscles.

Triceps and Chest

Select one to two ABLE Bodies strength exercises for arms. Triceps and chest muscles work cooperatively in many everyday tasks. Chest muscles do pushing movements and support the arms and shoulders (think of closing a heavy door). And triceps, with support of the chest and shoulders, are the muscles that most frail adults use to help them get up from a chair. I prioritize the triceps as important mobility muscles because they do help participants get up and go! Triceps should be one of your everyday selections, too.

Selecting Balance Activities

The balance section is the largest in this book, and its activities are subdivided into specific compartments of the balance toolbox: proprioceptive, visual, vestibular, and motor coordination. Within these lay interesting cubby holes for tools like Belly Button Training, Rhythm and Moves, Activities of Daily Living (ADLs), and Games. These many subdivisions are mainly for the benefit of personal trainers or physical therapists, who will want to select particular activities for specific needs of one client. Group instructors may feel more comfortable ignoring the subdivision titles and just begin combing through the activities to find ones most compatible with your teaching style and your participants. This will give you a wide range of program tools to use. Using a variety of balance activities will ensure you have offered many balance components and something for everyone. You can start at the top and just work down from there, if you like. As nearly as I could, all activities in each section go from easy to more difficult. Or you may want to use some of these ideas:

Themes

When selecting balance activities, consider using themes. Gait training, Walk the Line activities, Belly Button Training, Rhythm and Moves, and vestibular or somatosensory training all make great themes for a session. Games or ADL activities can also work well as themes (Teeter-Totter Chair Stands, It's a Reach). Tying activities to a theme creates a cognitive learning advantage for participants, because you provide multiple ways for learning one concept. Later you can tie this entrenched lesson to other activities. This is a wonderful added bonus reason for choosing themes.

Variety

Variety is important. Offering a variety of components is what makes ABLE Bodies multimodal. Adding a variety of balance tools means selecting a variety of activities from the balance sections. You can choose to add variety over several classes or in the course of one class. For example, pick two balance ideas, one from visual activities (tandem walking to encourage participants to use visual targets) and something from vestibular activities (an activity in a dim room with the balance pads and mats). On another day, you'd pick activities from two other areas. Isolating and engaging different sense receptors and balance systems is using variety to improve overall function and balance.

Ability

Appropriate training choices and supervision of your participants is your responsibility and those concerns should guide your choices in balance training. Training by ability has risks and benefits. Like the storyline in Goldilocks and the Three Bears goes, you don't want the activities to be too hard or too easy, but just right. We don't want participants bored or scared. To be maximally effective, the activity you select must be doable but challenging enough to keep participants interested, involved, and educated so they will want to do their best. It's a fine line; but getting their best effort on a regular basis gives you the best chance of making a real difference in their lives.

Matching activities with participant's ability will always require your full attention. Both parties (you and they) must consider the challenge to be safe and possible. Start with activities that will be safe and appropriate for the amount of balance safety your participants require. Consider offering different levels of classes, seated or standing balance for example. Aim for activities that suit the midrange of abilities in your class. Zoom in on and experiment with ways to modify or progress activities. Watch their body language and listen to their comments. You'll soon get better and better at matching activities for your group.

Class Size

Class size also will influence balance selections. Pick activities that will be safe and appropriate for your class size. Balance and mobility training in larger classes may need to be limited to seated activities. It is always better to be safe than sorry. For my largest assisted living group I principally select activities from chapters 4 through 6 (Flexibility, Posture and Core Stability, and Strength for a Purpose) and focus on seated sensory activities. Standing work is all done within arm's length of their chairs. Occasionally, I can safely add some of the team games; and have successfully done WalkAbouts with obstacles. I just make sure to position myself at key points or get extra staff to help.

If the group is large, be careful about which balance activities you choose; your participants need to be able to do the acitivity without you beside them. It's always safest to prepare classes with the frailest participant in mind. Keep participants within arm's length of their balance supports, such as walkers, railings, and sturdy chairs. For more complicated or riskier activities with big groups (Walk the Line or River Fun activities),

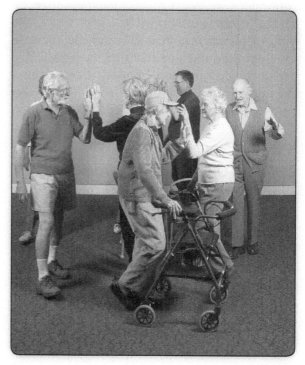

Every participant should have appropriate balance support to feel safe, comfortable, and willing to do the activity you choose.

have participants take turns or get staff to help out. Taking turns is great, actually! It adds a nice social component and gives participants little breaks. Participants rest in between turns while they watch, laugh, and learn from each other. And, you'll note that the person whose turn it is will almost always try a little harder when others watch. Any time you get a best effort is a good time. If for any reason a participant refuses a turn or an activity, honor and respect that choice, as you would any other good decision.

Selecting Cardiorespiratory Activities

Cardiorespiratory and muscular endurance in ABLE Bodies is the last component to gradually begin to fold into your balance training program when working with frail populations. It can begin sooner for more fit older adults (Mazzeo et al., 1998; Nelson et al., 2007). Cardiorespiratory and muscular endurance is the component that will best help build their stamina. If your group has developed sufficient muscle strength, joint stability, and balance to begin to tolerate some continuous exercise, light- to moderate-intensity aerobic training can begin.

Look for activities that will gradually increase the frequency and length of time they are active and moving continuously. The ACSM guidelines are to first build to frequency of at least 3 days per week and then gradually build duration up to 20 minutes (Nelson et al., 2007). Here are two options for meeting these parameters.

Option 1: Offer Cardiorespiratory Programming as a Separate Class

Offering a separate set of classes designated as cardiorespiratory classes is reasonable for more fit adults. Doing a separate cardiorespiratory class will yield the greatest aerobic results, of course, because of its specific structure and focus on aerobic variables. You might consider scheduling these cardiorespiratory classes before or after other ABLE Bodies classes you already teach that focus on flexibility, posture, strength, and balance. If classes are moderate, some participants will choose to do both and their program would be well rounded. Include activities for flexibility, posture, strength, and balance training in your aerobic programming.

Option 2: Make the Existing Programming More Aerobically Productive

With frailer groups or individuals, wherein one or more chronic conditions exist (including severe gait disorders, podiatric and orthopedic problems, visual impairments, dementia, and arthritis) and cause impairments for continuous walking, Option 2 is a better fit. As your ABLE Bodies participants improve their strength and balance, look for activities to make the existing classes more aerobically productive.

Option 2 is to begin creating combinations of appropriate exercises into short aerobic sessions of 3 to 5 minutes. If the aerobic portions are used consistently and are moderately challenging, these accumulated bits of cardiorespiratory training will begin to a make a difference in the stamina of your participants. This conservative option is like interval training, alternating periods of moderate to somewhat hard activities and recovery. For the sedentary frail adult, even small amounts of regular continuous activity can increase endurance, improve quality of life, have positive psychological outcomes, provide pain relief, and help with many disabilities (Mazzeo et al., 1998). Following are ways to add cardiorespiratory training to programming for frail adults.

Linked Exercises

Linking exercises is a creative way of creating moderate interval training. To accomplish linking, do two to four moderate-intensity exercises in a row without resting in between or until you see them tire a bit. Follow the exercises with a brief recovery time (perhaps stretching the muscles just used or doing an easy exercise), and then repeat the work cycle.

- Combinations of easy seated activities include Heel Raises, Crossed-Legged Knee Extensions, Seated Side Steps With a Thera-Band, and Rows With Check-Mark Feet and a Thera-Band. Do 8 to 15 reps of each, and then recover a bit while you stretch those muscle groups. Then do 3 or 4 more reps of the same, or another three or four moderate exercises. Keep an eye on your group or individual to see how they tolerate various combinations.
- Combinations of difficult seated exercises include Kayaking, Balloon Knee Squeezes, and The Up and Up. As participants improve their

endurance, include more difficult exercises in the rotations. Perhaps finish the combination with a few Teeter-Totter Chair Stands.

▶ Combinations of standing activities include Teeter-Totter Chair Stands, Heel Raises, Pendulum Legs, and Kayaking. Keep in mind that linking Chair Stands is especially pulse-raising and if done in combination should be paired with easier activities.

Hard Days, Easy Days

If you work with a group 4 or 5 days per week, consider offering hard days and easy days as a way to consistently plan for more aerobic activity. For example, two easy days I offer are Take It Easy Tuesday and Tai Chi Thursdays. Two and a half hard days are Back at It Mondays, Whole-Body Wednesdays, and Rhythm and Moves Fridays. Another suggestion for selecting activities by difficulty might be Two-For Tuesdays and Thursdays. On those days do double sets of exercises, or super sets (alternate agonist/antagonist muscle groups); and on Mondays, Wednesdays, and Fridays do single groups and more balance or flexibility. Some of these options emphasize strength training but the activities can still be linked for greater cardiovascular effect. Organizing classes this way works well for me and my participants. They know what to expect on which days. There are hard and easy days, a variety of exercises, and a variety of goals.

Exercises Overhead

If introduced gradually, exercises done at or above shoulder level can work well to increase cardiorespiratory endurance in seated classes. Overhead exercise is more difficult cardiovascularly because the heart must pump blood upward and through smaller vessels than when work is done at lower levels. As participants progress through linked exercise bouts, begin to increase intensity by including overhead work. A&Ws at the YMCA or any kind of reaching up are examples of increasing intensity by using overhead work. Intersperse the overhead exercises with lower exercise options so participants will better tolerate and adapt to the work.

Seated Marching

Legs are heavy! Marching is hard work, even when done seated. Start out with 12 to 16 marches per interval (each march is one knee lift). Increase the number of marches per interval over time. Work times will get longer and rest times can be a bit shorter. Watch your participants for tolerance. Are they getting too tired? Check with them to see if they have back pain. Do they know it's okay to stop and rest? Are they keeping their cores braced?

During seated marching activities, always cue participants to keep the abdominals braced and to keep their arms on the chair arms if they need additional back support. As they improve, they can take their arms off the chairs and add arm swings.

You can also vary marching patterns to use different muscle groups and to intersperse easier and more difficult work. Cues for varying marching patterns include "In, in, out, out" (narrow feet, wide feet) and "Big, big, small, small" (big knee lifts, small knee lifts).

More Time Standing

Weight-bearing upright exercise is wonderful for building stamina and specific for everyday mobility. Build up the number of minutes your group does standing exercises, from 3 to 5 to 8 to 10 minutes of standing exercises. Such exercises include Teeter-Totter Chair Stands; Standing Heel Raises; Clock Stepping; Knee Lift, Abs In; and Marching in Place.

Use Music to Set Work Intervals, Pace, and Rhythm

Adding a musical component to exercise can easily and happily increase the intensity and length of the work intervals. Enjoyable music lessens our perceived rate of exertion and does a great job at getting participants to move at a quicker pace than they normally would. The rhythm of music improves sequential coordination and provides pleasant external cues for cadence (Hamon and Kravitz, 2007).

Use Mobility Training

Motor Coordination/Agility training (exercise done moving) can be adapted for cardiorespiratory training, too. Consider using obstacle courses, games, relays, and activities like Walk and the Line, Puddle Jumping, River Fun, Kayaking, Bowling and Traffic School. All of these activities keep participants mostly up and moving for at least short amounts of time. If it's more movement than they usually do and they're doing it regularly, it will begin to make a difference in their endurance.

Encourage Walking

Encourage participants to walk and talk together outside of class. Discuss the parameters for building endurance (build up to walking on most days of the week for 20-30 minutes at a moderate pace). Encourage them to challenge themselves, even if it's just a bit, every time they go out. Suggest that to add challenge and balance training, they can use a different stepping pattern, walk faster, or use arm swings. On some days, perhaps you can find time to put down a simple chalk-line challenge by a handrail on a walkway for them. Even participants with walkers can find doable ways to walk more. They can walk the halls or get outside on nice days. Suggest that they focus on upright posture and walking closer to their walker. When they are ready for more challenge, they can put a big book in their walker and push that. They can even form a walking club, such as the WWWs (instead of World Wide Web it stands for Walkers With Walkers). Assure them that whatever they do on a regular basis, that as long as it is more than they used to do, will begin to make them stronger.

Give them other walking and cardiorespiratory suggestions and encouragement for what they can do outside of class. Could they use treadmills or bikes in the fitness center? Maybe they could play bocce ball, table tennis, pool, darts or Nintendo's Wii?

Before class is another good time to encourage walking. Walking will warm participants up, prepare them for exercise class, and build camaraderie. You can find time during class activities for walking. Have participants do relays or walk an occasional lap around the room, if they are willing and able. To add intensity, challenge them to change directions, take big steps, or use big arm swings.

Whatever keeps them active and moving continuously for at least short bouts of time will make a difference in their lives. The point is that you want them to become a little more active than they were previously. Ask your participants to keep you posted on how they do. Reward them with your interest and praise as they begin to make an effort and then begin to improve. Over time, perhaps your encouragement and guidance will help them build new healthy habits with their friends.

PROGRESSING ACTIVITIES

In the last section we discussed selecting activities or starting points within each component. In this section, we'll address how to progress through each component.

If I were to give you just two overall rules for progressing activities, the first would be to start simple and seated and go from there. Some of the simplest, seated, and easiest activities are the conceptual ones. In the Ball Game, for example, the hardest thing participants must do is close their eyes and guess which ball they have. It's a simple seated activity, but it will still build balance confidence and body awareness. Balance training can begin at that simple sensory perception activity and progress from there if it is well tolerated by your participants.

The second rule would be to pay close attention to how participants respond to your choices. This is how you will learn the way to pace and progress your training. Watch how your participants move, where they hesitate, where they excel. Watch their faces, their bodies, their attitudes. What do they enjoy? Which activities do they say are fun? Which ones do they talk about with their friends and families? At what activity do they try hardest? What activities do they request more often? Other signs for appropriate progressions are more physical. Signs of tiring are obvious if you look for them. Some participants will slow down or stop an exercise. You'll hear heavier breathing and comments such as "Whew!" or "It's getting hot!" If your group is doing standing activities, you'll notice a few of them sit down. They get clumsy or stumbly. They opt out of activities. Do you see pain in anyone's face? Are any participants putting a hand on their aching back? These are signs the class or an individual is beginning to tire and not tolerating the activities well. It's time to give them a rest and use easier activities. Let them recover for several minutes with easy activities or stretches. On the other hand if they look bored, watch the clock, aren't making an honest moderate effort, or seem to have plenty of energy to spare, chances are you can progress to more challenging activities.

Pacing and progressing activities is part science, part art, and part experience. The best instructors always seem to know which activities to add and when to add them. Their talent for this comes with their professional training, but also from hands-on experience. You will be no different and just as good if you are a good listener and passionate to learn. You'll learn progression from what you learn in this text (and others) and from experience; but also hugely from carefully and responsively listening to and observing participants. Notice how they respond to any of the tasks you give them. The goal is that it not be too hard or too easy. A good balance task or activity should capture their attention and challenge them, but not distress them or make them uncomfortable. Progressing exercises means creating fun, new experiences, and even generating laughter, camaraderie, and self-learning. These active listening skills will be your greatest friend for gauging appropriate progression. Proper progression is the art of you listening to *their* bodies.

Order of Components

Practically speaking, there is an order to the scheme of things in ABLE Bodies. ABLE Bodies balance and mobility components are presented in the order in which they should progress. These five components in developmental order are:

▶ Flexibility
▶ Posture and core stability
▶ Strength for a purpose
▶ Balance and mobility
▶ Cardiorespiratory endurance

Within each of these components, you'll find activities presented in order of difficulty. New instructors should start small, that is, at the beginning of each ABLE Bodies component list. Begin with flexibility and some of the conceptual activities, and then branch out as your group appears ready to move on to other components. Take your time working through these progressions, allowing participants to progress at their own pace.

Here is an example for new instructors. Start with flexibility, chapter 4. Spend the first few weeks teaching participants a basic feel-good routine. Guide your participants in experiencing good stretching, breathing, and posture. Use conceptual activities like Supple Spine to show how even gentle flexibility can improve everyday functions. The "Wow, that's cool!" response Supple Spine garners will keep them coming back for more. These early classes are also a good time to use simple seated somatic (learning from their body) lessons such as Coming to Your Senses.

These are seated, fun, and engaging activities with a subtle message about balance and listening to your body.

Over the next 3 to 6 weeks, begin adding posture activities. I suggest sprinkling in a few conceptual activities early on here, too, that demonstrate the value of core stability. I like to say that if you can convince their minds, their bodies will follow. Torso as a Cylinder or Feel-Good Posture are examples of conceptual posture activities that can be taught early. A little later add more active conceptual activities. The stepping and breathing in Posture Affects Function or Parts of the Whole are good self-learning, more active experiences that teach participants, hands on, how posture affects balance and function.

As they begin to understand and value the concepts of posture, begin to teach skills that will help participants achieve and maintain better posture. Teach them how to hold their abdominal muscles in and lift their ribs so their shoulders are over their hips, their shoulder blades are back and down, and their heads are pulled back to be held over their shoulders. Tall Sits or Rock the Pelvis (part of Supple Spine) are great activities for teaching good posture.

In weeks 5 to 8, you are ready to add exercises that will strengthen the muscles used to secure good posture, chapter 5. Posture exercises such as Thumb Rolls and Buddha's Prayer are recommended to underpin core stability. Conceptual activities from core stability include Torso as a Cylinder and When Push Comes to Shove, which are examples of experiential core stability activities.

Starting around week 8 and on, it is appropriate to include activities from Strength for a Purpose, chapter 6. Simple, seated exercises are taught first, such as Seated Toe Raises, Crossed-Legged Knee Extensions, Balloon Knee Squeezes, Rows with Check-Mark Feet and a Thera-Band, and Flag Salutes. About a month later, teach Teeter-Totter Chair Stands. These chair stands are one of the first balance activities and will no doubt become one of their favorites. You'll hear "Wow, that worked great!" as they get up using the suggested rocking motions and foot placement. Perhaps another month later, try Standing Heel Raises and a few other standing exercises.

Once you begin standing activities, you'll need to begin to allow for differences in abilities. You will need to pay attention and adjust to how your group adapts to standing activities. Give participants the option of doing activities standing or seated. Demonstrate options for both. You will soon be able to mix and match standing and seated activities to fit your group.

Progressing Flexibility Activities

There are both seated and standing versions of the stretches. Select seated or standing stretching activities, depending on your group's ability; if you are unsure when to switch, stick with seated. While standing activities add an element of balance, both seated and standing versions of activities provide effective stretches.

Cue participants to move slowly through each stretch. Remind them to use deep breathing as a rhythm to their movements. Coach them to draw their abs in and their spines tall as they inhale and to exhale while finishing a stretch. Get them to focus on their bodies, to notice where they feel each stretch, and how deep breathing can expand a stretch. When stretching is finished, they should feel relaxed, stretched, and wonderfully better. Drawing their attention to the feel-good part of stretching is a handy tool to help them enjoy exercise time and to love and trust their bodies. Just getting them to enjoy, relax, and notice how it all feels is a terrific first progression.

Once participants have good, tall posture and deep breathing when they stretch, add other progressions to the stretches. You can expand the stretches you currently do; reach arms higher and involve the ribs and shoulders more. Later you can add small twists and arcing movements (gentle, slow trunk rotations) if well tolerated.

Once your group is well accustomed to seated stretching consider progressing to standing stretches. Do only one or two standing stretches at first, then add more as participants show competence and comfort. For balance safety, of course, keep them in contact with, or within arm's length of their chairs. Remind them frequently that nothing in ABLE Bodies should hurt or make them feel frightened for their balance. Stretching should feel good and inspire your body to move.

Progressing Posture and Core Stability Activities

In general, beginning posture and core activities revolve around variations of the Tall Sit. In intermediate levels, Tall Sits become Genie Arms, then Genie Arms progress to Genie Arms With a Twist (torso rotations). These Genie Arms exercises lift elbows away from the body up to shoulder height, requiring more work from core muscles. Many of the core exercises also add arm movements that challenge a braced core. Advanced exercises for posture and core would start with the Tall Sit, or Tall Stand and braced-core position but add extended arms and perhaps a twist. These rotating movements are advanced and should not be done until participants show good posture and core stability and can do the activity without pain. Participants with osteoporosis would also be excluded.

Progressing Strength for a Purpose Activities

Frequency: The ACSM recommends that strength training be done on at least 2 nonconsecutive days a week. Two days will be beneficial and are enough to maintain gained strength, but 3 days will show faster gains and may be more appropriate for frailer adults (Mazzeo et al., 1998; Nelson et al., 2007). If you're working with a group multiple times a week, set a goal of strength training on 2 or 3 nonconsecutive days.

A Monday, Wednesday, Friday schedule is optimal and leaves a day off in between each workout to enhance recovery and focus on the other components: balance, agility, stretching, rhythms, tai chi, or other light activities. If you do not meet with your group multiple strength days, try assigning them strength training homework to do on their own or with a friend. Assure them that this additional strength training will help their balance. Perhaps someone in the group might even volunteer to lead a small-group session.

Repetitions of 10 to 15 (8 to 15 repetitions for frailer adults) are appropriate for this population (Mazzeo et al., 1998, Nelson et al., 2007). This is a broad range, which means you can progress according to the abilities and goals of the group and your sense of how they are doing. The first few times you do a new exercise, do 4 to 6 repetitions or fewer, working on proper form and keeping the activity pain free. Then build to sets of 12 to 15 repetitions for easier exercises. For more difficult choices, I think a range of 8 to 12 repetitions is about right, but sets of 6 or even 4 could also be appropriate. Doing multiple Teeter-Totter Chair Stands is an example of an activity that is very tough for many participants. Start with whatever number they can do, say 4, and gradually build from there. Watch them do these and gauge how they are doing as they approach the fourth repetition. If it appears they can keep going, go on to 6, and then decide if you should go on to 8. If you are doing sets of 10 in class, let participants know it is okay to opt out and rest a few repetitions. Some of my participants regularly do reps 1 through 3, rest during reps 4 through 6, and join in again for 7 through 8. If it works for them, it works for me!

We've not yet discussed intensity. Exercise to muscular fatigue is an appropriate intensity, even for older participants. Part of your role is to help them gauge what fatigue means. In ABLE Bodies training, fatigue does not mean totally exhausted. It means that when they stop the repetitions, their muscles should feel ready to rest awhile. There is a fine line between too easy and too hard. By the end of the 8 to 15 repetitions, participants should feel fatigue in the targeted muscle group. The right amount of challenge keeps participants engaged, focused, and progressing. During class or when working with a private client, demonstrate and discuss variations for adjusting exercise intensity to suit their individual abilities. They can, for example, tighten up on an exercise band, change an arm position, change their level of effort, do more or fewer repetitions, slow down, speed up, and so on. Overall, their goal for intensity is to notice and adjust their efforts so they can work tolerably hard at each activity.

Remember to be observant and learn to trust your perceptions of how the group or client is doing and then adjust the work accordingly. You want to get as much work from them as you can in each set, but you still want them to enjoy the activity and be successful at it. Be interactive with your class and respond to their needs. Reacting to how your clients respond will help you do a better job judging how far to push them.

Encourage Good Form

Whatever the exercise, help your participants learn the proper form first. Using good form means that each strength exercise is done with good posture and a stabilized torso. Proper posture and core stability comes before adding any progressions. Good form trumps all else. The tall sitting or tall standing position is the beginning posture for as many exercises as possible. Once participants show good form and then confidence doing an exercise, it should be safe to encourage them to add more resistance or some other difficulty.

Allow for Individual Differences

Allow for individual differences and encourage participants to develop self-awareness for those differences. Tall sitting (or tall standing) might be easily possible and pain free for one person but not for someone else. It is common, especially among frail populations, for crooked backs to be status quo. Ask them to achieve the best possible posture for them. Ask, where do they feel the effort? Is it comfortable? Does anything hurt? The best-case scenario is for participants to keep their torso stable and their backs and legs pain free during strength training. Self-awareness of individual differences will help participants maintain the best pain-free posture and will increase their understanding of what they need to do.

Allow for Individual Choice

Choice will always be a part of safe, effective exercise progression. It's a good thing to have different participants in one class do the same exercise in more than one way. For example, some participants might stand for Flag Salutes while others choose to sit at the edge of their chair; some may be more comfortable with their back against the chair and some might choose not do that exercise at all. A good instructor will show one or two suitable variations for almost every exercise and then let the participants pick their own challenge. Encourage them to make a choice; it keeps them involved and shows they are listening to their bodies. Reward their choices with a bit of praise. It always takes courage to be different.

Allow Time Between Progressions

Don't rush progress or be in a hurry to add on balance challenges. It takes time for strength to develop and for that strength to support balance challenges. Allow at least a couple of weeks, or even months, between progressions. These are conservative guidelines, but trust me; I have been there, and been there in too big a hurry. Participants need time to develop strength and skill. Expect significant improvement in strength to take 3 to 4 months of regular training. Take the time; it's a good decision that will avoid injury. Good things come to those who wait!

Types of Modifications

The ABLE Bodies strength exercises in chapters 5 and 6 will normally show two distinct progressions, following the original description of each exercise. The first modification suggests ways to make the exercise more difficult, or Take it Further, in terms of the amount of strength needed. The second modification, Give It More Balance, suggests ways to incorporate more balance challenge into the activity. Safe progression would be trying just the basic exercise first, and if it seems too easy, then work through the variations until you find a suitable starting point for your group or individual. Progress from there. Normally it is best to allow at least a couple of weeks or even a month before adding additional progressions. Take your time; it will be time well spent and it will allow your participants time to develop the skills and strength they need without experiencing overuse types of injuries.

Progressing from Beginner to Advanced Programs

Progress strength activities from easier, single-muscle activities to more complex motor patterns. The simplest, or beginning, ABLE Bodies strength activities are those that work just one muscle group at a time, and they are always listed at the top of each muscle grouping. Do these simplest activities first, without any added difficulty or balance progression. Help your participants master one exercise before progressing to another. A well-done exercise has proper form and breathing and can be done with good balance confidence. Early on, for example, if your group is quite frail, train the leg muscle groups separately (e.g., hamstrings and quadriceps are trained separately). This will build strength in that individual muscle group so that later it can contribute to a whole-leg exercise that involves many leg muscles.

An intermediate program of 8 to 10 mixed types of exercises would begin to add more difficulty to existing exercise selections and include standing exercises. Intermediate activities also begin to include simple, functional whole-leg activities, like Teeter-Totter Chair Stands. Consider adding intermediate work after 6 to 12 weeks of consistently working on the beginning exercises. Also consider having some of your participants do some intermediate back and arm exercises standing. Standing for upper body exercises can be a simple way to add balance and increase the strength of core muscles. I don't think you'll find it too disruptive to have some participants seated while others stand; rather, it's a nice way for people to feel comfortable doing what they prefer.

Finally (conservatively in months 5 and forward), move on to exercises that are more complex or that use various encumbrances. Examples of complex tasks and encumbrances are activities performed while moving, or with a narrower base of support, or that combined upper and lower body work, using dual tasks, heads-up or sunglasses, or otherwise requiring more balance. Complex strength exercises work several muscle groups at one time and may also involve standing or moving activities that keep time with music. Advanced functional activities are exercises such as modified lunges, clock stepping, and stepping up on steps.

Progressing From Seated to Standing Exercises

Seated exercises and a wide variety of core exercises will make up the greater part of your class for frail adults. However, because balance and mobility are the ultimate goals, some exercises need to be progressed to a point where they are done standing and moving, provided that participants are able. Learning to get up from a chair using an exercise such as Teeter-Totter Chair Stands can be an early link between seated and standing exercise. Standing Heel Raises are one of the best first standing exercises. As you begin to blend in standing work, you are transitioning the group from beginning to intermediate exercises. As time goes by, you will often find yourself mixing levels together. I think it is reasonable to strive to maintain your classes at the intermediate range. It may be that only a few star pupils would be able to do advanced levels, so in a group setting, meeting their needs would sacrifice the needs of the greater good. In any standing or moving situations, be sure everyone has adequate balance support to be safe.

Progressing Leg Exercises

Beginning-level leg exercises are seated, single-muscle-group exercises such as Seated Heel and Toe Raises or Heel Drags. But beginning exercises can be gradually progressed to also include some standing exercises. Teeter-Totter Chair Stands are in the beginning group because they are so functional and they are a good transition between seated and standing and between beginning and intermediate strength. Intermediate exercises begin with simple standing exercises, such as Heel Raises done standing and Weight Shifts. Intermediate begins to blend into advanced levels for legs by introducing more complex whole-leg exercises, including more difficult chair stands, Sidestepping with Thera-Bands, kayaking while walking, or walking with Heads-up glasses. Rhythmical activities done moving can be intermediate or advanced, because music makes movement easier. If you are unsure, supervise closely until you are sure.

Progressing Upper-Body Exercises

Begin upper-body activities seated with exercises that keep the arms at shoulder level or below. As participants' backs and shoulders become stronger and their postures improve, intermediate exercises will add overhead work. Make sure the activities can be done pain free. Advanced variations would include doing some of the exercises while standing or combining upper and lower body together, such as Pendulum Legs with arm raises.

Progressing Balance Activities

Progress balance activities as you would our other activities—conservatively and carefully. There's no rush. Begin with the easiest, most core-stable activities done seated and progress from there.

Safety, enjoyment, trust, and confidence are far more important to building successful classes and balance confidence than pulling out all the balance toys, because *you* can't wait. Here are a few guidelines that may help you decipher which ABLE activities are beginning, intermediate, or advanced. The dividing lines tend to blur a bit in real training, so it's best to think of the activities as being points along a continuum.

In general, think of beginners first doing seated activities and then progressing to activities that can be done with one hand on a chair. Intermediates still are standing by chairs quite a bit, but they are also able to do limited, closely supervised activities away from the chair. Taking turns, using handrails, and holding hands is still a big part of intermediate-level activities. By the end of intermediate training, participants are moving more independently and with more confidence. Advanced training is for participants who move about much more independently. It's not that you shouldn't still hover and hold hands, but these participants can and will feel ready to do things like Kayaking through Poles and lots of things with River Fun.

As early as week 2, select easy, seated, conceptual, and kinesthetic activities. Some examples of easy conceptual and kinesthetic (somatosensory) activities include Coming to Your Senses and the Ball Game. These seated activities target the sensory systems and get your participants listening to their bodies. When beginner level participants are ready to do standing balance exercises, pick the easiest standing activities first, such as Heel Raises, Marching in Place, or Clock Stepping. These can be done with hands on their chair. Opposing Circles, Heavy Hands, and Walking Sticks are a little more difficult because they are walking independently, but the activity is still quite easy. Single-Line Challenges under Walk the Line introduces activities that have a narrower base of support, but because these activities are done beside a chair, they'd be right on the line between beginner and intermediate work. Be sure you feel confident about your choices and always provide plenty of balance support for your participants' confidence and safety.

Moving on to intermediate activities, check out activities of daily living (ADLs). Many of the ADL standing activities can be done beside a chair, too. Traffic School is a good transition test for introducing intermediate activities. On days you have help, consider including group games, such as relays or River Fun. Puddle Jumping (where participants are asked to control momentum) would be on the difficult end of intermediates. Intermediates should be able to do some dual tasks, tasks with dim lights, easy tasks on balance pads, and so on, but they need lots of hands-on supervision by you.

Advanced activities would summarly be all the rest, of course, or just making intermediate ones more difficult. Kayaking through Poles, River Fun, and using balance pads and hedge hogs are not nearly so scary to these folk, anymore. But taking turns is still the way to go. That's why they have you!

The ACSM's position stand on balance training also gives useful guidelines for progressing balance training with frail elders; ABLE Bodies mirrors those progressions. The position stand says that while it is not currently known exactly what series of exercises will best improve balance, in general, "the use of progressively more difficult postures that gradually reduce the base of support, and require dynamic movements that disturb the center of gravity, stress muscle groups important to posture, and reduce sensory input conform best to the accepted theories of balance control and adaptation" is recommended (Mazzeo et al., 1998). To provide you with guidelines to work with those recommendations more readily, I have broken their list into categories with activity suggestions for progressively meeting the ACSM's list of parameters. Again, remember to take your time—months of it—moving through these suggestions.

Progress Activities From Stable to Unstable Positions

▸ Progress from seated with back against the back of the chair, to tall-seated away from the back of the chair, to tall-seated at edge of chair, to edge of chair with feet tandem, to tandem feet with heels lifted. Progress from seated on a chair, to seated on a balance disc with both feet flat on floor, to tandem feet, to heels lifted. (For one-on-one training use a stability ball on a holder next and progress to stability ball with no holder.)

▸ Strength exercises can be transitioned from stable to unstable by progressing from seated (see suggestions above that may be considered) to standing to moving strength activities.

▸ Balance activities, such as gait training or tandem walking, progress from moving quickly, to moving very slowly (because it's easier to walk quickly than very slowly), to maintaining an unstable position standing still.

▸ Progress from standing with feet shoulder-width apart, to a narrow stance, to an offset stance, to a tandem stance, to one foot, to standing on one foot with the other leg moving.

▸ Progress arm positions from arms down, to arms out to the side, to arms overhead, to arms moving. Progress from not using arm swings, to using arm swings, to exaggerating arm swings.

▸ Progress from standing on the floor, to standing on plush carpet, to walking on a lawn, to standing on a firm balance mat, to standing on a softer (less dense) balance mat or pad. On each surface, work through various arm and foot progressions. Use a variety of floor surfaces and balance mats and even shapes of mats, as well as poly beams or foam beams.

▸ Progress from easy movement patterns to more difficult patterns, such as from straight lines to curved lines, side steps to box steps, short steps to long steps, regular steps to high stepping marches, step-together-steps to step-together-step-turns to allemandes left and right. There's almost always a next step!

Challenge Their Center of Gravity

▸ Pick activities that perturb participants' center of gravity. This doesn't mean try to push them over, but it could mean to give them little pushes. Practicing dealing with these little perturbations helps them learn to recover and maintain balance control. There are many ABLE Bodies activities that will perturb your participants' balance. When Push Comes to Shove is a good first activity, and seated kayaking, High Fives, and tossing games (such as Bop the Hedge Hogs) are good activities for beginners, provided

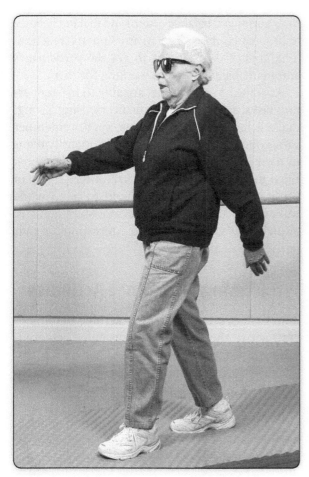

Unstable surfaces, such as balance mats, increase the balance challenge of many activities. Be sure to provide balance support, such as handrails, when using unstable surfaces. Also shown here are big arm swings and reduced visual input.

of inside-out type of somatic learning. Belly Button Training has a range of easy to difficult activities to try.

Target Muscles Specific to Balance

▸ Pick activities that stress important muscles for balance (legs and upright posture muscles). Progress these as discussed earlier, from single muscle groups when necessary to multiple muscle groups, and from seated to standing to moving. Strength for a purpose is detailed in chapter 6 where the target groups are addressed with specific exercises.

▸ For dorsiflexors (calf muscles), use progressive variations of heel raises (seated, standing, rocking, and moving). For the adductors and abductors (inner and outer thighs), use variations of sidestepping (seated, standing, Clock Stepping, Pendulum Legs). For quads work from Crossed-Leg Knee Extensions to Teeter-Totter Chair Stands to Modified Lunges. For quads and hip extensors progress from Seated Leg Press with Thera-Band to Teeter-Totter Chair Stands, Shallow Squats, and then Front Step-Ups.

▸ For muscles that help maintain upright posture, use various rowing actions (Bows and Arrows) seated then standing to strengthen shoulder blade retractors; and use Tall Sit variations and reaching-up activities for back extensors, like Push Up and Think Thin.

Encourage Use of All Sensory Systems

▸ Pick activities that engage and challenge the sensory systems for balance: Vision, somatosensory, and vestibular. For group settings especially, mix and match your choices with these systems so there is something for everyone.

▸ Some activities enhance how a person uses one system. The intermediate activities Eyes on the Prize and Follow the Light help participants use vision more effectively by using visual targets. Belly Button Training calls their attention to how they *feel* their balance within their bodies, thereby engaging and enhancing somatic perception.

▸ Other activities restrict one system in order to facilitate another. Most people rely primarily on vision for balance. So reducing some usual

there is plenty of balance support near by for standing activities. Marching in Place and Puddle Jumping are more intermediate examples of activities, because there is more balance risk or change in position.

▸ Perturb participants by using changes in direction, speed, or limb movement. Progress from kayaking seated, Heavy Hands, Traffic School, Words on the Wall in the Hall, walking with big arm swings, to kayaking standing in front of their chair, or games. Some more challenging center-of-gravity movement patterns might be Shake a Leg, Agility Grids, tandem walking (Walk the Line), kayaking moving, using balance pads, and so on.

▸ Belly Button Training also fits in this category as it gets individuals to notice and manipulate their center of gravity for a sort

visual input by dimming lights or wearing sunglasses or Heads-up glasses will cause participants to rely more on their somatosensory and vestibular systems. In dimmed rooms (seated activities for beginners or walking for intermediates), they will be more aware of the sensations their feet feel from the floor and their vestibular system is also challenged. Activities with closed eyes (done seated with beginners or standing with very good balance support for advanced) engage the vestibular system and somatic senses to assist with balance maintenance. Balance pads and mats are usually the most challenging activities for older adults; the soft mats restrict somatic input, and thereby engage the vestibular system. Balance mats with reduced vision are the most difficult of challenges.

▶ Use assessments to target specific deficits and select activities that can facilitate, challenge, and improve the participant's needs. Isolating and engaging different sensory receptors and balance systems can improve how those systems function. Balance instructors who have the skill and training to do assessments, can work with participants to improve their weakest link. If there is a system that is no longer operable, you can help a participant learn to cope with their loss. For example, some inner ear problems are permanent. No amount of closed eyes activities will restore function to their inner ear. But practicing slow head turns may help. Diabetics often have severe peripheral neuropathies; their feet already feel like they live on balance pads. In those instances, target the other sensory inputs and use activities like strength and gait training or activities for ADLs to help them cope.

Use Dual Tasks

Capable participants can try performing distracting secondary tasks to facilitate automatic balance. These dual tasks put the task of maintaining balance on autopilot, so to speak. It's like walking and chewing gum or using Debra Rose's Walkie Talkie Test (Rose, 2003). Dual tasks are verbal, cognitive, or motor tasks easy enough to do while standing still but are meant to be distracting while doing something else. These tasks distract participants from consciously maintaining balance, thus engaging their automatic balance system and making balance maintenance more like an involuntary reaction. The goal of dual tasks is to get the participant's automatic balance system working for them.

As some of your clients are able to master certain tasks, ask them to recite a verse, sing a song, make a list, answer questions, spell, remember cars, count backward by 3 from 75, identify items in their pocket by touch, or talk on a cell phone. Dual motor tasks could be carry a tray, a cup of water, or toss a ball from hand to hand while walking, or play catch while side stepping. Try to pick tasks appropriate and interesting for your particular client.

Progressing Endurance Activities

The first step to progressing aerobic endurance is to get to the point where sustained activity is tolerable for your participant. That means that choices for aerobic training must be well tolerated by participants, and strength, joint stability, and balance should be apparent before aerobic training begins (Mazzeo et al., 1998). For the frail or previously sedentary adult add endurance by gradually increasing connected minutes of exercise, as was discussed above for selecting endurance activities. For frail sedentary adults any connected minutes of exercise tend to increase their stamina (Takeshima et al., 2007). Begin by linking seated activities into 3- to 5-minute sections. Alternate length of work and rest times as tolerated. Gradually the work sequences can become longer and more closely connected as the rest time gets shorter. Over time, you can do the same with standing activities. Standing also increases the cardiorespiratory load. As activities become more challenging and connected and as more time is spent on their feet, your participants will build stamina. Then you could progress to what we think of as the more traditional aerobic training.

Cardiorespiratory activities should be progressed as recommended by the ACSM—increase frequency first (to at least 3 days), then increase duration (build up to 20 minutes), and finally increase intensity (progress from light to moderate workload). Aerobic activity should use large, multiple muscle groups. Always include a warm-up, a cool-down, and stretching (Mazzeo et al., 1998).

Consider how these activities and guidelines will best fit into your group. Remind participants to pay attention to how well they tolerate the activity. Nothing should hurt or make them dizzy, nauseous, or uneasy. Participants should enjoy the activity and describe it as moderate intensity. That means they can talk and sing while exercising. They should do only what they are confident they can do safely.

To summarize all of this progression information a bit, what order should any one class follow? For any one class, begin your classes with flexibility and posture so participants will be warmed up and in good alignment for the balance training. Balance activities should come next, before strength training—because balance training is complex and almost always mentally fatiguing, especially at first. You can expect participants to comment on how fatiguing it is to do balance work, especially early on. Participants will commonly remark something like, "It wasn't all that hard, but I'm tired!" You want them fresh for balance training and able to do their best. Then do your strength training. The final component, cardiorespiratory endurance, is folded in last, as well tolerated and appropriate for your group.

I've given you many guidelines and ideas for selecting and progressing ABLE Bodies activities. I hope that they will keep you organized, thinking, learning, and experimenting.

BECOMING AN EFFECTIVE INSTRUCTOR

We all remember great teachers we've had throughout our lives. The great ones had high expectations for us and inspired our best efforts. They drew out our best work and that best effort somehow brought about profound change in our life and our perceptions. Chances are you want to be that same kind of teacher. Being able to apply your skills and knowledge to bring balance and exercise into the lives of others with empathy and inspiration is a talent that is developed with time, experience, and a few good tools, like guidelines and methods that work. This entire book is meant to be those tools and methods you can use. But here specifically are some tools and methods that

can help you be a more effective instructor—one who will draw out the best and make a difference in the lives of others.

Be Professional

Dress for success means dress for the part. Dress professionally, appropriately, and conservatively; it will help you earn your participants' respect and attention. Be courteous, personable, respectful, professional, clean, and neat. Leave your troubles and your politics at the door. You are in their home and this is their time. Arrive before class early enough to set up and then relax and meet and greet your participants. This may mean arriving 20 to 30 minutes early. Bring your plan for the class, written out and ready to execute. Bring a roster of names, if you use one, and any other notes you may need. Have any supplies ready. If you are providing copies of homework, be sure you have those printed and ready as well.

Set up the classroom for clear view, activity flow, and safety. Set up your classroom so that each chair has a clear view of yours and participants have room to move their arms and legs. Some activities need a large, cleared floor space. Is there anything more to be done ahead of time? Double-check your activity list. For instance, you can set the balloons nearby or cue up the music and check its volume. Maybe you can put down masking tape and set up the obstacle course. Make a final safety check: Are there appropriate balance supports where they will be needed? Is the floor space clear and clean? Sturdy chairs and handrails? Room for walkers? Should you make any adjustments for lighting or temperature? Think the class through again, this time with your eyes closed. Imagine yourself having an enjoyable and successful time working with this group. Get ready to meet and greet your group with a smile and their name.

Welcome or acknowledge each participant personally with eye contact. Eye contact, a smile, a nod, or a hello are all personal greetings and show respect for their efforts in coming. Start and finish on time; that is part of what a good professional does. At the end of class, take a moment to summarize what you watched them accomplish. Pass out the homework and encourage them to complete it (homework keeps them involved between classes and enhances their fitness level). Put out some kind of "hook" that will entice them to come back for the next session. Then close on time, with a sincere thank-you for coming. Let them know you look forward to seeing them next time, and stay after a few minutes to answer questions and get to know them.

Make It Entertaining

An entertaining session is engaging, progressively challenging, and interactive. These are attributes anyone can add to their teaching style. Engaging means keeping things interesting, and challenging means participants have to try hard to see what they can do. An interactive teaching style means feedback is part of the learning process. Participants will get feedback from how you teach and observe. They will get feedback from their own bodies and they will even learn from each other. That is a good mix. Guide this process along and encourage discussions and fun. Participants will learn better balance and mobility skills when the process is engaging and challenging and they learn to use feedback from their own bodies, their minds, their environment, each other, and you.

Build bridges, be patient, and allow participants to learn for themselves. As instructors, sometimes we think we know all the answers for our students. After all, we are the ones trained and qualified to teach. We've worked hard at qualifying ourselves. We are able and motivated to help. But truth be told, people need to learn most lessons for themselves. The best teaching styles give people good information and guidance then allow participants to experiment with how the ideas work for them. Part of the process that helps them most is you learning from them and they learning for themselves.

If you have participants' attention, their bodies will follow. So it helps to entertain them a bit. Like it or not, classes need to be entertaining. Entertaining classes hold participants' interest longer and they will enjoy, remember, and share what they've learned too. This is surely doable in any ABLE Bodies class. Laugh, talk, share stories, and engage them on many levels; physically, socially, spiritually, and intellectually; all are possible.

I think ABLE Bodies training is successful largely because the activities are fun, interactive, at least a little challenging, and provide multiple ways to learn. Anyone will retain more of what they learn if the experience is fun and engages them on many levels. In ABLE Bodies classes there is a social element; participants interact socially with their peers. There is an intellectual element; we explain the theories behind the balance training and they enjoy the conceptual activities. Of course classes are also a physical experience, their bodies work hard and they learn skills. Finally, it's supposed to be fun. Entertaining, effective exercise—now that's exertainment!

Make It Interactive

Discussions connect people and help them further process what they have learned. Encourage questions and answer any you get. Ask questions to create discussion and gauge their response to activities. What did they learn the most from today? How did a particular activity feel? What worked best and why? Was it fun? Did they make a plan for each challenge? Do they feel like they are improving, and if so, why? These kinds of questions will add quality and depth to your class, make it more interactive, and keep lines of communication open. It will help participants process their learning.

Make liberal use of the cognitive prompts and cues provided with the activities. Verbal encouragement links mind and body and helps participants stay on track and pay attention to the goals. Encourage them to make a plan before each new challenge. Encourage problem-solving skills, and cue participants to recall prior knowledge about handling difficult situations. They will process more if they have to think things through.

Consider having a common theme that runs through several classes. For example, use music for tandem walking one week and use it the next week for stretching. Or, do the same activity a few weeks in a row, but do it a little differently or change the challenge. You might play Red Light, Green Light (see Traffic School) in a well-lit room and then in a very dim room the next time you meet.

You might also change environments from week to week. You could, for example, change locations. Teach in a different room or during nice weather hold one or two classes outside. Less dramatically, you could sit in different places in your regular room or change their chairs around. Use a guest instructor. Participants learn the same information but because the environment changes the learning will be *stickier* (Gladwell, 2000). The learning tool here is that when we learn the same information in different environments, the learning is better remembered. It has more places where it is attached to other information. It will be easier to re-access.

Set up the challenge. Their results will reflect their efforts, so your goal is always to get their best effort. The key to getting the most you can from your participants is finding the right challenge. You want something safe but one that also inspires them to make their best efforts. Trying hard with an ABLE Bodies activity is not about reaching for the moon; it's about getting participants to take that next step and then the next, until change and skill begin to surface. There's a fine line sometimes on which safe and effective challenges rest, so be careful and watch participants closely. See how they respond. Always give them a choice and an easy out. Good effort (from them) and smart training (provided by you) will get the best results.

Link and Layer Learning

Linking and layering means teaching one concept, then teaching it again in a slightly different way, or in a different context, or as an add-on to previously learned pieces. Linking and layering information is one of the most powerful tools an educator can use. It helps develop and expand the new knowledge by giving the learner more paths to access what they've learned and the ability to store it with other similar information. Grouping information helps the participants begin to see the *big picture*. In this way learning evolves and reveals itself to the person in the powerful "I get it!" kinds of ways.

In ABLE Bodies training, participants have many ways to learn: conceptual activities, various sensory systems, skills practice, exercise, and games; plus they will learn from you, from others, and from trial and error. All of these are layers of learning and they all work synergistically. It is toward that point that we say, no ABLE Bodies element is meant to stand alone—each tool for learning can help develop another element (i.e., layering). And it helps the learning process to bring past information forward again (i.e., linking). Linking and layering give the information

and learning another place to sit, so to speak. When mind and body learn together, like ABLE Bodies curriculum seeks to do, the learning is multi-dimensional. It is composed of many layers, overtly and covertly, linked by experiences. When accomplishment is paired with understanding, it can lead to mastery. Helping students experience these kinds of connections is a powerful strategy. It not only reinforces what you teach but more importantly it will create a solid foundation of confidence that can bring about change in your participants. Help your participants attach new experiences to previous ones, and use previous experiences to help master new challenges. Facilitate this special kind of learning with discussions, reviews, repetitions, and the powerful teaching moments that inevitably will present themselves.

Homework is a way to link and layer information, too. Doing homework gives participants the opportunity to use newly learned information on their own and their active effort empowers them to effect changes in their own lives. Linking, layering, repeating, and developing material in these kinds of ways will make a big difference in your teaching outcomes for participants' bodies, minds, and behaviors. It's the ultimate win–win outcome. Here are some other practical ways to accomplish this.

Coach participants to connect their experiences in balance class to movement skills they use outside of class. Teeter-Totter Chair Stands is a good example. In learning Teeter-Totter Chair Stands, participants will discover the usefulness of momentum with both their bodies and their minds, and then they will begin to use this discovery at home, too. Soon they will have mastered that previously difficult skill. There's nothing that builds confidence like mastering something that has been difficult!

Link new learning to previous learning. The core stability participants use in When Push Comes to Shove will help them later with standing, tandem balance, and balance pads. Venus de Milo Arms will encourage better range of motion for stretching or strength activities. Connections to somatic sensations like in Belly Button Training are endless; you can tie this concept to swaying, one-legged standing, stepping up and crossing the river, and more. Visual targeting can be used almost any where and it is also a powerful balance aid, especially for gait and balance challenges. And finally, "Abs in, ribs lifted, shoulder blades back and down, core braced, head retracted, chin level, and knees soft," is a mantra they will know by heart by session 8 and use in almost every activity.

These connections between body and mind will keep your classes engaging, fun, and memorable. And they will help participants integrate classroom learning with movement and balance outside of class. Integrated learning happens when learning is connected to many senses and to your understanding the world. It is about layering information and connecting mind and body in memorable ways.

Know Your Comfort Level

You will learn many new ways to do balance training in this book. Determine now that you will use only what is comfortable for you. If you are only comfortable with half the activities, so be it. It's a good start, and more importantly, it's the right start for you. You need to be comfortable with ABLE Bodies techniques and activities before you will ever be comfortable teaching them to your group. The same is true with possible balance toys. Use only the equipment you are confident will work for your group. You are the best judge of their abilities and the layout of your facility. Add new materials to your classes slowly. Build skills and concepts progressively, layering them together. Know yourself and your group.

Always take your time preparing to teach these new kinds of balance classes. Spend time learning and thinking about ABLE Bodies concepts before you begin teaching them. Read the instructions for selecting and progressing activities in this chapter, as well as the instructions provided for each activity. A clear understanding of the information can greatly improve your effectiveness and confidence, and preparation will help you spot and solve problems even before they occur.

If you need help, ask. Asking for help is not a sign of incompetence; rather, the opposite is true. Getting help and seeking new information or strategies for class demonstrates that you have the interests of your participants at heart. Supervisors, other staff, peers in your field, the Internet, libraries, books, journals, seminars, and other activity classes are all sources for learning and adapting your classes so that they are little better, or safer.

You don't need to be perfect, just capable of finding answers. Consistent effort and growth is the mark of a caring and gifted professional.

As your skills and confidence grow, expand what you teach. Rehearse new activities before you try them with participants. As you master early materials, you will naturally find yourself interested and ready to try new activities. When you plan to teach participants a new activity, review the suggestions for making that activity safer. Then practice the activity a few times, first on your own, and then with a friend or colleague. Your level of confidence and your work will be better for your efforts.

There's a well-known saying that goes like this: "If you always do what you've always done, you'll always get what you've always gotten." To really improve or change a system or an individual, there needs to be a change, a tipping point for change, or an added stress that begins a change in the system. Be a bit adventurous and unafraid to move out of your comfort level a little. With growing knowledge, ideas, and experience your "What if?" and "I think I can" thoughts will turn into a plan that you picture working. Then those experiences and plans lead to thoughts such as, "I'm starting to do it," "I will do it," "I need to alter it this way," "I'm going to do it!", and finally "I did it!" All of these realizations are signs of a changing person, reaching out to try new ideas. As a professional who is always learning new things, you are in a fantastic position to create change. I hope you will go for it!

Build a Career Path

Since our study was completed (Scott and Rosenberg, 2005), university interns from the ABLE Bodies classes have used these lesson plans to set themselves up as instructors and personal trainers in their own communities working with special populations. Offering a comprehensive balance class is a great way to get your foot in the door at similar facilities in your community. The several months you spend teaching the balance class will give you the opportunity to develop relationships with your participants and the facility. The participants will appreciate the skills you have taught them and will be pleased that their facility offered these classes.

Instructing these classes will showcase your personal and professional skills and give you something unique to offer. Personal trainers in particular will find that these classes will open up other opportunities for personal training. I hope you will send me e-mails about how ABLE Bodies training works in your career. You can write to me at renewablefitness@comcast.net.

Experienced Group Instructor

If you're an experienced group instructor, you probably need less guidance in how to use this book. I hope that many of these ideas will further your career and help you make positive differences in the lives of your clients. Add your favorite ABLE Bodies activities to your own training toolboxes, or use the book as a resource.

Here's one final idea for group instructors. Pretend each session is a wonderful five-course meal. You will be serving tasty treats from all five components of the training at each meal. For each class, pick one or two activities from each course to make the whole meal. Blend them together for the perfect meal—to suit your class: The hors d'oeuvres are the warm-up and flexibility activities. The fruits and vegetables might be the posture and core stability. Meat and potatoes are strength and balance. Dessert is the fun and conversations you'll have. Instead of the tool master, you've become the chef!

Experienced Personal Trainer and Physical Therapist

Working one-on-one is much different than working with a group. Say you need some new ways to improve vestibular or somatic function in a particular client. Check out the ABLE Bodies toolbox and borrow a few tools to help your program. Or perhaps my ideas will be your springboard to creating your own new ideas. E-mail me what you think of the ABLE Bodies tools and how you use or adapt them (renewablefitness@comcast.net). We are professionals and colleagues in this field together. We're lucky enough to be doing what we love, and sharing will help us all become better at what we do.

Personal trainers will find these materials more useful if they are trained and experienced at testing and evaluating balance tests. The information gleaned from testing will enable you to more successfully select the proper tools to meet specific balance deficits in your personal clients. If you are not experienced with balance testing, it would be helpful to have your client assessed by a physical therapist. Then you can follow the therapist's lead in the design and progression of a program beneficial for your client. Your skills and understanding of balance will set you apart from a typical group instructor and from less qualified personal trainers.

TAKE-HOME MESSAGE

Every challenge you choose should have the ability to capture your participants' interest and improve their skills. You will add your own inimitable style to this program. That is how it should be and what will make this program yours. Will they learn something new? Will they do something they never thought they would? Maybe they will hear a great story or get a great laugh trying some activity. Make your class one that they enjoy and look forward to attending each week. It will make a difference.

3

Ensuring Safety in ABLE Bodies Training

Safety is no accident, especially in balance training for older adults. Safety is job one and nothing supersedes it. Instructors must pay careful attention to a wide range of details. Falls are extremely serious. They are the leading cause of injury deaths in people over 65 and account for two-thirds of the deaths from these injuries (Kochanek and Smith, 2004). In the United States, one in three people aged 65 and older and living independently falls at least once per year. This proportion increases to one in two for those over 80 years of age (Chang et al, 2004; Rubenstein and Josephson, 2002). Not only does the incidence of fall-related injuries increase with age, but the severity of these injuries becomes more devastating (O'Loughlin et al., 1993; Tinetti, Speechly, and Ginter, 1988). So be careful! Your participants should expect that they will be safe in your care. Meeting these expectations will be easier if you can recognize and address potential problems in advance. The aim of this chapter is to help you construct safe, effective, and fun ABLE Bodies classes.

Participant safety takes planning. The setting must be safe with adequate balance support. Instructors need to know when to stop an activity and how to make adjustments for special populations or health concerns. Instructors should also encourage participants to do only what they feel comfortable doing. Tasks must be clear and well understood. Instructors need to be comfortable with policies for medical clearances, and they must have a plan and know how to respond to emergencies. Understanding what is expected of you and managing your classes to address safety concerns will give you confidence that you are offering a safe and effective program.

There will always be situations not covered by this manual. Your own perspective, common sense, and responsible behavior are necessary to a safe program. Discuss safety with participants and any staff who work with you frequently so they will be careful, too. Always allow participants to take their time, and take the time you need to do things safely.

MAKE A PLAN FOR ALL CLASSES

Good planning is essential to a quality class. Take time to properly prepare for each class you teach. Participants will notice and appreciate your effort. They will feel more confident that you are well prepared each time they see you have a written plan.

Lesson Plan

Lesson plans lay out the decisions you have made ahead of time for what you want to teach and why. For each class, make a written plan to follow. Select the activities you want to teach and organize them so that they flow well for your group, making sure to intersperse easier activities with more difficult ones to allow time to rest and recover. Think through each planned activity to discover what problems you might encounter and how you will solve them. Print the plan out in a large enough font that you will be able to read while teaching.

Equipment Plan

Make a list and check it twice. Write out a list of all equipment needs on the side or at the top of your lesson plan so you won't show up without something important. Keep these lists on your plans for repeated classes.

Clutter Plan

Know how you'll place and manage the equipment you've brought—neatness counts. Thera-Bands, balls, balloons, and hurdles can easily become tripping hazards. In addition to equipment, other potential tripping hazards can be cords, carpet edges, throw rugs, removed shoes, purses, sweaters, and walkers. Plan ahead how you'll deal with any kind of clutter. Develop a sense for when clutter happens. Vigilantly monitor your workout spaces until class is over and people have left. Remind participants each time they get up to watch for any floor clutter, and always keep an eye out for it during classes.

Floor Plan

A prepared setting builds in safety by design. Plan the room layout or floor plan before class starts. This will make the class go much more smoothly and safely.

- ▶ The room should be large enough to accommodate the number of participants you expect and the activities you have chosen.
- ▶ Plan the routes to follow for warm-ups and challenges done moving. Consider if there will be tripping hazards that may happen along the chosen route.
- ▶ Plan how and where to provide balance supports. Will participants need handrails for any activity? Will chairs work as hand holds? For tall participants, would double-stacking chairs be better?
- ▶ Plan how you will set up the chairs: where in the room, how much space between, does each chair have a clear view of yours?

- ▶ Is there any setup you can do ahead of time for special activities? If so, plan to do that ahead of time.

Chair Plan

Chairs should be sturdy and neatly arranged in a predictable order. Spacing should also allow participants to maneuver between chairs with their walkers. Each chair should have a clear view of your chair so that participants can clearly see and mimic your movements. Create personal spaces around each chair so participants have room to move their arms and legs without smacking their neighbors. There should be room on all sides of each chair to allow for standing activities. Sometime double-stacked chairs are a better height as a balance support for taller participants. If you do stack chairs, be sure they are stable stacks, not wobbly.

Lighting Plan

Making a lighting plan sounds more like a Hollywood production than a balance class, but lighting is important for both learning and safety. Any room you use should be well lit and comfortably warm. If there is natural light from windows, it should come in on your face, not theirs—they will see you better if bright light is not shining in their eyes.

If you are planning to dim the lights to create a balance challenge, turn the lights down ahead of time to test just how dark the room will be. During class, tell the participants ahead of time that you will be turning down the lights. Some people will not want to be in a darkened room. When you do turn down the lights, make sure all your participants are comfortable by asking them, before proceeding. If they are not comfortable, respond accordingly by adjusting the light, stopping the activity, or allowing the uncomfortable participants to leave.

Plan for Class Size

The greater the class size, the greater the fall risk because there is less supervision. If your class requires high amounts of supervision, the class should be smaller. A small class of 10 or fewer is ideal for ABLE Bodies training. If classes are larger, use different activities for larger class sizes. For large groups I use many more seated activities. Even seated activities can greatly benefit core strength, flexibility, and aspects of balance, including posture, core strength, and kinesis. Seated activities present little balance risk and therefore are appropriate for almost any large class.

There are also some activities that can be done standing or moving, even in large groups. Use greater caution. Sturdy chairs or handrails must be available for balance support. Movements should be kept simple and participants should be kept near the chairs or a handrail. Balance pads, beams, and River Fun activities are all examples of work that should be attempted only with close supervision in small groups.

Stick to It

Once you make a plan, stick to it. Without a doubt, it is the unplanned activities that present the greatest fall risk. Spontaneity compromises safety. Say you remember a fun idea, such as adding a step-turn to a side-step activity. You call out for your group to carefully add a step-turn to the activity. But they aren't partnered up, or some are too far from safety supports. Someone may stumble and even fall. Because safety wasn't planned for ahead of time, the error may be yours. Once you make your safety plan, stick to it. This is not to say you should never adapt a plan. You will need to do that, but do it judiciously.

ESTABLISH RULES

Having a few rules establishes a safety net. I try not to have too many rules, but I do have a few. Here are my top four.

Nothing Should Hurt

My number one rule is about pain. It's a simple rule: If it hurts, don't do it. Participants should never get the idea they should just grin and bear it. Nothing should hurt, cause physical problems, or even make participants feel uncomfortable or anxious. They should stop or go to plan B. This is only exercise class. If something hurts, they should stop—no exceptions. Remind them of this rule every class.

Many of your participants will have worked hard all their lives, growing up during a time when hard work and personal sacrifice were a badge of courage. They may still harbor messages

such as "No pain, no gain" or "What doesn't kill me makes me stronger." You want them to replace those messages and listen to their bodies. Here are two examples. A participant experiences pain during a stretch. She may have stretched too far or too hard, or the joint simply doesn't take well to the stretch. She should stop what she's doing and let you know. Depending on your own skill level as an instructor, you might coach her to ease off on the stretch or to change her body position a bit so that the stretch is comfortable. Or, you may be able to recommend a different or modified stretch. If no comfortable, safe way can be found, she should skip that particular stretch altogether, at least for the day.

Another example happens during weight-bearing activities. Many of your participants are dealing with worn-down knee cartilage, replaced joints, old injuries, arthritis, and other everyday 80-year-old problems. During an activity, a participant makes a move and yells "Ouch!" You should step in and let him know that sharp pains are body language for "Stop, now!" If it hurts, he should stop, or modify, or wait.

Arm's-Length Rule

Whenever participants are not sitting, they should be no farther than an arm's length away from a balance support. That support will usually be their sturdy chair, but it could also be a walker or cane, handrail or counter, partner or assistant, or your hand. Make no exceptions, and take turns if necessary.

Ninety Percent Rule

Succeeding at a task that was once difficult is hugely effective at building self-confidence. Struggle and effort make the reward sweeter and more uplifting. You want your participants to do their best and gain the self-confidence that goes with that effort, but you want them to do it safely. The 90 percent rule says participants should attempt only what they are 90 percent confident they can do safely—that is, what they're pretty sure they can do. In the face of great enthusiasm, this provides a wider margin of safety. When people are ready, they believe they can do it, and chances are that is the beginning of when they can. Whether it's a game, a challenge, a timed activity, or any other activity, participants should feel 90 percent certain they can do it safely. Give participants encouragement, tools, and all the room they need to make their own decisions. The challenge and the choice will more safely build their confidence and keep them engaged in the learning process.

Choose or Refuse Rule

Participants can refuse to do anything they do not want to do. They are not obligated to give you a reason for refusing. Participation is always their choice. If any activity makes them uncomfortable, advise them to stop or wait until they do feel that needed bit of confidence. A participant may choose to stop for any reason. Here are some common nonmedical reasons participants may refuse to do an activity:

- They don't feel well enough at the moment.
- They are reluctant.
- They feel anxious, insecure, or embarrassed.
- They don't understand what is expected.
- They just can't picture themselves doing the activity.
- They think it is dangerous or silly.
- They worry about incontinence. (Sometimes physical activity triggers an urge to urinate or causes leaking.)
- They refuse for any reason.
- They refuse for no reason.

Give participants control over class choices for themselves. Encourage them to do their best, but show respect if they back off. They may refuse an activity in week 8, but in week 12 they just might try it. Hooray for them! That shows growth and a progression in their confidence and skills. It all contributes to helping them trust their own bodies, judgment, and perceptions. Choosing or refusing activities and experiences is another way for them to be interactive with and listen to their body.

MENTAL AND EMOTIONAL SAFETY

Emotional safety ensures participants feel they are in a safe place and that their choices will be supported. When instructors are supportive and respectful, participants will feel safe and valued. There are many ways to show respect for participants in your classes.

- Ask for their input. When you involve them in the process of selection, it helps keep them in their comfort zone.
- Respect their decisions. They need to be comfortable and believe the activity is safe and effective as much as you do.
- Make eye contact.
- Listen. Ask about them, and listen to their stories. This is good for both you and them.
- Explain the benefits of the activities you choose. Share your knowledge with them; they are wise and experienced. They will appreciate learning from you.
- Say please and thank you. It sounds small, but at least a few times each session, be sure to add in some pleases and thank-yous to your directions. It honors their effort, time, and compliance.
- Tell the truth. Make your praise and comments specific and honest.
- Respect and guard their privacy. As their instructor you will likely learn about their medical conditions or they may confide other information to you. Keep it to yourself.

Your ethics as a professional should guide your decisions and conduct toward others, every day in every way.

PHYSICAL SAFETY

We've already talked about creating plans and constructing a safe setting for each class. Here are other aspects of ensuring participant safety.

Signs to Stop an Activity Immediately

Ask participants to tell you if they experience any of the following symptoms. These symptoms are reasons to immediately stop any activity.

- Dizziness or nausea
- Shortness of breath
- Unusual fatigue

- Heart racing or pounding
- Uneasiness or anxiety
- Blurred vision or slurred speech
- Pain or tightness in chest, jaw, or arm
- Sudden paleness or clammy skin

Familiarize yourself and your participants with these contraindications. If they experience any of these symptoms, it may constitute a medical emergency. The participants should be advised to talk with their health care provider. Do not alarm them or embarrass them by publicly discussing private concerns. If there is a medical emergency, you should know and follow the response plan for your facility.

Fall Prevention

Falls happen in an instant, and any fall can easily become a worst-case scenario with debilitating long-lasting or even permanent consequences. Make your activities as fall proof as possible. Participants need to know they will be safe from falling in your class. For each activity you plan, you should feel confident that you have addressed the fall risks for your particular class working in that particular environment. Here are suggestions to keep participants on their feet.

Just Say Whoa! and Take Turns

Anytime balance toys are out, participants will clamor to try the toys. You'll look up and have five people in the river of balance. That's way too many. Sometimes you just have to say, "Whoa!" Keeping control of your classes is your responsibility. Anytime the participants are beyond an arm's length away from a balance support, they should take turns with you by their side or you should have extra staff. This program is designed for the frail elderly. Do not risk a fall. You will need to supervise and hold hands anytime they are not directly by their chairs or a handrail or with their walkers. Taking turns slows the pace a bit, but it's fun and social. They learn from and enjoy each other. As an added bonus, the waiting participants get extra time to observe, plan, and build their confidence.

Take Your Time

Take your time introducing new activities. As a motivated instructor, it's tempting to want to move fast—but don't. Take your time. Get one skill down well before moving on. Teach whole movements in parts, first. Practice a little longer. Give lots of explanation. Get a feeling for their readiness. If in doubt ask them, "Are you ready?" They will tell you. Listen and watch their eyes and body language, too. Be patient. Spread the balance and strength work over many months.

Provide Plenty of Balance Supports

Plan to make ample balance support available. A balance support is something sturdy they can grab or hold on to should they feel the need. Easily available items like handrails, counters, sturdy chairs, or walkers work well. For some activities with more able participants, partnering participants works for balance support. Here are some good basic balance supports.

Sturdy Chairs

A study chair is the best backup safety system for participants in a classroom setting. If they lose their balance, the chair can help. Touching a chair or walker is a reliable way for participants to steady themselves. Chairs should be sturdy enough for participants to use to steady themselves or lean on a bit when standing. If a participant normally uses a walker, have them use the walker while standing instead of a chair. Whenever they are standing, suggest that they maintain some contact with the chair or their walker. Sturdy chairs are a must if you do standing activities. A lightweight chair can tip easily when leaned on, and chairs on rollers can move quickly. If you are doing standing activities near a chair, here are some more ideas for positioning participants around chairs.

- Stand behind a chair. Participants can stand behind their chair for activities such as heel raises. This is probably the safest standing position. When participants are standing behind their chairs, they can hold on tightly or lightly with one or both hands as needed.
- Stand beside a chair. For activities with forward and backward swaying and rocking, such as Clock Stepping, or when more leg and knee room is needed, participants can stand to the side of their chair. Position them so their hips are in line with the back of the chair. That way their hand can rest comfortably on the

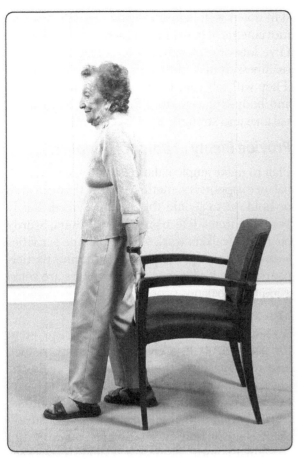

Strong, stable chairs are an excellent balance support. Encourage your participants to touch their chair on a regular basis. Keeping at least one leg touching the chair will help them keep their balance when standing.

back of the chair (the chair back's height is appropriate for a hand rest). When standing to the side, they can hold on to the chair with only one hand.

▶ Stand in front of a chair. You may want participants to stand in front of the chair for activities, such as chair stands, squats, and side-stepping. If they lose their balance, they can simply and safely sit down. This position will be much safer still, if you advise them to keep at least one leg in contact with their chair. It's amazing how well this works. Try it yourself. Also, have them reach back with a hand to touch their chairs on a regular basis. These two ideas will do a good job keeping them placed in front of their chair; otherwise, my experience has been that they tend to wander too far away for arm's-length safety.

▶ Holding on. Let participants choose how tightly to hold onto their chairs: two hands, one hand, or just fingertip touches. I like to cue them to hold on tightly or lightly or just hover their hands over the chair.

Walkers

Any participants who normally use a walker should use the walker whenever they are standing in class and for the balance challenges. Walkers prevent participants from leaning too far forward or too far to either side. However, the back side is always open, meaning they could fall backward during an activity. Place participants with walkers in front of a chair or so that their backs are to a wall. This way, if they feel weak or wobbly, they can simply sit down or touch or lean against the wall. Remember that the chair should be very sturdy and not on wheels. If it is on wheels, it should be backed against a wall.

Walkers make great supports during standing activities. Make sure participants firmly set their brakes on wheeled walkers for all standing activities. Walkers provide good balance support for moving activities, too, whether walking along a tandem line, balance beam, or pad. The first few times participants do a tandem line or beam, you might suggest that everyone use a walker, and ask participants to share. It's fun and much safer.

Handrails and Countertops

Handrails provide good balance support for moving or walking activities. They work well for sidestepping, tandem walking on lines, steps, heel raises, and heel–toe foot patterns, as well as work on half-rounds. Obstacle courses used as warm-ups should be placed by handrails or a row of chairs. Secure railings and ballet bars or counters can be used by several participants at the same time. Also it gives them a safe place to hold on, if they are waiting for their turn. Challenge participants to hold on as needed (with two hands or one hand, firmly or lightly touching with fingertips).

Countertops work like handrails. In the home they are common balance supports. When you ask participants to practice sidestepping on their own, remind them to do so using a countertop.

Corners

Corners are great balance support! Participants can stand with their backs into a corner. This position provides balance help on both sides and from behind. A participant conceivably can drift to either side or backward and not risk falling. In these situations, I also recommend placing a walker in front of clients positioned in a corner. It's a great extra precaution that helps them feel safe and secure and ready for the challenge.

Corners are good for balance challenges, including sways, heel raises, arm lifts, dim light activities, head turns, balance pads, and catching balls. There are only so many corners in a room, so it may be that corners work best with small classes, circuit classes, or personal training.

Partners

Two participants may be able to act as each other's balance support while standing. For example, waltzing to music is a natural activity for partnering. Tight Tandem Walking on a Line can be done with two lines and two participants holding hands. Partnering provides a nice social and physical connection, too.

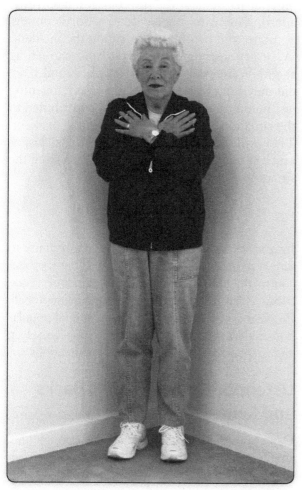

Corners provide additional support for your participants. A participant conceivably can drift to either side or backward and not risk falling. For an extra measure of safety, place a walker in front them. You should stay close, as well.

Extra Helpers

Extra staff to help with your class is always nice, if that can be arranged. Staff members, caregivers, and occasionally family members can all help. But often facilities are busy and staff is spread thin. Consider recruiting local high school students who need community service credits or invite participants to ask their grandchildren for a special occasion.

Make Sure the Task Is Understood

Being a good communicator is essential to safety in teaching. When you introduce new materials, make certain each participant knows exactly what you're asking them to do. The task needs to be very clear. Here are some ways to achieve that kind of clear communication:

- ▶ Tell participants the purpose for doing the activity. Knowing the reason provides motivation and clarification.

- ▶ Demonstrate the task. Include verbal descriptions with the demonstration using words you want them to associate with the skill or activity. The familiar words become part of the memory pack for that skill.

- ▶ Invite them to try it. Never insist or *bug* them till they do.

- ▶ If they have trouble, break complex activities into smaller parts. As they work their way through the skill, cue them to use skills or concepts they already know. For example, remind them to use core stability (keep shoulder blades back and down) or spot a visual target they can use to keep their path steady.

- ▶ Have them do the task again. Watch carefully—is there something else that would help? Can you help them self-discover? Praise successes, paying specific attention to the skills you saw in action.

- ▶ Practice, practice, practice. Practice always helps ingrain motor patterns. Have them repeat new movements or tasks several times. Once the activity feels comfortable to them, you can add progressions.

- ▶ Consider naming the activities and tasks. Typically, an ABLE Bodies task is an integrated movement. That means the task is a set of skills rather than one discrete movement.

Naming a task combines many skills into one succinct memory pack, which makes the skill easier to remember and repeat. Naming the task will give a clear picture of a complex task.

Speak Clearly

Some of the best advice I ever received for public speaking came from the famous playwright Danny Simon. He attended my classes for a few years. His great advice was, "Finish each word you speak." He said that I should hear myself say the last letter of each word I spoke. It's been great advice! It works for me and it has made me a better speaker. Full enunciation will slow you down a bit, but overall, going a little slower will be of benefit, too.

A little consistent effort on your part will significantly improve the clarity of your words and style of teaching. Here are suggestions to help shape your communication skills:

▶ Speak your words clearly, each one succinctly. Finish each word you speak.

▶ Pause between phrases and between sentences. Slow down for effect.

▶ Keep the pitch of your voice low. A low-pitched voice is easier for older adults to hear than a high-pitched voice.

▶ Explain the task in more than one way, using different words or examples.

▶ Try a conceptual activity.

▶ Watch the faces and body language of participants for signs that they understand your instructions. Are they puzzled? Squinting? Interested? There are many clues available if you watch.

Know the Fall Policy

A fall policy tells you what to do if someone falls in your class. Knowing the fall policy at your site will make these scary situations a little safer and more predictable. Most commonly, facilities want the person who has fallen to remain on the ground until facility medical staff can assess the situation.

If participants fall, resist the urge to run over and pick them up. Moving them may cause greater pain or injury, and you could even hurt yourself. Instead, take a deep breath to calm and organize your thoughts. Assess the environment for your safety and the safety of others. Designate someone to alert other staff or the facility emergency team, and then keep the person as calm and as comfortable as possible. If you have current cardiopulmonary resuscitation (CPR) or first aid training, perform as you were trained. Stay with the participant until relieved by medical personnel or trained staff. You will likely be asked to write a report for the facility immediately afterwards. Do so as soon as possible; write what you actually observed, accurately and fully.

Following an incident, take care to respect the person's privacy; never share details without permission and not with anyone inappropriate. Talk with your supervisor; get their guidance. Show genuine concern for the injured. Check on your participant the next day and later on as appropriate. After the incident, be forthcoming, accurate, and helpful in evaluating the incident. What actions might prevent it from happening again? Were safety supports in place, and if so, did they work as expected? What was happening just before the fall that may have contributed to the situation? Again, work with your supervisor. They will want to develop a better plan, just as much as you want to improve and learn from the situation yourself.

HEALTH CONCERNS

Instructors do not always have the opportunity to screen participants from their classes, but they can control the activities offered. In these kinds of classes, consider the limitations of some as guidelines for all. Please review these suggestions for special populations and consider how they can help you plan, select, and adapt activities for your special populations.

Osteoporosis and Fragile Backs and Spines

Osteoporosis is common, especially among older, smaller women. Bones become brittle and can break easily, sometimes even without obvious insult. The spine, hip, and wrist areas are especially vulnerable. Participants who have osteoporosis require extra precautions during exercise. Suggest that those participants talk with their doctor and physical therapist about pain management and safe movement. Encourage them to follow their doctor's advice, avoid exercises in your class that are contraindicated for them, and do the exercises recommended by their doctor or physical therapist.

In addition to osteoporosis, there are chronic, painful back conditions that merit special adaptations. *Stenosis, scoliosis, kyphosis,* and *lordosis* are common in this population. Their presence can cause pain and make normal posture, movement, and gait difficult or impossible. Use these precautions for all participants:

▶ There should be no unsupported forward or sideways bending of the spine. Whether sitting or standing, the back needs to be supported and the movement needs to be gentle. They should keep their shoulders over their hips, as able. When participants lean forward, backward, or sideways the movement should be done gently with back support provided. Coach them to move slowly and gently and to put their hands on their laps, legs, or chair arms for back support. You may ask them to round their back for a stretch, but they should do it slowly and gently. When doing Gentlemen's Bow, our basic modified hamstring stretch, be sure to remind them to support their back by placing their hands on their legs or chair when leaning forward. Also cue them to lean forward from the hip (a hip hinge motion) not by bending through the back (spinal flexion).

▶ All stretching should be done gently. Nothing should hurt. Cue participants to move slowly and thoughtfully, mindful of how their stretch feels and progresses.

▶ Focus on breathing to help participants relax and respond to the stretch.

▶ Use deep breaths to gently expand the rib cage during a stretch.

▶ Use balance supports generously, including walkers, rails, and arm holding.

▶ Keep the area free of clutter and any tripping hazards.

▶ Instruct participants to avoid anything that causes pain. Pain can be especially common among those with osteoporosis and spinal abnormalities when reaching upward with their arms or when trying to sit, stand, or walk tall. Tell them

they need only accommodate the most upright posture that is comfortable for them. Remind them that pain is a reason to stop and adjust. They need to be comfortable.

Fragile Hips and Hip Replacements

Hip and knee replacements are also common in this age group. For the first few months following surgery, the patient should do only supervised exercises with a specialist. This is a circumstance when their doctor should clear your participant for class. Talk with these participants before class to make sure they understand what the doctor or therapist says is safe for them to do. Ask for written medical recommendations or have them sign waivers regarding their decisions to exercise. In classes with open enrollment it is often not possible to preclude participants from joining a class. That is why it is important to stress that exercise should not hurt or make them feel dizzy, nauseous, uncomfortable, or otherwise cause increased discomfort.

▶ Participants with hip replacements should avoid crossing their legs until cleared by their doctor to do so. Crossing the legs may destabilize a freshly repaired or new hip.

▶ Coach gentle flexibility for all stretches.

▶ Nothing should hurt or cause increased discomfort.

Parkinson's Disease

People with Parkinson's disease have trouble initiating and maintaining movement. They can get stuck or *frozen* in one spot, unable to initiate the next move for a moment. When they begin to move they may stutter-step (festinate). Or they may have difficulty keeping a motion going smoothly for more than several steps. They often have trouble with sequential coordination and can be quite rigid and stiff, especially in the core muscles. They often display a stooped posture. Sometimes they can have cognitive impairments as well.

The abundance of external cues (visual targets, rhythm, counting) used in ABLE Bodies training seems to benefit these participants by helping them initiate and maintain movement. Also, with their permission, light touches on their shoulder or leg may help them initiate a movement. Here are some other guidelines:

- Use generous amounts of balance supports such as walkers, rails, and arm holding. Stay close when the person is having trouble standing or moving. Have participants take turns doing activities so you can give one-on-one support.

- Exaggerate movement. Coach them to *think big* when they move. Maintaining the size of repetitive movements is easier if they are trying to exaggerate each movement.

- Visual targets are very helpful. Coach them to look at the goal. You can also place agility dots on the floor as stepping stones for them to follow.

- Strengthen back muscles used for posture, as well as spinal extensors, which help the trunk to rotate and lengthen.

- Stretch often, especially flexor muscle groups like hip flexors and chest muscles.

- Their posture is generally stooped and many joints are rigid. Stretching the chest and shoulders on the anterior side and the muscles on the back of the leg (calves, hamstrings, and gluteal muscles) will help those constraints.

- Make sure your tasks are clear and well understood.

- Keep work areas free of clutter and tripping hazards throughout your class.

Diabetes and Peripheral Neuropathy

The popular lyric "Ground control to Major Tom" from David Bowie's song, "*Space Oddity*," is a fun analogy for the role feet play in balance. Sensations from the feet provide us with ground control. Sensory receptors under our feet and in our ankles communicate all kinds of surface information to the brain. The ankles and feet can tell whether the ground is uneven, inclined, soft, or slippery. Pressure sensors can communicate to the rest of the body just how balance is distributed over the feet. This is all important feedback. It's so important that lessened sensations in the feet

or lower legs, common in diabetes and peripheral neuropathies, seriously compromise balance and agility.

Can you remember a time when your feet felt like ice cubes? Maybe you were playing in the ocean or were out in the cold too long. Do you remember how clumsy you felt when your feet had no feeling? The loss of sensation from your feet is what made you clumsy. Try this idea with your friends. Place your feet in an ice bath for about 5 minutes. When your feet feel like two ice cubes, take them out, get up, and try to walk. Are your coordination and agility affected? Rub your feet gently to warm them up, and then walk again. Better? This experience is similar to how loss of circulation or poor innervation feels to participants. A loss of sensation in lower extremities is fairly common with age, especially among people with diabetes and those with peripheral neuropathies. Participants will say it's as if they can't feel their feet, or that their feet feel like two bricks. Be cautious doing standing, moving, or balance activities with this population. They get little information from their feet and ankles. Here are some guidelines I use.

- Keep these participants on firm surfaces. Balance pads are soft compliant surfaces. They are not appropriate or as effective as hardwood floors.

- Require they keep their shoes on when they are on their feet. Their feet will be safer from injury and they will have better balance because a shoe provides larger surface area.

- Offer ample balance supports, such as walkers, handrails, and arm holding.

Cognitive Impairment

Some class members may have difficulty following instructions, making good decisions, or maintaining awareness. This impairment will be a distraction and a safety hazard to themselves and others. Many people who struggle with cognitive impairment may have trouble remembering basic information, such as how far away they are from their chair or what they are doing at that moment. At minimum, participants must be able to follow verbal instructions to benefit from and be safe in ABLE Bodies classes. Their ability to learn both knowledge and new skills is important for their placement in a balance training program.

If such participants are placed in your class, keep them seated and ask for the assistance of a caregiver. They should be able to safely do seated activities for strength, flexibility, and posture.

If you do plan to work individually with this population, they will do best in situations where they enjoy themselves. Simple activities are best. Avoid adding variations or making anything too busy. Keep it simple and enjoyable. Consider using familiar music with the activities; it may help to bring back associated motor skills.

Medications

Prescription medicines are ubiquitous among older adults. Medications can cause dizziness, sudden changes in blood pressure, altered alertness, weakness, fatigue, and other fall risks (Rose, 2003). Older adults taking four or more medications are four times more likely to fall (Campbell, Borrie, and Spears, 1989). Suffice it to say, medications are a major reason why ample balance support and the arm's-length rule are important to ABLE Bodies training. Talk with your classes about medications in general so they are aware of the risks. Get them to pay attention to how medicine works for them and respond accordingly by being careful what activities they choose. Medicine can mean good days and bad days for balance skills. If you are given specific information about their prescription medications, treat that information as confidential. Never give medical advice!

Hygiene and Illness

Here are a few tips to ensure your participants stay healthy while in your class.

▸ Remind them to wash their hands before and after class. Chair arms, handrails, Thera-Bands, and other shared equipment can spread germs and illness. Participants can better avoid the flu and colds when everyone practices good hygiene.

▸ Advise them to stay home if they are not feeling well. They will do much better when they feel better, and nobody wants to catch what

they may have. My rule of thumb for when they should return to class is this: When they are sick, they should stay home. When they feel better, they should wait one more day and then come back. Being conservative may help avoid a setback and they will feel that much stronger.

This list of health concerns is partial. Low vision, poorly functioning vestibular systems, and many other major illnesses have not been addressed in this chapter. Overall, how a person tolerates the activities is your best guide. Be careful, err on the side of caution, progress slowly, monitor your participants, and talk with them about what feels good and works for them. When possible, always seek recommendations or medical clearance from their doctors or other health specialist.

MEDICAL CLEARANCES

To screen or not to screen? That is the question—and it's a good one. In most class settings, facility management does not prescreen participants for their medical fitness to exercise. This policy leaves instructors working with whoever comes to class that day. Normally, that means all kinds of medical and cognitive conditions are present.

Generally, participants with medical conditions are fairly well informed about their condition and know to follow their doctor's advice. They can tell you, for example, how their particular condition or medicines affect them on a daily basis. They usually will know what is okay to do. In these regards, participants can be responsible for their decision to join your class. For our part, as group instructors in open enrollment setting, using conservative programming and exercise tolerance as guiding principles should work well in group settings. Safe, moderate, and gentle exercise is the goal.

Having said that, it would still be preferable that all participants receive a signed medical clearance to exercise from their doctor or specialist. Additionally, an informed consent and waiver may protect you and your facility against unwarranted legal actions. Examples of forms for preexercise health screening, informed consents, and waivers are available through www.ideafit.com and other professional publishers. A sample form for medical clearance is shown on page 56.

Recommendations for Supervised Exercise Program

Physician: _____ Date: _____

Clinic or address: _____

Phone: _____ Fax: _____ E-mail: _____

Patient: _____ Date of birth: _____

_____

Your patient, _____, wishes to participate in an exercise program to improve _____ (insert goal, i.e., flexibility, posture, strength, balance, and endurance). This exercise program will be closely supervised by an _____ (insert professional certification). The program may include or gradually build up to the following:

- Progressive, moderate-intensity, supervised exercise sessions, 30 minutes, 2 to 3 days a week

- Flexibility, strength, and functional training activities

- Light resistance devices (bands, tubing, weights, balloons), standing, or walking

All training is administered only as apparently well tolerated and follows guidelines of the _____ _____ (Insert your certifying agent).

Please list any recommendations or concerns appropriate for your patient's participation in this exercise training program: _____

_____

_____

_____

☐ My patient may not participate in the exercise program as described.

☐ My patient may participate in the exercise program as described.

Please list any medications that may limit or reduce exercise tolerance, heart rate, or blood pressure response during exercise: _____

_____

_____

_____

Physician's signature _____ Date _____

From S. Scott, 2008, *ABLE bodies balance training* (Champaign, IL: Human Kinetics).

Doctors generally advise their patients to exercise as tolerated. That is, if participants feel they are doing well with the exercise or activity (no pain and are comfortable physically and emotionally), then they likely are okay to continue. However, any changes in physical activity should be discussed with their doctors, who can best advise them if there are any specific moves or activities they should avoid.

Personal trainers should seek and follow recommendations for their clients from the primary health care provider, medical specialist, and physical therapist, as appropriate for their exercise program. Getting these kinds of recommendations will open important lines of communication that will benefit your client.

EMERGENCY PROCEDURES

Here is a story I will tell on myself. It is about knowing what to do during an emergency. It's a funny story, but only because it turns out well. Today, the experience is filed under the lived-and-learned department of my life. If you remember my lesson only because it makes you laugh, too, that's also fine by me.

I was teaching a group class at an assisted living facility when an earthquake rocked our city. On the Richter scale the quake was only a size 3.6, but it lasted several seconds. I didn't feel the first shock, but one woman in class did. She looked up at me and said, "Did you feel that?" I hadn't, so I thought she was experiencing dizziness and I rushed to help her sit down. It was about that time when we all began to realize it was an earthquake!

It went on for a while and shook us all pretty good. As it continued, I realized I didn't know what I was supposed to do. What was expected of me as their leader? Should I yell for help? Lead them outside? Or just "duck and cover" and save myself?

Thankfully, no decision was needed. The earthquake ended and all was well. But from then on, I made it my business to know the emergency policies at each facility where I work. Knowing the emergency plan should be your business, too.

▶ Always have a phone available for your use during class.

▶ Make sure a written copy of the emergency plan is posted where you can easily access it.

▶ Maintain current CPR and first aid certification, and regularly review and practice.

▶ Write down emergency numbers; don't rely on your memory.

▶ Rehearse the predetermined emergency plan at your facility.

▶ Establish regular review dates to update and verify emergency information.

▶ Reviews and mock practices really do better prepare you for the real thing. Participate in these events; you'll be calmer when you need to be.

Know how to activate emergency procedures in case of a medical emergency or a disaster. Know what is expected of you during an emergency and be prepared to do your part. Every facility should have a written, posted emergency plan for disasters, medical situations, and other emergencies.

TAKE-HOME MESSAGE

Appropriate supervision is mandatory for safe balance training. No doubt about it. Their safety is in your hands. Have a written plan for each class or session that outlines each activity, the flow of the class, the classroom environment, and the equipment used. Provide ample balance support and minimize clutter. Activities should be well tolerated by participants. Always be cautious; it's better to be safe than sorry.

Heath status, medications, mood, stress, strength, and balance all affect tolerance. Select activities that suit the mid- or lower range of your class. Know how to make activities easier or more difficult, and know when to stop an activity. Your instructions need to be clear and understood. Get participants to listen to their bodies. If you need help, ask! Have a plan for falls, and know and rehearse emergency procedures. Enjoy yourself, use common sense, and be careful out there!

II

ABLE Bodies Balance Training Activities

If this book is to be your balance training toolbox, then part I is the instruction manual and part II contains the tools. In part II, these tools (activities) are assigned to a chapter according to where they best fit into the five ABLE Bodies components:

Flexibility

Posture and core stability

Strength for a purpose

Balance and mobility

Cardiorespiratory endurance

Chapter 4, Flexibility, covers the first ABLE Bodies component. You'll learn both seated and standing versions of stretches for all major muscle groups. There are some great whole-body stretches (such as Carry the Baby, Farmer's Stretch, and Lunge Stretch), as well as some wonderful conceptual activities that will help participants explore flexibility and the ways it affects their everyday life (don't miss Supple Spine and Venus de Milo Arms).

Chapter 5, Posture and Core Stability, offers activities to improve posture and core stability. It begins with conceptual activities that are very somatic and interactive; they will help participants self-discover posture and core principles from the inside out. Concepts have a remarkable way of continuing to teach, even when class is over. Following the conceptual activities are more than 20 ABLE Bodies exercises and their variations that focus on progressive strength for core and postural muscles. As much as possible, the core strength exercises progress in the chapter from the easiest and most basic exercise (such as Tall Sits) to core exercises that are more complex and involve back extensors (such as Tap and Catch a Balloon).

In chapter 6, Strength for a Purpose, you will discover nearly 50 strengthening exercises for better balance and mobility. They are organized by muscle group and then by level of difficulty. Progressions are shown to add more difficulty or greater balance challenge.

Chapter 7, Balance and Mobility, offers more than 70 balance activities for your perusal. They are categorized under two main umbrellas: sensory activities (which include visual, somatic and vestibular activities) and motor coordination activities (which cover gait, ADLs, games, and other integrated movements). These assignments to one category are somewhat arbitrary because in real life, most activities overlap many categories. Other tools, such as dual tasks, are used alongside almost any activity when appropriate.

Chapter 8, Cardiorespiratory Endurance, is handled a little differently than the others. Cardiorespiratory endurance may be addressed indirectly by linking groups of exercises (see chapter 2 for suggestions to link activities together and facilitate cardiorespiratory training). Gradually, as balance and strength improve, begin to increase endurance exercise and fold in chapter 8 activities that include, WalkAbouts and more time spent standing. Chapter 8 will give you many ways to incorporate cardiorespiratory training into existing classes.

Delve into these next five chapters to find the tools that you'd like to use. These physical activities, specific to balance and mobility, alongside the guidance from part I and your own wisdom and experience, will help you to create ABLE Bodies training for your classes and individuals.

CHAPTER

Flexibility

Everyone knows that the leg bone is connected to the hip bone, which is connected to the back bones, and so on. But why is that relevant to flexibility? It's relevant because the flexibility between these connections affects how we function and balance. Think of a playing with a puppet. Pull a few strings and the puppet straightens right up; add a few twitches of your hand and it dances. Pull a few more strings and the doll flops over to take a bow. It's easily apparent that the person pulling the strings provides the motion. But what may not be so apparent is that the motion is limited by how the doll is made. Movement for any human is much like that of the puppet. Muscles are the puppet strings, but it's the joints that allow the movement.

Wherever muscles span a joint, the connected bones move toward each other when the muscles contract. The two bones can only move in a path allowed by the structure and health of the joint. For example, knees can flex and extend because that's what they're designed to do; they don't twist or bend backward because their construction doesn't allow for that. All joints have similar structural constraints. They move the way they were designed to move. Flexibility, then, is limited by joint structure.

It is also often limited by joint health. Arthritis, wear and tear, deformation, disease, pain, and tightness all can limit range of motion. These constraints related to joint health would be analogous to wrapping duct tape around key joints of our puppet. It can't dance the same way, not at least until you take the tape off. Improving flexibility in older adults is like removing some of that duct tape. Flexibility can help restore function and enable more efficient movement.

People whose joints are in good working order and get regular activity have greater freedom of movement. They can stand tall and straight, walk without a forward lean, and extend the knees in a normal gait pattern while walking. However, when key joints are affected by pain or other limits, major changes in posture, movement, and balance follow. Painful, stiff joints make people understandably less able. In many intricate ways, improving range of motion with flexibility training can change the lives of your participants.

The most basic ABLE Bodies exercise, the Tall Sits, involves pulling the spine into a tall, upright position. This requires suppleness and flexibility along the entire spine and in the pelvis and hips. Supple spines allow for better posture, freer movement of shoulders, and greater ease when reaching or pulling. Tight hamstrings can also affect posture and back health. Shortened, tight hamstrings tilt the pelvis and spine backward, resulting in flexed knees and a bowed low back. Flexibility can improve the mechanics of standing, moving, and balancing. Research shows that flexibility reduces fall risk, enhances posture and function, and facilitates more efficient movement (Alexander et al., 2001; Liu-Ambrose et al., 2004; Rose, 2003).

The activities in this chapter will help create suppler spines, more moveable hips and shoulders, and greater range of motion in hamstrings, calves, and gluteal muscles. These actions will improve posture and function. They should be a part of every session with your participants.

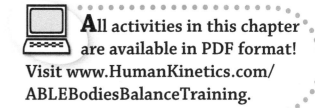

All activities in this chapter are available in PDF format! Visit www.HumanKinetics.com/ ABLEBodiesBalanceTraining.

Quick Reminder

Hold stretches for 10 to 15 or even 30 seconds, as well tolerated by participants. Repeat key stretches twice during each class. Encourage participants to relax with the stretch and focus on feeling it in the targeted muscle. Use deep breathing during stretches to expand the chest wall and increase the effectiveness of the stretch. A good stretch should feel tolerable, not too tight but tight enough to feel it doing its job. It should be an enjoyable tightness, as opposed to a painful strain. When a muscle is stretched too far or too fast, the muscle is more likely to tighten than relax. Teach participants how to stretch in meaningful ways that let the body relax while they breathe and reach a little farther.

As always, progress only as well tolerated by your participants, which means that nothing hurts and participants are willing and able to continue and show no signs of dizziness, nausea, or excessive fatigue. Also make sure that participants can do the stretch using proper form before progressing. Provide balance support for standing stretches.

VENUS DE MILO ARMS

Getting older adults to extend through their trunk or lift their ribs can be difficult. This imaginative exercise invites participants to pretend they are the famous sculpture, Venus de Milo—which has no arms! Without their arms they'll certainly appreciate their torso a little more as they discover untapped ranges of motion.

Benefits))

- Showcases trunk and shoulder flexibility in a fun and memorable way.
- Enhances body awareness and appreciation for the human body.
- Engages participants' imagination and body together for long-lasting learning.
- Helps with the everyday skill of reaching.

How to Do It))

The Start

Ask participants to pretend for a moment that they have become Venus de Milo, the famous statue that has no arms. Participants can fold their arms on their chest or place one arm on their waist in front and one at waist level in back. Then ask them to sit tall, away from the back of their chair.

The Moves

- Imagine a light cord is hanging just above you and you need to reach for it without arms. You can only reach with your right shoulder.
    - How high can you reach?
    - Can you feel your ribs lifting and stretching, too?
    - Can you feel your skin moving and stretching?
    - How much of a reaching distance do you get from just lifting the shoulder?
    - Nice try.

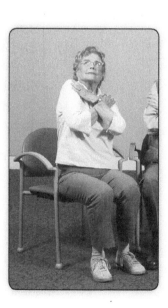

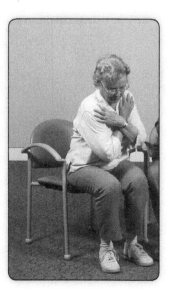

- With the arms still against the torso, reach for a book on an imaginary table in front of you. Again you can use only one shoulder.
    - Do you notice how much forward distance your shoulders can give you?
    - Reach with the other shoulder.

⊙ Now reach backward, as if you are reaching for a pair of sunglasses on a table behind you. With arms still against your torso, reach backward with one shoulder.

- Reach with one shoulder.
- Reach back with the other shoulder.

⊙ Find the circumference for how far your shoulders can reach.

- Reach up, down, and backward with your shoulder. Do it again.
- What are you beginning to notice about shoulder flexibility?
- Did you notice that increased range of motion in the shoulder can extend reach 4 to 8 inches?

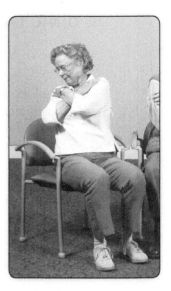

⊙ Put your arms back on—pop, pop.

- With your arms back on, reach one hand up, toward the imaginary light cord.
- Use your Venus de Milo arms to reach even farther, stretching with your shoulders to extend how far the arm will reach.
- Did you get more distance reaching with Venus de Milo arms?
- Did you notice your ribs and shoulders also lifting upward?
- Reach forward and use Venus de Milo arms to add inches to your reach. Is that better?
- Reach back, Venus de Milo style. Is that better?

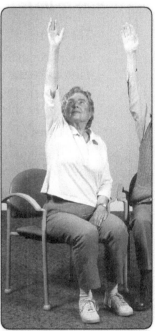

Live It))

Flexibility and function go arm in arm. Do your participants notice how much more distance they can get using the functional flexibility in their shoulders? That's the take-home message.

EXPLORING JOINT STIFFNESS

This activity provides a quick exploration of how even one joint can throw the proverbial wrench into how the body moves and functions.

Benefits))

- ◉ Stresses the importance of flexibility.
- ◉ Explores how each joint matters in a quick, fun, easy activity.
- ◉ Shows problems associated with decreased range of motion.

How to Do It))

Ask for a few volunteers to role-play some simple examples of what happens when a particular joint freezes up. Pick participants one or two at a time to demonstrate the following:

- ◉ Walk with stiff, arthritic knees.
- ◉ Walk with one knee suffering from a sprain or strain.
- ◉ Pretend one hip just won't be getting out of bed today. Walk with one hip stiff.
- ◉ Stand on both feet when a thorn is stuck under the left big toe. Try Walking.
- ◉ Walk with an aching, stiff back.
- ◉ Be seated. Pretend one shoulder is stiff and sore. Try to reach a bottle of ibuprofen on a top shelf.

Ask what did they learn from each other? Did joint stiffness limit motion? Was balance trickier with just one stiff knee or hip? Are joint limitations important when it comes to walking, moving, seated activities, and weight bearing?

Live It))

The ways in which participants can move and position their joints affects how they move and balance. Greater flexibility means more efficient, safer movements.

FLEXIBILITY

Many times when older people look over their shoulder they turn their whole trunk. The danger is that if they turn their whole trunk while walking, the turn will alter their path. Try it yourself—stand up and look over your right shoulder. Do you turn only your head, or do you turn your shoulders and torso, too? Do the same test walking. When the entire torso turns while you are moving, it usually alters your route. Maybe you've had a similar experience on a bike. You look behind and without realizing it, you've also turned the handlebars in the same direction. Participants with stiff, tight, or sore necks, shoulders, or chests are more vulnerable to this kind of oversteering. Flexibility can make a difference, and this activity helps them experience that difference.

Discuss with them that this activity gets a little more flexibility out of their neck by using their eyes. Provide some background. Demonstrate yourself walking with a stiff neck. Whenever you turn your head to look at something, turn your body, too. Show and tell them that turning the trunk with the body alters the direction in which they walk. Walk a distance, look left, and start walking to the left. Look right and wander right. They'll quickly get what you mean. Talk to them a bit about driving and head turns. Will a head turn alter their route? Would a stiff neck keep them from seeing something important?

Benefits))

- ◉ Uses eye movement and visual targeting.
- ◉ Improves neck, shoulder, and trunk range of motion, useful for everyday movements.
- ◉ Separates head turns from torso turns.
- ◉ Increases participant safety while walking and driving.

How to Do It))

The Start

Begin and follow this activity with shoulder rolls and chest stretches. It will help and feels great.

The Moves

Use the following cues.

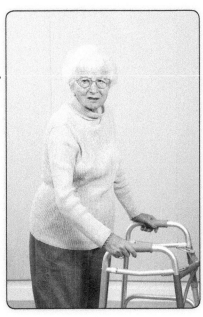

- ◉ Turn your head to the right as far as is comfortable. Note how far to the right you can see without pain.
- ◉ Turn just your eyes farther right. Does the head follow?
- ◉ When the eyes look farther right, the head can turn farther right.
- ◉ Turn the head left.
- ◉ Look a little farther with just the eyes. Then see if your head will turn a little further to follow.
- ◉ Look forward again.
- ◉ Did that work? Were you able to turn your head a little more using your eyes?
- ◉ Repeat with the other side.

- Can you *feel* how it works? Can you see how it works (i.e., look and see flexibility)?
- Repeat one or a few more times: Turn, look, turn more.
- Now, add the torso and arms to the turns. (Note: Trunk rotation may not suitable for participants with osteoporosis.)
    - Turn the head.
    - Turn the trunk and keep the abs braced so the trunk moves as a unit.
    - Reach back with the same-side arm.
    - Look down the outstretched arm. The palm of that hand is their visual target.
    - Turn a little more through the trunk, if able. Notice that looking down the arm gives you a little more rotation.
    - Look and see.

Keep It Safe))

The head turns in this activity may cause dizziness. Participants should stop if they feel dizzy. Do head turns slowly and gently. Don't hold a head turn longer than a few seconds; each gentle turn should take no more than 3 to 5 seconds. Nothing should hurt.

Live It))

Visual targets can add a little more distance to neck turns. In small ways, this activity will help participants achieve better neck flexibility to walk and drive better and be safer.

WORDS ON THE WALL IN THE HALL

Words on the Wall addresses neck stiffness and some aspects of gait (walking with head turns). It builds on concepts learned in Look and See Flexibility, adding walking, dual tasks, and more head turns. Turning the head without turning the body takes awareness and flexibility.

Benefits))

- ◉ Enhances neck flexibility.
- ◉ Builds awareness for safety during head turns.
- ◉ Practices staying on path when turning the head.

Set It Up))

First, you'll need some words to put on the wall. They could be words from a familiar nursery rhyme or oddly spelled common words such as *NV* for *envy* or *t42* for *tea for two*. I've used favorite funny license plates, Dr. Seuss poems, and "The Owl and the Pussy-Cat." Print the words or short verses on one page using very large letters, such as 72-point font. Add pictures from clip art and use bright, fun colors for a nicer presentation and better comprehension.

Before class, tape these pages to the walls of the room, spreading them out and taping them up in order. For example, if you were using "The Owl and the Pussy-Cat," you would place the first sheet on the right side of the hall ("The Owl and the Pussy-Cat"). The next page goes on the left side of the hall ("went to sea"). The next page goes on the right again ("in a beautiful pea green boat") and so on, until you have created six to eight head turns. Then consider if you want to put one or two verses on the ceiling, or maybe hang them from the ceiling on a ribbon if ceilings seem too high for participants to look up at safely. Looking up while walking presents a greater balance challenge. The point is to get a variety of head turns.

How to Do It))

The Start

Begin with a flexibility session. Include shoulder rolls, head turns and tilts, chin dips, and chest and neck stretches. Add a little show and tell. Discuss how stiff necks can create problems getting around by causing the whole upper body to turn when the head turns. If they do this whole-body turning while walking, they may veer off course or stumble. A ripple effect may be extrapolated to driving. Show participants your version of whole-body turning in a humorous way.

The Moves

Use the following cues.

- ◉ Do head turns while sitting. Get them turning just their heads instead of their heads and trunk.
- ◉ Practice head turns standing in front of the chair or with a walker. (Ask participants if anyone is dizzy. If all clear, go on to walking.)
- ◉ Practice walking along a handrail with head turns. If no handrails are available, then consider holding participants' hands or walking beside them.
- ◉ Do head turns every third or fourth step at most to start. (For the frailer, do less.)

Now you're ready to take them out in your prepared hallway for Words on the Wall in Hall.

- Start walking.
- Turn only the head to the right. Be like an owl.
- Read the words out loud. Look forward again and keep walking.
- Turn only the head left.
- Read the words out loud. Look forward again and keep walking.
- Keep a straight path and pay attention to balance and the path.
- Continue looking right and left until the entire nursery rhyme has been read.
- At the end, turn and walk back, reading the poem from the last lines to the first. (Participants are still walking forward, not backward. Going back through the poem, participants will be less able to predict the next line and will have to pay more attention to the printed material they are reading. Distraction is good for balance training, too.)

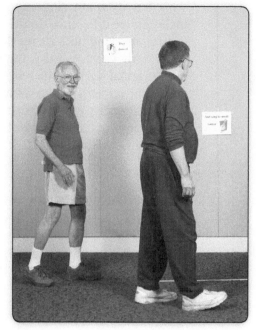

Keep It Safe))

The head turns in this activity may cause dizziness; talk about the possibility in advance. Participants should stop if they become dizzy. The dizziness may stop if they slow the head turns way down. If that works and they are comfortable, invite them to continue.

Be especially cautious about looking up. Watch them more closely and remind them to be careful. This is a good activity for taking turns. Walk beside the participant, and hold their hand the first time through, especially if you are having them look up to the ceiling. Stretching the chest, shoulders, and neck first will help.

Live It))

Stiff necks can cause problems with posture, balance, and function. Keeping the neck and shoulders flexible will help maintain mobility. Participants should be aware of their surroundings and stay on track when turning the head.

SUPPLE SPINE

This activity is amazing—and it's one of my favorites. The gentlest of motions can make a huge difference. In the beginning, participants are asked to spot a point on the ceiling, marking how far up they can see without pain. Then as their spine becomes suppler, they discover that they gradually can see farther and farther up, well beyond their original mark on the ceiling. Another plus for Supple Spine is that it uses only very gentle movements of the spine and pelvis, including flexion, extension, and rotation. The difference participants will experience with just a little more suppleness in their spine is unforgettable. I like it because participants experience the changes immediately and because it is so gentle. It's a lot of work to learn to teach, but it's worth it.

Benefits))

- Ties function to flexibility.
- Causes participants to notice how the spine is affected by both head and pelvic motion.
- Uses gentle, relaxing spinal flexion, extension, and rotation to increase function.

Set It Up))

Supple Spine is a complex, multipart activity that requires practice to teach. The sequencing is important, and so is your choice of cues for guiding participants through the sensations. Allow yourself several practice sessions to get it down. Practice with friends and family. Everyone who tries it sees a difference, so chances are your friends will enjoy doing the activity, too.

How to Do It))

Tell participants they will be asked to do some gentle stretching of the back and neck. They should look and move only as far as they can without straining or causing pain.

Mark the Spots

Use the following cues.

- Sit up comfortably.
- Look up at the ceiling, slowly and comfortably, without any strain or pain in the neck.
- Look forward again.
- Look up again. This time, notice exactly how far up the ceiling you can see without any pain or strain. Make a mental note of that spot for later.
- Look left and make a mental marker there.
- Look right and make a mental marker.

Rock the Pelvis Backward

Ask participants to sit tall on the edge of their chair with their feet flat on the floor, shoulder-width apart. Abs should be in, ribs lifted, shoulder blades back and down. The chin is parallel to the ground and head retracted a little. (This beginning position will be used in other exercises in this sequence as well.) Use the following cues.

- Place hands on the hips, thumbs to the back. (This hand placement will give participants a better feel for how to rock their pelvis.)
- Take a deep breath to prepare. Exhale and slowly tilt the pelvis backward so the lower back rounds toward the chair. Your hands are on your hips; use them to help roll the hips back toward the chair.

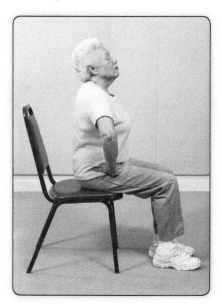 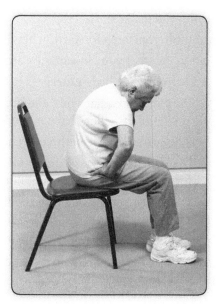

- Hold the position until you've exhaled completely.
- Inhale and return to tall sitting. Relax.
- Repeat the backward roll, but this time drop the chin to the chest and look down.
- Hold the position.
    - Do you notice that the back rounds into a *C* shape?
    - Do other changes occur when the hips tilt back?
    - Do your shoulders roll forward and come closer together?
    - Does this posture make you a little shorter?
    - Do you feel your weight shift toward your tailbone?
    - Is your breathing restricted?
- Return to tall sitting. Repeat if desired.

Rock the Pelvis Forward

- Sit tall with hands on the hips, thumbs in back.
- Blow out your breath.
- Inhale and begin to lift your chest forward and up, pulling back the shoulders.
- Use the thumbs on the hips to tilt the pelvis (hips) forward.
- Exhale and return to starting position.
- Inhale and repeat the activity, but this time look upward and lift your chin to the ceiling at the end of the movement.
- As you tilt your hips forward, what do you notice?
    - Do you feel your lower back arch a little?
    - Do you feel a little taller?
    - Do you sense that your chest feels more open and your shoulders have moved backward?
    - Is breathing easier with your chest expanded?
    - Do you notice that your body weight moves forward toward your sitting bones?

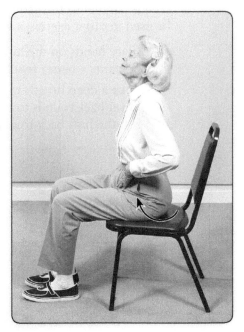

- Repeat. This time look up on the ceiling again, as far as you comfortably can.
- Can you see farther than at the beginning?
- The movement should be pain free and without strain. Remember to keep your abdomen, back, legs, and chest relaxed.

Combining Head, Eye, and Pelvic Movements

- Sit tall on the edge of the chair, feet flat on floor, hands on the hips.
- Cast your eyes downward to the floor. Keep the gaze down, no matter what.
- Inhale and slowly lift the chin toward the ceiling. But keep the eyes looking down—don't lift them no matter what. Soon you'll be at a spot where you can lift the chin no higher without lifting the eyes.
- Return to neutral posture and then repeat this gazing option one more time.
- But this time allow the pelvis to tilt forward and the chest to rise. Try to keep the gaze downward until the very end.
    - Do you notice that your gaze limits the movement of your head?
    - Was there any tightness in your back?
    - Do you feel a stretch in your abs and across your chest when you rock the hips forward?

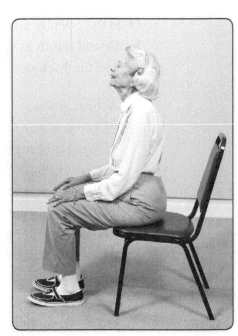

- Return to neutral posture and then repeat this gazing option.
- At the end, when you cannot lift your chin any higher because your eyes are limiting the head movement, let the gaze go. Look up, slowly and gently, all the way to the ceiling.
    - Can you see farther than the last time?
    - Was the movement easier when the eyes could move with the head and neck?
    - When your eyes, head, neck, and torso all contribute, is your range of motion clearly better?
    - Did the gentle stretching and rocking of the spine, hips, and neck make a difference in your overhead view?

Take It Further))

- Start with the beginning position.
- Exhale and rock the pelvis backward.
- Inhale, rock the pelvis forward, and begin to lift and rotate the chest and trunk up and to the right by lifting the right shoulder.
- Look up to the right. Lift the chin and right side of the face up and to the right.
- Return to the beginning position.
- Inhale and rock the pelvis forward. Lift and rotate the chest and trunk up and to the left by lifting the left shoulder.
- Look up to the left. Lift the chin and left side of the face up and to the left.
- Return to the beginning position.
- Turn the head right, then left.
- Compare how far you can see now compared with the beginning. Can you see farther than when you started? You bet!

Keep It Safe))

Stress that these movements are simple, gentle, undulating movements of the spine. Nothing should hurt.

Live It))

Even gentle stretching improves function.

Based on Zemach-Bersin, Zemach-Bersin, and Reese, 1990, Healthy spine. In *Relaxercise* (New York: Harper Collins).

SEATED WHOLE-BODY STRETCH

Stretching should feel great the entire time you're doing it. A good stretch is an enjoyable tightness across the desired muscles. Nothing should hurt. Deep breathing can make a stretch work and feel better. There are many types of seated stretching, several of which are outlined next. I always prefer to start with toes, feet, and ankles and work up from there. Remind participants that they should follow their doctor's advice and do only what feels comfortable.

Benefits))

- Stretches key joints for better posture and balance.
- Prepares participants for exercise.
- Draws participants' focus to their body.
- Feels good.

How to Do It))

This gentle whole-body stretch starts with the ankles and feet and moves upward from there. Participants begin comfortably seated, their hips and back against their chair.

Ankles, Feet, and Toes

Use the following cues to guide participants.

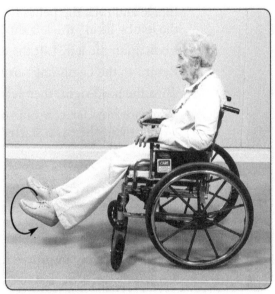

- Lift both feet forward and up off the ground.
- Point and flex both ankles a few times
- Hold the pointed position a few moments, and hold the flexed a few moments.
- Draw big, relaxing circles with the feet.
- Try to bring the bottoms of the feet together (supination).
- Lift outside borders of the feet upward (pronation).
- Do a few ankle alphabets (pick a participant's name to write in the air).
- Wriggle, scrunch, and spread out the toes like starfish (you can do hands and fingers at the same time, if you like).

Knee Hugs

This activity is good for gluteal muscles and hips. Use the following cues.

- Start with the back and hips against the chair back.
- Slide the hands under one knee and lift it toward the chest.
- Hug the knee closer to the chest, wrapping hands or forearms around it.
- Breathe, relax, and give the stretch time to develop; hold 10 to 15 seconds.

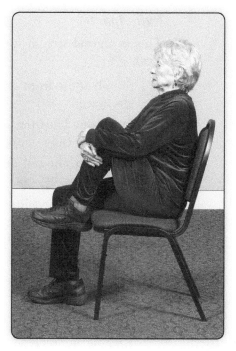

Crossovers

This is a good activity to stretch the outer thigh (hip abductors). Participants with a hip replacement or recent surgery should have their doctor's clearance to do this stretch—it pulls on the joint in a way that may be destabilizing to the joint.

- Start with the back and hips against the chair back.
- Use the hands to lift one knee up and cross it over the other knee, as comfortable.
- Tilt the crossed legs over to one side so that the top leg begins to stretch.
- To progress, use both hands to pull the top leg gently across the chest, toward the opposite shoulder.
- Breathe, relax, and give the stretch time to develop; hold 10 to 15 seconds.
- For more stretch, pull the back away from the chair and sit tall, holding the knee close.

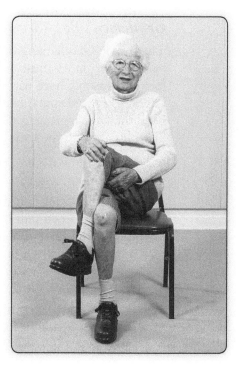

Pull-Aparts

This is a good stretch for the inner thighs (hip adductors).

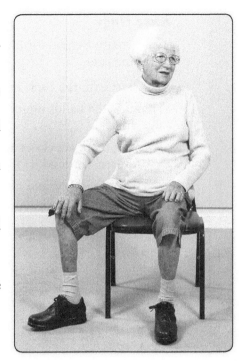

- Sit tall at the front of the chair, shoulders over hips, abs braced.
- Draw one knee out to the side; keep the knee and ankle vertically stacked.
- Repeat this in-and-out motion a few times to warm up the joint.
- Hold the out position a few moments.
- Gently press the knee out a little more with one hand to increase the stretch.
- Sit a little taller and breathe in (adds to the stretch).
- Exhale and turn the upper body away from the knee (adds to the stretch).
- Turn back to center.
- Breathe and relax.

Gentlemen's Bow (Seated)

The bow in Gentlemen's Bow involves forward leaning. It's a good stretch for the hips, hamstrings, gluteal muscles, and low back. Be sure to cue for back support. During the forward leaning, have participants rest some of their upper-body weight on the bent knee. Also avoid spinal bending during the forward leaning. Cue participants not to bend their back but to lean forward from their hips. The bow should occur at the hips, like a hinge, with the back held tall and straight and with core muscles braced.

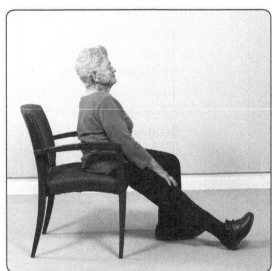

- Sit tall at the front of the chair, both feet flat on the floor, legs parallel.
- Extend one leg out and place the heel on the floor. Then pull it back under the knee. Repeat this knee flexion and extension three to four times to warm up the knee. After the last extension, leave the heel out on the floor with the knee as straight as is comfortable.
- Sit tall again to start the stretch. (This makes a nice hamstring stretch.)
- Draw in the abdominal wall and slowly begin to lean forward from the hips. Place one arm on the opposite leg for back support. Continue to lean forward in a movement that looks like a slow, graceful Shakespearean bow over the straight leg. Allow the stretch to develop; hold 10 to 15 seconds.
- To progress, reach the long arm out in front and lift the arm and trunk slowly until the arm is reaching toward the ceiling.

Proud Mary

Hip flexor muscles cover the front portion of the hip joint and play a key role in upright posture. When hip flexors are overly tight, posture appears bent over at the hip and standing up straight and tall is difficult. These muscles are commonly tight in older adults from leaning forward when they walk or use a walker. An effective hip flexor stretch that can be done seated is challenging to find. Proud Mary is my best attempt at a seated hip flexor stretch. Some of my participants have a hard time getting the foot turned under. See how it works for you. If you find one you like better, then please e-mail your suggestion to me (renewablefitness@comcast.net).

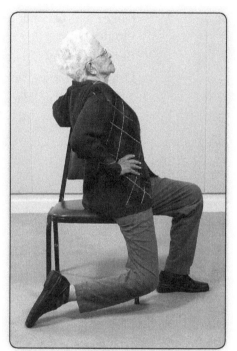

- ◉ Sit sideways on a chair, outermost leg off the chair, knee hanging toward the floor, in a half-kneeling position, foot turned sole up, so its top side is on the floor.
- ◉ Begin with the back tall and straight, one hand on the chair, the other on their hip.
- ◉ To stretch the hip flexor, push the outer hip forward and gently draw the outer leg back.
- ◉ Look proud! Lift the chest up and out, draw the shoulders back, and take a deep breath to fill the lungs and expand the stretch.
- ◉ Keep hand on the hip to keep stretching.
- ◉ To progress, pull the upper body back slightly.

Sunbursts

This activity stretches the chest and shoulders.

- ◉ Begin from a Tall Sit position.
- ◉ Extend both arms out to the side at shoulder height.
- ◉ Spread the fingers out.
- ◉ Slowly lower the arms toward the chair until a stretch is felt across the chest and front of shoulders.
- ◉ Like the sun coming up over the horizon, lift the arms laterally back to shoulder height and beyond, as comfortable. Stretch should be felt across the chest and shoulders.
- ◉ Bend the elbows in and place the hands behind the ears.
- ◉ Draw the elbows back and take in a deep breath.
- ◉ Lift the chest and face upward to expand the stretch.
- ◉ Exhale and bring the arms down gently.

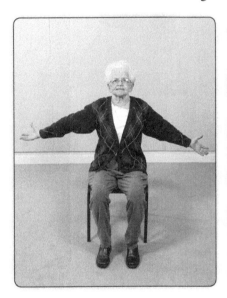 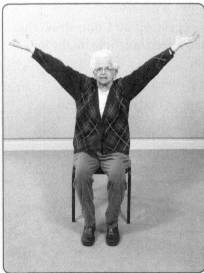 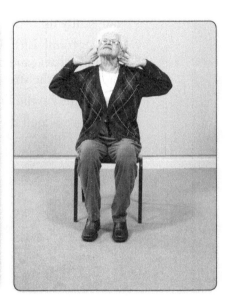

Hands Up!

This is a variation of Sunbursts for internal and external shoulder rotation.

- ◉ Lift both arms forward at shoulder height.
- ◉ Pull the elbows back and then lift the forearms (looks like a robber who's been told "Hands up!" by a police officer).
- ◉ Inhale and hold the position.
- ◉ Exhale and rotate the forearms downward. Keep the upper arms at shoulder level, if able.
- ◉ Repeat and rest.

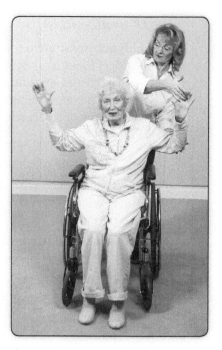

Inside-Out Arms

This activity stretches the upper back and posterior shoulders and begins from a Tall Sit position.

- ◉ Extend both arms out to the side at shoulder height.
- ◉ Bring them both in front still at shoulder height.
- ◉ Intertwine the fingers and turn the hands inside out.
- ◉ Round the back gently without leaning forward.
- ◉ Pull the arms back and sit tall again.
- ◉ Roll the shoulders backward a few times to help recover good posture.

Wrist Pulls

This activity stretches the back and shoulders.

- ◉ Inhale and reach for the sky with one arm, reaching up as far as possible. Exhale and return to the starting position.
- ◉ Inhale and reach up as far as you can with the other arm. Exhale and return to the starting position.
- ◉ Now reach both arms straight up in the air, fingers reaching.
- ◉ Inhale and one hand should grab the opposite wrist and pull gently. Allow the trunk to arch a bit to expand the stretch into the shoulders and ribs. Exhale while holding the stretch.
- ◉ Breath in deeply again and repeat the pull on the other wrist. Allow the trunk to arch a bit to expand the stretch into the shoulders and ribs. Exhale while holding the stretch.
- ◉ Wriggle the fingers while bringing both arms down to rest, hands on lap.
- ◉ Roll the shoulders and relax.

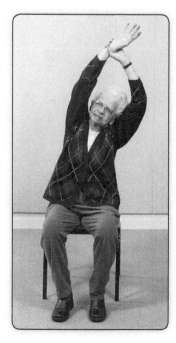

(Parentheticals)

This activity stretches the lateral sides, ribs, triceps, and shoulders. The resultant body position looks like parentheses; you'll make one to each side. Technically, they're side bends, but the amount of side bending should only be slight. Provide back support by placing the opposite arm on the chair or chair's arm. See if you can get participants to notice how deep breaths help the stretch.

- Sit tall and place one arm on the chair for back support.
- Inhale and reach up as far as possible with the other arm.
- Exhale, and gently arch the trunk slightly so that the stretch is felt through the ribs and shoulder. (This will look like a parenthesis).
- Inhale and bend the reaching arm at the elbow. Try to place that hand on the opposite shoulder.
- Exhale and gently arch ribs over the supporting arm.
- You can add to the stretch by continuing to lift the elbow overhead. Imagine the rib cage gently spreading as the elbow pulls.
- Gently bring the arm down.
- Do the other side: Inhale and reach up; exhale and bend the elbow. Inhale and arch over; exhale and come down.

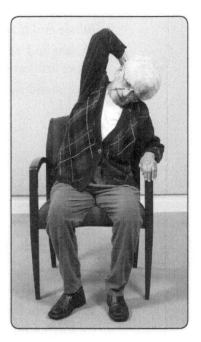

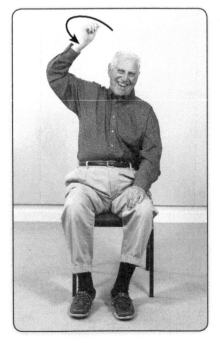

Lariat Arms

Pretend you're a cowboy getting ready to lasso a calf. The rope hand swirls out to the side, then forward, then over the head and back. These are big, rolling shoulder circles. Perfect.

- Do big, rolling arm circles with one arm—out to the side, then forward, then over the head and back.
- Repeat with the other arm.

Shoulder Rolls

- Begin with a series of slow, big shoulder rolls. (Always roll the shoulders backward.)
- Do both shoulders together.
- Stop at the top (shoulders pulled to ears); stop again with shoulders pulled back (extra chest stretch).
- Do some rolls alternating shoulders.
- Take deep, slow breaths while doing these to expand the chest wall.

Head Tilts and Rolls

- Sit tall with the chin level. Draw the head back as far as possible; the goal is ears aligned with the shoulders. Inhale.
- Exhale and draw both shoulders down.
- Tilt the left ear toward the left shoulder.
- Drop the chin forward to the collarbone.
- Roll the chin along the collarbone to the left shoulder.
- Lift the head and inhale.
- Repeat on the other side in the other direction.

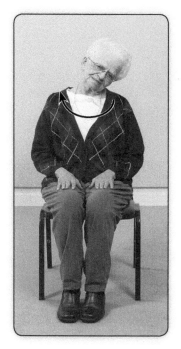

Head Turns

- Sit tall. Pull the head back so the ears are more over the shoulders. Inhale.
- Exhale and turn the head to the right, as is comfortable for the neck.
- Hold just a few seconds.
- Turn back to center and inhale.
- Repeat on the other side.

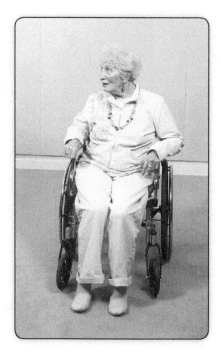

Chin Dips

- ⊙ Sit tall and draw the head back (ears in line with shoulders, chin level). Inhale.
- ⊙ Place two fingers on the chin.
- ⊙ Exhale and gently press the chin to the neck.
- ⊙ Try to maintain the Tall Sit position.
- ⊙ Hold the neck stretch for 10 to 15 seconds, as tolerated.

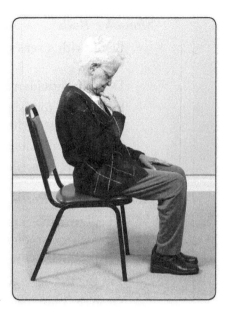

Live It))

Taking time to do a whole-body stretch prepares participants for exercise and gets them to focus on their body. Seated Whole-Body Stretch can be done by just about anyone, anywhere.

FARMER'S STRETCH

This is a wonderful stretch for the whole front of the body. It stretches the hip flexors, abdominal wall, chest, and shoulders. It reminds me of a farmer surveying his fields, with his hands in his suspenders and his shoulders drawn back with pride. His back may be aching from the day's work, but he's thinking, "What a beautiful sight my fields are!" See if you can get participants to notice how deep breaths help the stretch. If the stretch hurts, participants can try standing with offset feet (instead of parallel).

Benefits))

- ◉ Stretches the frequently tight hip flexors.
- ◉ Stretches the abs, chest, and back.
- ◉ Strengthens the postural muscles that bring the shoulder blades together.
- ◉ Provides some relief for sciatic pain.
- ◉ Includes an element of balance because it is done standing.

How to Do It))

The Start

Participants should stand in front of their chair with the back of their legs touching the chair. Feet should be wider than shoulder width, and hands are on the hips, if possible.

The Moves

Use the following cues to guide participants through the stretch.

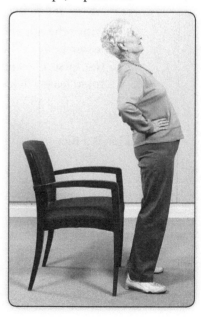

- ◉ Inhale and push the hips forward enough that you feel a stretch across the front of the hips and abs. Exhale and hold the position.
- ◉ Tighten the gluteal muscles.
- ◉ Inhale again, and pull the elbows and shoulders gently back until you feel a stretch across the shoulders and chest.
- ◉ Exhale while holding the stretch.
- ◉ Draw the shoulder blades together and look up a little.
- ◉ Hold for 10 to 15 seconds, as tolerated and pain free.
- ◉ Return to the starting position, being careful for balance. March in place a bit to relax the legs.

Give It More Balance))

A modification of this stretch is to use offset feet; stand with one foot forward and one back. The hip flexors of the back leg are stretched. So do one side and then the other.

Live It))

This is an energizing stretch. It feels great when participants have been sitting a lot or when their back is tired. Squeezing the gluteal muscles really gives the sciatic nerve a rest.

FARMER AND THE HULA

This is a variation on the Farmer's Stretch. It adds more flexibility for the hips and some reciprocal motion to the activity, which is nice for balance training.

Benefits))

- ◉ Loosens low back and hips.
- ◉ Requires whole-body coordination (reciprocal motion between hips and torso).
- ◉ Participants discover that hips and torso are separable body segments that can be moved reciprocally about each other.
- ◉ Adds an element of balance because it's done standing and involves movement.

How to Do It))

The Start

Participants stand in front of their chair with the back of the legs touching the chair. Feet should be wider than shoulder width, and hands are on the hips, if possible. This is the same position used for the Farmer's Stretch.

The Moves

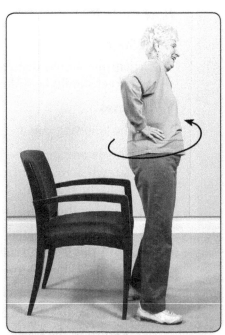

- ◉ Gradually begin to circle hips with big, circular motions.
- ◉ Change directions.
- ◉ Move in a figure-eight pattern.
- ◉ Move the upper body in the opposite direction of the lower body. When the hips are pushed to the right, the torso goes left; when the hips press forward, the torso leans backward; and so on.

Live It))

This is a nice, relaxing, yet invigorating stretch.

LUNGE STRETCH

This standing lunge stretch is another variation of Farmer's Stretch. However, it's done standing behind the chair with feet in an offset foot position. One side is done at a time.

Benefits))

- ◉ Progresses Farmer's Stretch.
- ◉ Adds elements of balance (standing, offset feet, reaching).
- ◉ Provides a whole-body stretch (hip flexors, anterior trunk, shoulders).

How to Do It))

The Start

Participants stand behind their sturdy chair with both hands on the back of the chair and feet parallel. Ask them to step one leg back in a big step, about 18 to 24 inches (46-61 centimeters). They keep the heel of the rear foot up off the floor during the stretch. The feet should still be shoulder-width apart and both hands still on the chair.

The Moves

Use the following cues.

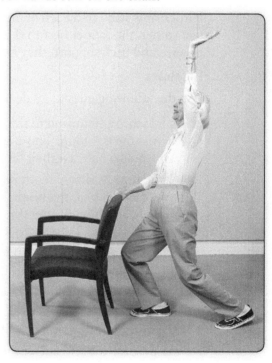

- ◉ Lower the back knee toward the floor until you feel a stretch in the hip flexors of that side.
  - - It looks similar to a curtsy.
  - - Do not lean forward, but rather drop straight down.
  - - The front knee will stay over the front foot, if done correctly.
- ◉ Add to the stretch by gently pulling the upper body back, as comfortable. Hands stay on the chair.
- ◉ Add even more to the stretch by slowly lifting the same-side hand as rear leg off the chair and reaching that arm up and over the head, sort of like a one-armed Arabesque.
- ◉ Hold any of these positions or a combination for 10 to 15 seconds, as tolerated.
- ◉ Relax, place both hands back on the chair, and bring the feet back to parallel.
- ◉ Do the other leg.

CARRY THE BABY

Carry the Baby begins from the position that parents use when they set their baby on their hip. It's an effective stretch for the entire side of the body, from triceps to tensor fasciae latae. Carry the Baby is done standing, but there is also a seated version, (Parentheticals), described on page 80. Provide back support for the side bending by having participants place the down arm on their chair back.

Benefits))

- ⊚ Stretches sides of ribs, hips, and shoulders.
- ⊚ Helps participants feel the connectedness of the whole body.
- ⊚ Involves both the upper and lower body.
- ⊚ Adds an element of balance because it's done standing.

How to Do It))

The Start

Participants stand to the left of the chair, hips aligned with the chair back and with offset feet so that the foot closest to the chair is in front and the outside foot is in back. For balance and back support, they hold onto chair with the chair-side hand.

The Moves

Use the following cues to guide participants.

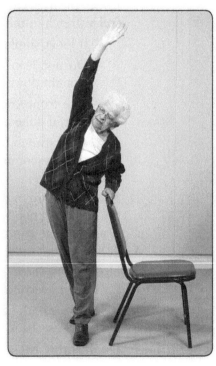

- ⊚ Slide the right hip out to the side until you feel a stretch across the right hip. This motion is similar to how parents hold a baby on their hip.
- ⊚ When ready, slowly reach the right arm out to the side and then up over the head. The arm is overhead and a bit left, reaching for the sky.
- ⊚ Inhale deeply and allow the ribs to arch slightly left. Feel the ribs lift and spread out like a fan. Exhale while holding the stretch.
- ⊚ To progress, bend the elbow and reach the hand toward the opposite shoulder.
- ⊚ Hold this position for 10 to 15 seconds, as tolerated.
- ⊚ Repeat for the left side of the body.

Live It))

These big, gentle, arching side bends that focus on breathing and relaxing feel best when participants are feeling tight or tired.

GENTLEMEN'S BOW (STANDING)

This is a standing version of Gentlemen's Bow, described earlier (see page 76). Be sure to provide support for the upper body during the forward lean, or bow.

Benefits))

- ◉ Stretches entire posterior leg and hips.
- ◉ Adds an element of balance because it's done standing.

How to Do It))

The Start

Have participants stand sideways behind a sturdy chair or other balance support. They should rest the chair-side hand and forearm on the chair back or on a handrail for back support. Feet should be parallel, shoulder-width apart.

The Moves

Use the following cues.

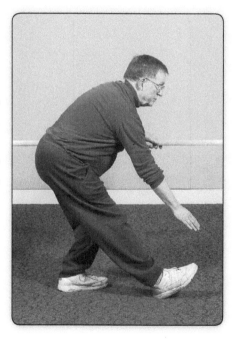

- ◉ Extend one leg out and place the heel on the floor. Keep the knee as straight as is comfortable.
- ◉ Draw in the abdominal wall and take a bow, slowly leaning forward from the hips over the straight leg. Allow the stretch to develop; hold 10 to 15 seconds.
- ◉ To progress and involve the lower back, extend the free arm and reach up to about ear level. Then reach out a little more.

5

Posture and Core Stability

Posture is how the body aligns itself over the earth. This alignment affects your balance whether you're standing still or doing any number of everyday activities. Core stability braces and sustains posture so participants are less perturbed by jostling crowds or other unexpected changes. Potential balance disturbances for the frail elderly can range from simply turning their head while walking to being bumped in a crowd or lurched about by a walker that sticks on a threshold. Good posture and the steadying power of a strong core will help your participants feel stronger and better balanced.

There are additional benefits to improved posture and core stability. Enhancing core strength and consistently using more symmetrical and balanced postures can often reduce chronic back pain. Better posture also makes many everyday functions easier, including walking and reaching. These many benefits may allow participants to become more active and independent with better posture and core stability.

Quick Reminder

The majority of the ABLE Bodies activities in this section can be done seated, thereby enabling participation by those with a wide range of abilities. Participants who are not mobile or able to stand also benefit from improved posture, core strength, and balance. Core strength and balance make transfers easier and can provide relief from back pain in nonambulatory adults. Seated activities also work well for large classes or whenever standing safety is a concern.

As always, progress only as is well tolerated by your participants, meaning nothing hurts, they are willing and able to participate, and they show no signs of dizziness, nausea, excessive fatigue, and so on. Participants should be able to do the exercise using proper form before any difficulty is added. Please review chapter 3 for more information on safe progression.

All activities in this chapter are available in PDF format! Visit www.HumanKinetics.com/ABLEBodiesBalanceTraining.

FEEL-GOOD POSTURE

Posture affects how you feel. Stand tall and upright and you'll feel proud and strong; cower in a corner with your face covered and you'll feel at least a little afraid. This charades-style posture activity gets participants to start connecting posture with how they live and feel.

Benefits))

⊙ Acts as a good icebreaker and mixer for new groups.

⊙ Demonstrates the link between posture and body language.

⊙ Illustrates connections between mind and body in a fun way.

⊙ Allows everyone to participate—it's easy and almost free of balance challenges.

Set It Up))

Before class, make a list of easily conveyed emotions or characters that participants can portray, such as happy, proud, ferocious, scared, shy, runway model, the winning boxer in a ring, and the other boxer in the ring. Put your suggestions in a hat, bag, or bowl.

How to Do It))

Tell your class this game is similar to charades. Begin the activity yourself.

⊙ Demonstrate fatigue. Stand in front of the class and assume a fatigued posture. Show it with your whole body. Head, back, shoulders, knees, eyes, mouth, even the way you breathe—do the whole works.

- Ask them to guess what feeling your posture portrays.
- Ask them what clues gave it away. (Was it slumping shoulders, bent knees, or the frown?)

⊙ Now it's their turn. Ask them to show you their most tired posture possible. Ask them to show you tired with their back, neck, eyes, mouth, knees, and mind. You want them to connect posture with mind and body. Once they look fatigued, ask them these kinds of leading questions:

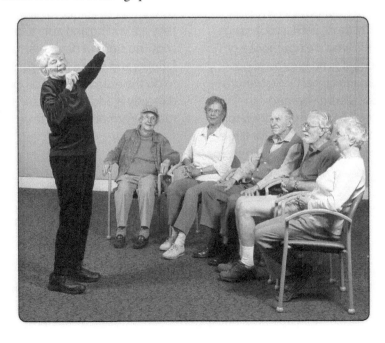

- How do you feel physically?
  Emotionally?

- How do you look? Are you taller or shorter?

- Is it hard to look up? Does your back hurt?

- Do you sense any shift in your attitude?

Pull out your cache of easily conveyed emotions or characters.

◉ Ask for a volunteer to pick an emotion or character and then demonstrate it. The other participants will try to guess the answer by reading the body language.

◉ Once the emotion is guessed, another volunteer selects a piece of paper and the activity continues.

◉ As each emotion is displayed, observe and discuss with your class what changes happened with the postures.

- Proud. (Do taller postures feel more capable?)

- Ferocious. (Do certain stances feel bolder?)

- Fear or shock. (Can posture affect how we feel?)

- Ask them all to take a bold, proud stand. Then ask them to take a bow.

- Ask a volunteer to show a bent over person walking down the street.

- Ask another volunteer to be a runway model. (Ask your participants if certain postures feel younger or older.)

- Did they do a good job of expressing their assignment using only body language?

- Did they begin to feel how they looked?

Keep It Safe))

Never insist on participation, but always invite it. Some people are shy, especially in new classes. Let the willing ones go first. They'll get some laughs and this will help everyone feel more comfortable.

Live It))

Posture is powerful stuff! It affects how participants feel, look, and even portray themselves. Good posture can take a few years off their age, add confidence, and help them understand how others are feeling.

This activity encourages inside-out learning. Participants are invited to experiment with their own posture and then discover how changes in posture feel. Manipulating their posture into exaggerated positions lets them discover and appreciate the in-between positions. Hopefully they will compare these ideas with their own habits and become more aware of how posture affects them.

Benefits ⟩⟩

- ◉ Helps participants feel their body's response to changes in posture.
- ◉ Helps them monitor their posture.
- ◉ Invites self-discovery for personal preferences.
- ◉ Introduces neutral, in-between positions.
- ◉ Builds social ties within the class.
- ◉ It's fun to watch and listen as everyone tries new things.

Set It Up ⟩⟩

No props are needed, but practice helps. Knowing the options and their order, as well as the cues to use, will make this activity go more smoothly and productively. For the pelvic section it may help their visual perception if you are wearing pants with a belt for that class.

How to Do It ⟩⟩

This series of activities starts at the feet and ankles and works up, so begin with the participants standing. If your group is unable to stand, start with the head and neck and work down as far as the hip. They can shift their weight on their chair.

Feet and Ankles

For each change in foot position, ask how the change feels. Then ask which position feels best.

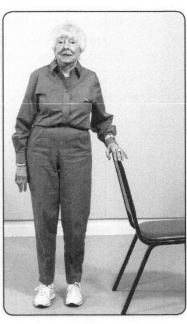

- ◉ Have them place the feet a few inches apart and parallel.
    - Where do they feel their weight under their feet? Is it mostly under their heels? Their toes? Along the sides? A little of each?
    - Can they lean a little forward and feel their weight shift toward their toes?
    - Have them shift back again and see if they feel a more even distribution now.
    - Ask them to push out one hip and rest their hand on it. What pressure changes happen under their feet now?

⊙ Duck feet: Ask participants to turn their feet outward, like a duck's feet.
- What changes?
- Does the duck stance strain the arches of feet?
- Do they notice that the ankles roll in? Can they feel that?
- Can they feel any changes on the inner side of their knees with duck's feet?

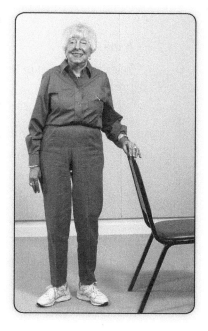

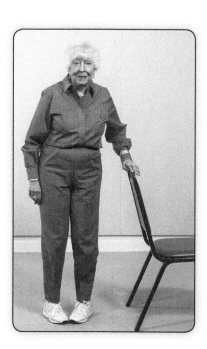

⊙ Pigeon toes: Ask participants to stand pigeon-toed, turning their toes in.
- What changes?
- Can they feel any strains in the outer knee?
- Go back to parallel feet, a few inches apart. Does that feel better?

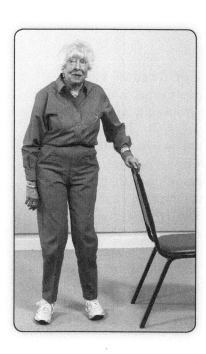

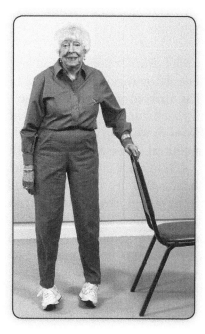

⊙ Ankle rolls: Ask participants to roll their ankles in and out. To roll in, lift the outside of the feet, and to roll out, lift the inside of the feet.
- Do it again. Ask them to feel the changes.
- What changes?
- What hurts?
- How are their knees affected?
- Find a middle point, feet flat on floor.
- Ask what's best for them.

Knees

For each change in knee position, ask how those changes feel and which positions they prefer.

- Flexed knees: Get them to bend their knees and hold the position for a moment.
    - Do their legs tire quickly?
- Soft knees: This is a slightly flexed standing position.
    - Does this feel better? Less tiring?
- Locked knees: This is a hyperextended, or super-straight knee, position.
    - Does this cause their hips to tilt forward?
    - Does it change where they feel the weight under their feet?
    - Do they feel any changes in their back?

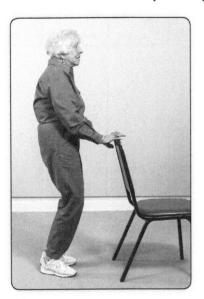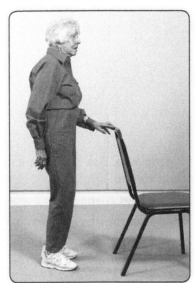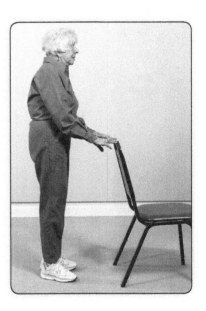

- Which of these three options feels best to them?

Pelvis

The word *pelvis* comes from the Latin for "basin," or a large bowl. A neutral spine or pelvic position can be found easily by rocking the pelvis. Imagine the pelvis is a basin filled with water. Tilt the pelvis forward and water spills out the front side. Tilt it backward and water pours from the back side. Hold it level and no water spills. This no-spill position is a neutral spine. If you're wearing a belt, it clearly displays whether the hips tilt forward or back or are in neutral. In neutral position, the belt will be level.

While standing (or sitting tall on their chair), ask participants to place their hands on their hips, thumbs in back, fingers in front. Show and tell them how they can direct their hips into a forward tilt by pushing forward with their thumbs. If they were a basin, water would pour out the front side. They can tilt the pelvis backward by pushing back with their fingers. Their low back will round and water would spill out the back. After your demonstration, let them try. Their hips should be level to start, tilting neither forward nor backward and not listing to either side. For each change in the pelvis, ask participants to notice how the change feels and then which positions they prefer.

- Backward-tilting pelvis: Ask participants to tilt their pelvis backward, pushing their pelvis backward using their fingers. This motion rocks the pelvis backward. To some it feels like tucking their hips under their shoulders. If they were pouring water from their basin, water would pour out from the back.

  - What changes do they notice in their back and chest? (Cue them to notice that the back and shoulders round forward, chest muscles shorten, and chest flattens.)
  - What happens at their knees? Do they bend a little more? (Yes.)
  - Any other changes? (Head is lowered.)
  - Is their breathing restricted? (Slightly.)

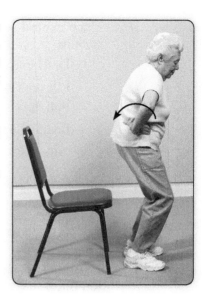

- Forward-tilting pelvis: Now ask them to tilt their pelvis forward. To do this, they should push their pelvis forward with their thumbs. This will rock the pelvis forward. If they were pouring water from their basin, it would pour from the front. Ask them questions about how this feels:

  - Do they notice that their tailbones lift upward?
  - Can they feel a hollow develop in their low back?
  - Can they feel this especially in their low back?
  - Do they feel a slight stretch across their abdominal wall?
  - Which way do their shoulders move this time?
  - What else changes? Are there any changes to their knees? Do they hyperextend?
  - Do they notice how the changes are opposite to the backward tilting?

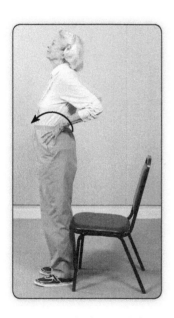

Ask them if they notice how their pelvis is a link between the upper and lower body. (This activity illustrates it well because the spine connects the two.)

- Rock the Pelvis: Now participants will rock their hips back and forth. Ask participants to place one hand on their abdomen and one hand on the middle of their low back, just above their buttocks.

- In a simple rocking motion, have them pull the abdominals in and up with the front hand and push the hips down and under the torso with the back hand.

  - Do they feel how this rocks their pelvis under and in line with their shoulders?

- Do it a few more times for effect. Have them rock the pelvis backward and forward using their hands.

  - Allow time for them to find a comfortable in-between position that feels good and that keeps their pelvis centered under their shoulders.
  - This comfortable in-between position is neutral spine for their low back.

POSTURE

- Once neutral feels good, have the participants secure the position with core stability.
    - Draw in the abdominal wall.
    - Lift the ribs to lengthen the spine.
    - Pull the shoulder blades back and down.
    - Breathe in; stand (or sit) tall!
    - Nice work. Good job. Ask them, how does that feel?

Shoulders and Midback

This section can be done seated. Your participants may be tired from standing.

- Ask participants to draw their shoulders up toward their ears.
- Have them push their shoulders down toward the floor. Repeat.
- Have them find an in-between position for the shoulders that feels level.
- Call it their level best. (Get it? Level is best!)

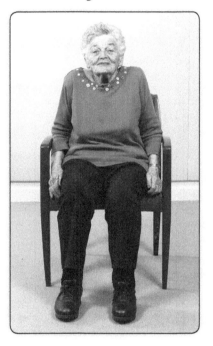

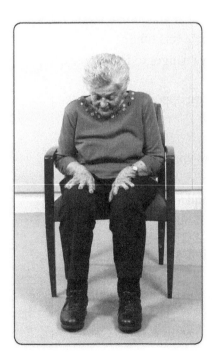

- Have them roll their shoulders forward.
    - Have them try to take a breath in this position.
    - Can they feel that their breathing is restricted with the shoulders forward? (It is.)

- Now, ask them to pull their shoulders back by pulling the shoulder blades together.
    - Have them take another breath. Was this breath much easier? (Much!)
    - Ask them if this chest-out position feels natural. (Probably not quite.)
- Ask them to find an in-between position for their shoulders, somewhere between back and forward, up and down. The best position is when the shoulders point directly out to the sides.
- Once they find the sweet spot for their shoulders, continue:
    - Lift the rib cage and spine into a tall sit.
    - Hold abdominals in and up a bit.
    - Bring shoulder blades back and down.
    - How does this feel for stable and tall?
    - This should feel great!

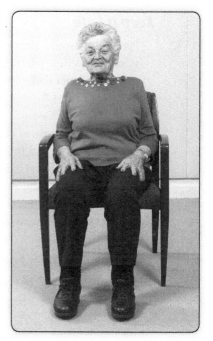

Head and Neck

Participants can be seated or standing. Begin with some background information about the head. Heads are heavy! They weigh 10 or more pounds (4.5 kilograms), balanced at the top of their structure. Any change in head position is hard work for the body to support.

- Lift the chin and look up. How does that affect the chest and back? (Lifts chest and arcs back.)
- Lower the chin and then drop the head. Can they feel these changes in their neck and back? (Do it again to compare kinesthetic learning.)
- Hold the chin level, parallel to floor. How does that feel? Is it better in between?
- Tilt the head right, then left. Discuss how that feels. Can they feel a stretch? Ask them if one side feels tighter than the other (it usually does).
- Center the head. Is this another in-between position?
- Can they notice the weight seems easier to support when the head is centered?
- Head like an Egyptian or head on a silver platter (head retraction and protraction):
    - Beginning from a level chin, ask participants to use their neck and shoulder muscles to slide (retract) their head directly back. Their tendency will be to lift their chin, but we want them to keep the chin level, and slide the head directly back as if it were on a platter. At the end of this motion, the ears should be in line with their shoulders, or as close as possible.
    - Next have them jut the chin forward, in an Egyptian-looking head movement.
- Ask which of these forward and back positions felt best.
- Ask them to find an overall in-between position for their head. (That's neutral head position.)

Keep It Safe))

Nothing should hurt or make them uncomfortable. They can stop or refuse any suggestion. When participants are doing Parts of the Whole standing, provide balance support as needed.

Live It))

Improving posture is a compilation of many positions. Being aware of all the possibilities is the first step to making smart changes. Rocking the pelvis can help participants find their neutral spine. They should stand tall with the knees soft, feet parallel, and hips tucked under just a bit. Abdominals should be in, ribs lifted, shoulder blades back and down, and head lifted and retracted. Good posture takes an almost constant effort over a long time. It also takes desire, awareness, and lots of practice. Hopefully this activity will contribute to positive change.

SMELL THE COFFEE

We all know how to straighten our posture when we want to get a whiff of some wonderful smell, whether it's perfume, an ocean breeze, or cinnamon buns. The sense of smell is one of the keenest senses. Over long periods of time, its memory is the most accurate of the senses. Here is an example that compares visual memory with olfactory (smell) memory. Most people remember what their old grade school looked like, but when they go back for a visit they find it's much smaller than they remembered. That visual memory wasn't quite accurate. But smell is different. Over many years we remember smells well, and we remember them accurately. Mom's fresh baked bread? Kindergarten lunches? Fresh mowed lawn, or hay? An ocean breeze? We recognize those smells quickly and right as rain.

For this activity, it's the smells of fresh-brewed morning coffee that participants want to find. Smell the Coffee is a fun, quick, and easy activity that marries deep breathing and a natural back-lengthening movement. It will help participants lift into tall, ribs-lifted posture, with abdominals braced and head and shoulders retracted and aligned. This combination enhances posture and core stability. Use it for those times at the beginning of class when you look out at your participants and they don't seem quite ready for exercise. Maybe they're slumping and not yet smiling . . . it's as if they need a wake-up call. Smell the Coffee can come to the rescue and whisk away those doldrums. Pretty soon, participants may start liking this activity better than actual coffee!

Benefits))

- ◉ Helps participants achieve tall sitting posture.
- ◉ Uses memorable cues to evoke an ingrained sequence for tall sitting.
- ◉ Begins posture exercises in a fun, easy, and social way with a warm and fuzzy feel.

Set It Up))

Come up with a list of smells that would be easily recognizable by participants. Talk with your participants about their memories of favorite smells. Maybe laugh about some awful smells we remember just as well. Share some of your own favorite smells or smell memories. Then invite participants to do a little imaginative smelling.

How to Do It))

Use the following cues.

- ◉ Close your eyes and take a deep breath. Try to find a favorite smell. (Mention some of the responses they said earlier.) Smell deeply. Can you smell it?
- ◉ Did your posture change with your deep breath? Are you sitting taller to catch that smell?
- ◉ Again, image the scent drifting by on a breeze. Can you smell it?
  - Ask them to notice their posture.
  - Did they sit up tall?
  - Did they pull their back away from the back of the chair?
  - Did they lift their ribs, their head, and their spine?

Now they are ready to try the activity again. This time they'll have the concept in their mind and will know what they're doing for posture. You might say something such as, "Okay everyone, wake up and smell the coffee! Give me a tall sit and take a deep breath in!" Here are some cues to use:

- Bring your back away from the back of the chair.
- Breathe in and pull yourself up tall.
- Abdominals in.
- Ribs . . . spine . . . lifted.
- Smell the coffee? Enjoy the great aroma and smile.
- Exhale slowly and pull the shoulder blades back and down.

Progress the activity by adding some flexibility. Give the stretches a morning theme to fit with smelling the coffee. The next stretch can be a good-morning yawn. They reach up with one arm and breathe in deeply, as if yawning and stretching, and then reach with the other. They can push their arms out and around their back. It's their morning coffee with you!

Keep It Safe))

Although this activity should be safe and fun for just about anyone, too many deep breaths in row may leave some participants out of breath or even dizzy. Remind them to take their time and be gentle.

Live It))

Smell the Coffee—three simple words that cue participants to sit tall and breathe deeply. It has a way of marrying deep breaths with tall, centered, and balanced postures. It feels natural and benefits participants greatly!

POSTURE AFFECTS FUNCTION AND BALANCE

This activity provides three hands-on activities, Breathe Easy, Anchors A-Sway, and Bent Over Posture, to show participants more ways in which posture can affect ordinary aspects of their lives.

Benefits))

- Reveals how posture affects breathing.
- Explores how posture affects tipping points.
- Shows how posture affects needing to take a quick step when walking.

How to Do It))

Breathe Easy

- Take a breath from a slouching posture.
- Participants round their back, drop their head, and roll their shoulders forward.
- Ask them to take a deep breath.
    - Can they? (It's a little difficult.)
    - Is their breathing restricted by this slouching posture? (Yes.)

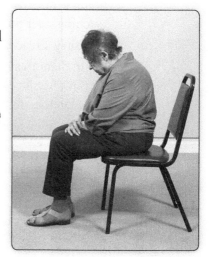

- Take a breath using tall posture. Coach them from their slouch into a tall sit.
- Ask them to sit tall and pull their head back.
- Ask them to breathe in deeply.
    - Was that a little easier this time? Noticeably easier? (Yes.)
    - Did posture seem to make a difference?
    - Have them do it again for effect and their own personal reference.

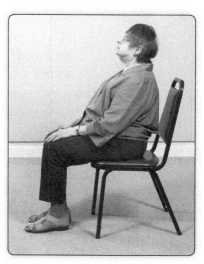

Anchors A-Sway

This activity helps participants find their tipping point and feel how it relates to posture. The feet are their base of support. How they position their body parts over the feet has an immediate effect on balance stability. Some postures set them up for a fall; leaning forward is one of the more precarious positions.

⊙ A walker, handrail, or instructor needs to be in front of each participant for this activity. Put down a line of tape on the floor in front of the participant (or use a line in the carpet or flooring). The line serves as a visual starting point for participants to stand behind. Set up a line for yourself, too, so you can demonstrate.

⊙ Stand behind the line on the floor and demonstrate for the group. Lean forward from your ankles and reach out with one arm until you must take a quick step forward to avert a fall. Tell them that's your tipping point, and now you'd like them to play with theirs.

⊙ Invite willing participants, one at a time, to stand behind their line and try just the reaching. Get them to reach forward, with one or both arms out, just a little.

⊙ Can they already feel their tipping point move forward?

⊙ Invite them to sway or lean forward from their ankles, going just far enough that they start to feel their tipping point.

- Do they feel the tendency to tip?
- Do they feel their toes digging in?
- How far can they lean before they think they need to take a step?

⊙ Have participants bend their knees and push their hips backward a bit. See if you can get them to bend their knees in a way that drops their hips backward behind the position of their feet. Now have them lean forward again.

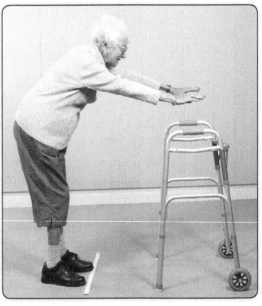

- Does this change their tipping point? (It will.)
- Why do they think this is so? (More of their body weight is behind them as an anchor when their hips are back).

⊙ Have participants stand with the feet in an offset position so that the feet still are shoulder-width apart but one foot is forward and one back.

- Can they reach farther now without tipping?
- Do they feel much safer?
- Why do they think this is so? (The feet are offset in the direction of the reach, providing a wider base of support.)

⊙ Assume the bent over posture (see the following activity).

- Do they notice some forward leaning as they assume the position?
- What if they were to stand just a little taller? Can they feel that change?

Bent Over Posture

Slouched, forward-leaning postures can slow the quick initiation of a needed step. For example, in the previous activity, Anchors A-Sway, once a person reaches the tipping point, a quick step may be needed to arrest a fall. Individuals who habitually slouch forward may not be able to bring their quick stepping foot out to stop their fall as quickly as someone with tall posture. In other words, poor posture can be a fall risk. Bent Over Posture literally takes Anchors A-Sway to the next step.

The Bent Over Posture also affects our tipping point, as they just experienced. But it also affects how participants walk, shortening stride length. Long strides work better with a tall posture. The emphasis for this activity is for them to feel how posture affects their tipping point and the mechanics of taking a quick step.

- To start, demonstrate what a quick step looks like. Stand in front of the class and assume what you call the bent over position.
- Display a forward lean, with rounded shoulders that hunch forward, a slouching back, a lowered head, and bent knees. Then tip yourself forward until a step is needed to prevent your fall.

Take a Step with Bent Over Posture

- Each participant should have a walker, a handrail, or an instructor in front. Do this activity by taking turns. They will watch each other and learn that way, too.
- Have participants assume the bent over posture—head lowered, back rounded, and knees flexed. They don't need to lean.
- At your command, have them take a quick, self-arresting safety step.
- Ask them to remember how fast they were able to get that stepping leg out in front.

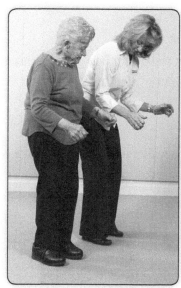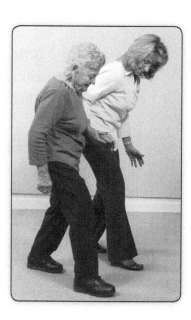

Take a Step From a Tall Posture

- Now, tell them to stand with a younger, taller posture: Take a deep Smell the Coffee breath, lift the spine tall, bring the shoulders over the hips, and brace the abdominals. They should keep their weight equal on both feet.
- Invite them to lean toward their tipping point just a bit.
- Now ask them to take a quick self-arresting safety step.
- Was it much quicker to step from a position of upright posture? (Lots quicker.)
- Repeat the two postures for clarity.

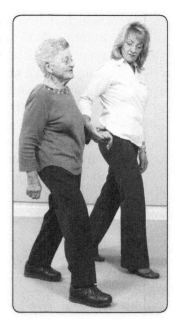

Walk With Bent Over Posture

- Participants begin walking. Have them assume the Bent Over Posture.
- Ask them to notice how their leg swings feel. Are leg swings easily initiated? (Not really)

Walk More Upright

- Ask participants to walk tall and upright, as a younger person.
- Do they feel younger and stronger?
- Ask them to notice how their leg swings feel now. Are they easier?

Alternate Bent Over, Up Tall

- Focus on ease of leg swings; that's the biggest change they will feel.
- Do a couple repetitions of each posture.
- Ask them for their thoughts on which posture they prefer and why.

Keep It Safe))

Not all participants will be comfortable leaning until they are close to their tipping point, and that's fine. They don't have to lean; they can just change their posture and the activity will still work. The point is not to make them nearly fall, but to feel how posture affects them. As always, provide modifications and balance supports (e.g., walkers, sturdy chairs, handrails) so that as many as possible will give it a try. Those who don't try will still learn from those who do.

Live It))

Good posture affects how we breathe, feel, and move. Breathe Easy means breathing is easier with good posture. Anchors A-Sway allows participants to experience how posture affects their tipping point, and Bent Over Posture helps them feel the changes in the mechanics of stepping and walking. Taking a quick step and walking are easier with upright posture.

TORSO AS A CYLINDER

Common structures can be related to the structure of the human body. A column in a building is much like the torso in a human—tall, strong, and straight supports the structure best. This activity is all demonstration. Participation consists of watching and thinking about what they've seen.

Benefits))

- Demonstrates functional relationship between posture and core stability.

- Provides an easy activity without balance risks; it's all observation and thinking.

- Lets the instructor be dramatic. Its fun to be dramatic!

Set It Up))

Have these items ready ahead of time:

- Small, heavy ball, about the size of a grapefruit and 2 pounds or less (in fact, a grapefruit works great, as does a bocce ball or even a light-weight medicine ball)

- Piece of paper

- Small piece of tape, just in case

How to Do It))

Introduce the group to your props. They are both simple items; however, one of them will become an extraordinary item of great strength!

The Ordinary Becomes Extraordinary

- Show your group the single piece of paper. Flap it around in the air to show how flimsy it is.

- Show the heavy ball. Toss it and catch it as if it were an ordinary ball. "But wait!" you say. "It's not so ordinary."

- Pass the ball around. See if you can surprise them with how heavy it actually feels. Maybe a careful toss will do the trick. Make comments such as, "Pretty heavy ball, isn't it? Can you feel its weight?" If you are using the grapefruit, you can also talk about its texture, softness, and smell, just to build tactile awareness.

Can the Paper Hold the Ball?

- When you get the ball back, ask, "Who thinks this piece of paper can hold up the ball?" Set the ball on it and watch it fall off right away.

- Let them talk and guess. It's okay if someone gets the right answer.

- Begin to roll the paper to form a column. Roll it up from top to bottom. (A short column will create a stronger, stouter column.)

- Use a very small piece of tape only if needed to get the paper to stay rolled up. (It is so much cooler to have it work without the tape, and some days it will.) Place the ball on a table in front of you.

- Tell them this is a surprisingly strong structure. With any luck, they'll ask, "How strong is it?"

POSTURE

- Place the ball on the cylinder. The rolled-up cylinder should support the ball.
- Make your point—it was the shape of the structure that gave it strength. A column is a cylinder, built to support. The paper went from flimsy to strong and supportive just because you changed its structure.

Crinkled Cylinder

Tell them, "Suppose the column is 80 or 90 years old. It's bent over and feels pretty old."

- Crumple up the column so that it's bent and sad looking. Set it back on the table.
- Ask them, "What happens now? Will this cylinder hold up the ball?"
- Place the ball on top.
- Timber!

Is All Lost?

You've given them a problem. Age and frailty seemingly have led to a loss of strength and structure. However, this column is about to become an ABLE Body. It has begun to do a little regular strength training, with lots of awareness and practice for posture and core stability.

- As you talk, begin to smooth the cylinder back out.
- Ask, "Who thinks those lost attributes might be renewable?"
- Place the ball back on the cylinder. It should hold the ball.
- Tell them it's a renewable structure; it just took a little strength training, posture, and core stability. By standing tall and erect, again the paper supports an amazing amount of weight. They are no different—they can renew their strength and posture.

Live It))

The human torso is much like the cylinder. The torso provides strength and stability in the same way. Bracing the torso and using good posture makes participants much stronger and more stable. Posture and core stability are renewable strengths.

WHEN PUSH COMES TO SHOVE

This activity teaches participants that a braced core will keep them more stable in situations where their balance might be jostled. In this activity, participants are partnered up. One partner will challenge the other's ability with little pushes and shoves. The partner being challenged will play the role of Lucy Goosey who has almost no backbone or the Mountain Man who remains immovable. Success is to be the Mountain Man, unmoved by the little shoves and pushes. Participants will learn a way to stay balanced under challenging conditions by using good core stability. When Push Comes to Shove is fun, social, and interactive, and it gives participants a good sense for the value of core stability.

Benefits))

- Participants experience *loosey-goosey* posture and its effects on their balance stability.
- Participants experience core-stable mountain posture and its effects on their balance stability.
- Participants and instructors interact with each other in hands-on, fun, and memorable ways.

Set It Up))

No props are needed, but do let them know ahead of time that you or their partner will be giving some of them little pushes—call them *perturbations*. It's such a nice word. The activity is voluntary, of course. They should watch a demonstration with you and a volunteer first.

How to Do It))

Demonstrate both the loosey-goosey and mountain scenarios outlined next. Tell them you'd like them to take their pushes standing up. However, it would be easy to do a seated version of these ideas. Demonstrate taking perturbations seated, if that would be more suitable for your group. For seated versions, have participants sit at the edge of their chair. This will make the perturbations more effective.

The Start

- Partner up participants by counting them off 1, 2, 1, 2; or let them pick partners themselves. If appropriate, have them stand up. Arrange for walkers or sturdy chairs to provide balance support for the Lucy Gooseys and the Mountain Men. If there is an extra person, that person will be your partner.
- Have the partners designate one to be the challenger who will do the pushing and shoving and the other to play the roles of Lucy Goosey and the Mountain Man.

The Moves

Introduce Lucy Goosey

- Participants stand beside a sturdy chair or with a walker, feet shoulder-width apart. Have every Lucy become loose all over. Cue them to stand totally relaxed and slumped. You've used this posture before, so they can probably find it easily.
- Walk up to one of them and demonstrate a small shove against one shoulder.
- Can the group see that from even your gentle shove, the whole torso reeled backward, with a bit of a twist?

- Say, "It didn't take much of a shove, did it?"
- Now they should try it. Have the Challengers give their Lucy Goosey a firm, gentle shove on one shoulder and notice what happens.
- Do it again and observe again.
- Push them again from the front, the side, and even the back. Push at the hip, too. Always use little shoves. Watch, observe, and let them learn.

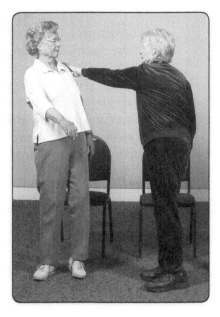

Challenger Meets the Mountain Man

- Now the Lucys will turn into the Mountain Man. Cue them to stand tall. Their shoulders should be over their hips, abdominals braced, and spine lifted. Cue them to keep their knees soft and feet parallel, shoulder-width apart.
- Ask the Mountain Men to take in a deep breath.
- As they exhale, cue them to draw their shoulder blades back and down while they push their arms down toward the ground. Cue them to imagine that with their exhalation they are planting themselves into the earth—humph!
- When they have blown all their air out and look stable, have the Challengers give their new partner a firm, quick push on one shoulder.
- Ask, "How'd that go? Any difference?" Discuss the outcome.
- Get them to do a few more perturbations, pushing from the front, side, and back and at the hip.
- Watch, observe, and let them learn.

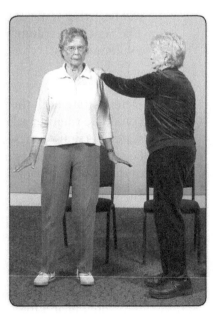

  - Ask them which character would do best in a crowded mall.
  - Ask what makes them stable. (It's the braced torso, soft knees, aligned posture, and determination.)
  - Are they beginning to sense the value of core stability?
  - Partners switch roles and repeat the activity. Both partners will learn from the experience this way.

Lucy Goosey Goes to the Beach

An alternative to When Push Comes to Shove is to pretend that they've all gone to the beach as their Lucy character for a party. Lucy Goosey has been sipping piña coladas and watching the palms trees swaying gently in the ocean breeze. Soon they'll become the palm tree.

- Participants can stand with their walkers or sit at the edge of their chair.
- Tell them they're going to become the palm trees.
- With Lucy Goosey palm trees, everyone sways with no core stability. Their forearms can be the palm branches that sway in the breeze. Keep the arms low (arms too far overhead can be a fall risk because they may sway too much). Have the trees sways left. Have them sway right. Torsos stay loose.
  - Cue them to pay attention to how this feels, especially to their back.
  - Ask that they remember these sensations.

Lucy Switches to Iced Green Tea

- Maybe some of the sways might have felt a little too loose? Try a different style.
- Suggest that they've decided to wise up and switch to a nonintoxicating beverage, such as green tea.
- Now, everyone assumes the Mountain Man posture and then begins to be palm trees again. Have every palm tree sway left, then right.
  - Ask them to tune into these new sensations.
  - What was different from the Lucy Goosey sways?
  - Did their backs take the swaying a little better? (Probably.)

Keep It Safe))

Before anyone does any pushing, demonstrate what you mean a few times. Remind them to be gentle with their perturbations—quick, firm, but gentle little shoves. Always provide adequate balance support. They should be able to use their walker in front and a sturdy chair behind, or be near a handrail. The activity will benefit them whether they watch or participate—let it be their choice.

Live It))

Core stability helps participants every day in many ways. A stable, strong core helps steady the body against all the little perturbations that life seems to toss its way. In everyday situations, it helps to steady them against everyday simple perturbations such as turning the head while walking (have them try that), swinging the arms, or little missteps.

WHOOH, WHOOHH, WHOOOHHH!

This one is fun and kind of silly. Even so, purposeful exhalations will strengthen core muscles and improve awareness of core stability.

Benefits))

- ⊙ Improves core stability.
- ⊙ Links breathing to core strength.
- ⊙ Strengthens core muscles, especially the abdominal wall.

How to Do It))

The Start

Participants sit with their back away from the chair back. The hips can touch the back of the chair, but the back should not. Feet are flat on the floor, shoulder-width apart. Sit with shoulders over the hips, head retracted slightly, and chin level. Ask participants to place their hands on their abdomen.

The Moves

- ⊙ Participants take 3 seconds to inhale deeply and slowly through the nose. As they do so, they pull into a tall sit.
- ⊙ Exhale slowly through pursed lips ("whooh") until they have blown out all their breath. The exhalation should take 3 to 5 seconds.
- ⊙ Repeat. (Can they feel bracing in their abdomen during the exhalations?)
- ⊙ Inhale again through the nose, slowly. Cue it as, "Big breath in."
- ⊙ Exhale through pursed lips again, but this time blow out short, quick, little puffs of air with each "whooh, whooh, whooh!" (Can they feel their abdominals brace with each puff?)
- ⊙ The last puff should be a long "whooohhh," lengthened to expel the very last of the breath.
- ⊙ Repeat four to six times, as tolerated.

Take It Further))

- ⊙ Do a few more repetitions.
- ⊙ Do more whoohs or longer whooohhhs.

Give It More Balance))

- ⊙ Progress from parallel feet to offset or tandem feet.
- ⊙ Add simple upper-body activities, such as Waist Whittlers (see page 123).
- ⊙ Do while standing.

Keep It Safe))

Remind participants to maintain a tall sit with abdominals pulled in gently. If they get dizzy, they should stop and breathe normally.

Live It))

It's nice to see how breathing ties to core stability. The long, slow exhalations help participants hunker down and get stable.

POSTURE

CUPS AND RELAYS

Relays are a blast! There are lots of varieties that your participants might enjoy. This one helps teach the value of core stability. The task of carrying something is also a distraction that is an appropriate challenge for the automatic balance system. You can have them carry cups filled with water, cotton balls, wrapped candy on long wooden spoons, or trays with objects on them. The challenge here is to give them something to carry that they need to hold balanced and steady to transport it safely.

Benefits))

- Demonstrates the usefulness of core stability.
- Introduces a dual task to a mobility task.
- Helps connect people through fun teamwork.

Set It Up))

Think about the logistics ahead of time. For any relay, you will need plenty of space and you'll need chairs set up in a way that is conducive for the relay—chairs at both ends, the right number of chairs, and so on. One team member at a time races as safely as is comfortable from one side of the room to the other. The mission is to spill as little booty (water, cotton, or candy) as possible while getting to the other side.

- You'll need measuring containers for each team to score the results at the end. Each team also needs whatever they will carry the booty on or in. Trays, wooden spoons, cups, whatever. Team members carry the booty back and forth on or in these items. The most booty properly accounted for at the end determines the winning team.
- If you're using water in cups, Styrofoam or plastic pill cups work best; paper cups get soft and leak quickly. For the most challenge, fill each cup all the way to the brim with water or booty. Don't use water if it will make the floors slippery.
- If there are four people on each team, have four chairs on each side of the relay path. If you plan a square or circular route, you will not need double amounts of chairs, but do place teams on opposite sides. This keeps traffic cleaner.

This is a relay in which participants carry something, so you'll need some rules for people using walkers. Participants with walkers that have a seat can carry their items on the seat. Unfortunately, the no-seat walkers won't work. You can grant them an exception—they don't have to carry anything, but their team still will need their participation crossing the field. You could make sure both teams have the same number of walkers.

How to Do It))

- Divide the group into teams, making sure there are equal numbers and abilities on each team. This is tough to do fairly, so just do your best. Then divide the teams in half and station the half-teams at opposite ends of the relay.
- For this example, I am using four pill cups filled with water and placed on trays for each team. The first team member takes the tray and carries it across the room to his teammate as quickly as he can without spilling any of it.
- When the first racer gets to the other side, he hands off the tray to the next team member and sits down.
- Once he's seated, that's the signal for the next member to cross the room with her booty. This continues until all team members have completed the relay.

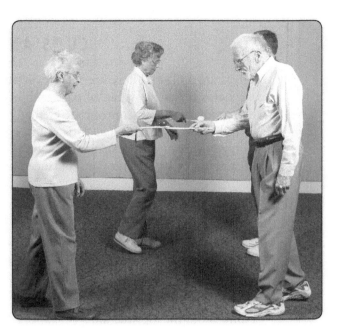

- At the end, combine each team's containers to see which team collected the most booty. The team with the most booty wins. Maybe something like chocolate kisses or candy gold coins would be good prizes.

Progress this activity:

- Racers hold the booty with both hands.
- Racers hold the booty above their shoulders or keep one hand behind their back.
- Make the route a little more circuitous (use agility cones to make the route like a slalom course or tape on the floor to make wavy lines like Holiday Lines (see page 316).
- Require change in plans or in direction (chairs on course can mark corners to turn around like a short maze).
- Make the path a little more perilous. Add an obstacle or two (such as soccer balls made of wadded up paper, one or two hurdles, a step, or a beam) to step through, over, or across. Keep the perils simple and small.

Keep It Safe))

It always amazes me how fast people want to move in a race. We don't necessarily want that. But they will want to go as fast as possible for their team. Remind them that this is about core stability and to only go as fast as they feel safe moving. They will end up with more booty that way anyhow.

When the games involve candy, everyone should get a piece, one way or another. It is only a game. For many games, having fun will be enough of a reward; don't feel you always need prizes. Make sure nothing they carry can become a tripping hazard if dropped. Water on a hardwood floor would be an example of an unsafe idea. On hard surfaces, like wood, tile, or linoleum choose a dry, soft booty to put in the cups.

Stay in the runways of your battle fields to hold a hand if needed or pick up anything that may be a hazard. Consider getting extra staff to assist on game days.

Live It))

Core stability has many benefits. The more stable they hold their body, the more booty they will get.

POSTURE

TALL SITS

Tall Sits is the most basic ABLE Bodies exercise. It serves as the basis for all tall posture activities and is the form from which most of the exercises begin. While doing a good tall sit, if participants were looking in a mirror, they should be able to see a clear difference in their height. Between their relaxed slump and the Tall Sit there should be a height difference of 2 to 4 inches (5-10 centimeters).

Benefits))

- ◉ Improves posture and core stability.
- ◉ Strengthens core muscles, especially the back extensors and abdominals.
- ◉ Teaches neutral spine.

How to Do It))

If you can provide mirrors for participants to observe themselves it may be helpful for this activity. Many facilities have a room with mirrors or mirrored closets. Some variations need a balloon or a balance disc.

The Start

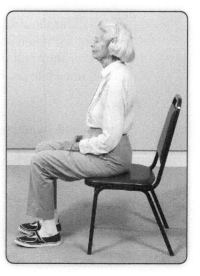

- ◉ Sit all the way to the back of the chair, but without resting against the chair back (the hips but not the back should touch the chair back).
- ◉ Sit with shoulders over hips, head retracted slightly, and chin level.
- ◉ Place feet flat on the floor, hip-width apart.

The Moves

- ◉ Inhale and lift the ribs to lengthen the spine.
- ◉ Pull the abdominal wall in and up tightly to help brace the midsections.
- ◉ Exhale, staying tall and pulling the shoulder blades back and down.
- ◉ Hold this tall sitting position 3 to 5 seconds, while exhaling.
- ◉ Relax and slump a bit.
- ◉ Repeat the exercise four times and build up to doing eight repetitions, as tolerated.

Take It Further))

- ◉ Do fewer repetitions, but hold the Tall Sit position longer, for 10 to 15 seconds and up to 30 seconds. Continue to breathe fully while holding the Tall Sit.
- ◉ Add simple arm movements.
    - Genie Arms: Cross the arms and hold them away from the chest.
    - Hold arms out to the side.
    - Single-arm overhead reaching: Starting with hands on knees, pull one arm up until reaching overhead. Do the same with the other.
- ◉ Add small knee lifts with one knee and then the other.

Give It More Balance))

Draw participants' attention to what they are learning from their body. Ask them what differences they feel in their posture when sitting taller. Do they notice how much their spine lengthens with each tall sit? Are they able to lift their ribs? Did they feel themselves bracing their core muscles? Try these variations to add more balance.

- ⊙ Sit closer to the edge of the chair; balance and core stability become a little more challenging with less back and leg support.
- ⊙ Sit at the front of a chair and place feet in an offset position (shoulder-width apart, one forward, one back).
- ⊙ Sit at the front of a chair and place feet in a tandem position (heel of front foot touches toe of back foot).
- ⊙ Use the tandem or offset position with the heels lifted off the floor.
- ⊙ Add slow head turns, with the emphasis on maintaining a Tall Sit.
- ⊙ Tap a balloon back and forth between hands while maintaining a Tall Sit.
- ⊙ Place the feet on top of a balloon or balance disc on the floor.
- ⊙ Tall Sit on a balance disc in a chair with arms.

Keep It Safe))

The Tall Sit should be pain free. Cue participants to lengthen the spine by lifting their ribs, not with their shoulders. There is a tendency for participants to hold their breath whenever they pull in their abdominal muscles; encourage them to practice breathing in and out while tall sitting.

Live It))

Participants should feel and see a clear difference in their height as they sit tall. Between their relaxed slump and the tall sit there should be a height difference of 2 to 4 inches (5-10 centimeters). It's amazing! Practice tall sitting daily.

TALL SITS WITH A BALLOON SQUEEZE

This activity is a progression of a Tall Sit. Participants will squeeze a balloon, pulling it in against their chest, to engage back muscles essential to posture.

Benefits))

- Improves posture and core stability.
- Strengthens back extensors and scapular retractors.
- Uses colorful balloons or balls as resistance tools.

Set It Up))

You will need one 12-inch (30-centimeter) balloon per person and a few extras, just in case. Balloons are fun and inexpensive tools to use in class. Balloons really brighten up a classroom! They generally cost about a dime each and you can change colors with the seasons and holidays. For best results blow up the balloons a day or two before class. The first day you blow up the balloons, they tend to be tight and slippery—they're better the next day and after. If you have a bigger budget, consider buying Slo Mo balls on Web sites or in equipment magazines. They stay blown up much longer, meaning less work for you. Some variations require a balance disc or an extra balloon.

How to Do It))

The Start

- If possible participants sit with their back away from the chair. The hips can touch the chair, but their back should not. They are sitting tall, with shoulders over hips, head retracted, and chin level. Feet are flat on the floor, hip-width apart.
- They place a balloon on their chest and cross their forearms over the balloon like the Genie Arms position.

The Moves

Use the following cues.

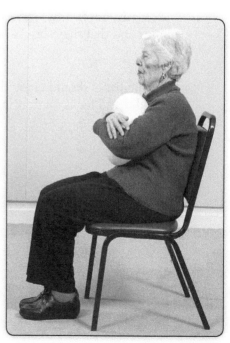

- Inhale and pull up into a tall sitting position (ribs lifted and torso long, lengthened by the spine).
- Exhale for 3 seconds and squeeze the balloon firmly, pulling it in toward the chest. The pull is done with the arms, back, and shoulder blades.
- Cue to draw their shoulder blades back, down, and together.
- Hold each squeeze for 3 to 5 seconds, while exhaling, and then relax.
- Inhale, sit tall, and do it again.
- Repeat four times and build to eight times, as tolerated.
- Stretch the midback gently and do a few shoulder circles when done.

Take It Further))

- Increase hold times while continuing to breathe fully.
- Add leaning during the exhales; but always return to the Tall Sit before the repetition is finished.
  - Lean a little to the left. Return to the center and sit tall.
  - Lean a little to the right. Return to the center and sit tall.
  - Lean a little forward and backward. Return to the center and sit tall.
  - Make small circles or figure eights with the torso. Return to center and sit tall.

Give It More Balance))

- Discuss what participants felt and learned. Could they feel the muscles between their shoulder blades come together? Did exhaling while they squeezed help? Do they notice that when their back is held strong and stable the entire spine works as a single unit (there's no flexing or bending up and down the spine)? Nice job! Here are some more balance variations:
- Sit at the front of the chair.
- Use an offset or tandem foot position.
- Use an offset or tandem foot position with the heels lifted off the floor.
- Place one foot or both feet on another balloon on the floor.
- Stand to do this exercise.
- Sit on a balance disc, in a chair with arms.
- Squeeze the balloon while walking.

Keep It Safe))

Pressing a balloon against your chest compresses the ribs. Cue squeezes by saying, "Gently, but firmly," instead of "tightly" or "hard." Remind them that nothing should hurt and that they should be comfortable throughout the activity.

Live It))

Participants should enjoy this progression to Tall Sits. It will make them work a little harder and focus on drawing the shoulder blades back and down.

THUMB ROLLS

Rolling the shoulder blades toward each other stretches the chest while strengthening the back. Both actions can help improve rounded-back postures, common in frail adults. I've named it *Thumb Rolls* because of the way you cue participants to roll their thumbs backward with straight arms. It seems to accomplish the shoulder-girdle movement better than when you cue them to roll their shoulders back.

Benefits))

- ⊚ Strengthens posture muscles, especially the scapular retractors.
- ⊚ Improves shoulder-girdle function and flexibility.

Set It Up))

You will not need any special equipment. Some variations require a balloon or a balance disc and a chair with arms.

How to Do It))

The Start

- ⊚ Participants should sit with their back away from the chair (the hips can touch the chair, but the back should not). Shoulders over hips, head retracted comfortably, and chin level. Feet are flat on the floor, hip-width apart.
- ⊚ Arms should be straight and down by the sides.
- ⊚ Thumbs face forward or in.

The Moves

Use the following cues.

- ⊚ Roll the thumbs from facing forward to facing backward as you are able without pain.
- ⊚ Squeeze the shoulder blades closer together.
- ⊚ Hold the position 3 seconds. Relax.
- ⊚ Repeat 4 times and progress to 12 times, as tolerated.
- ⊚ Stretch the midback gently and do a few shoulder rolls when done.

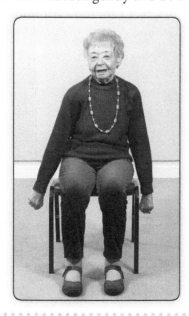 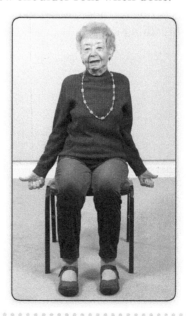

Take It Further))

- ⊙ Increase the hold times while continuing to breathe fully and deeply.
- ⊙ Combine it with the Tall Sit.
- ⊙ Add backward wrist circles to Thumb Rolls; it will recruit a few more posterior shoulder muscles.

Give It More Balance))

- ⊙ Add slow head turns.
- ⊙ Use an offset or tandem foot position.
- ⊙ Use an offset or tandem foot position with heels lifted, as shown in the picture to the right.
- ⊙ Use a chair with arms and place feet on a balloon.
- ⊙ Sit on a balance disc in a chair with arms.
- ⊙ Stand for Thumb Rolls.
- ⊙ Do them while walking tall.

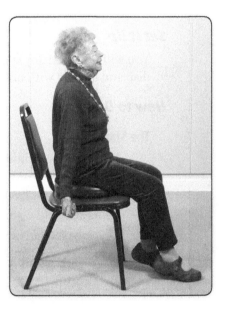

Keep It Safe))

If the activity is not comfortable for the back, try using a gentler motion. If that is not helpful, they should not do the exercise.

Live It))

Thumb Rolls is one of those feel-good exercises that lifts and expands the chest and makes deep breathing easier.

SHOW ME THE MONEY

Show Me the Money sounds a lot more fun than Scapular Retraction. This great posture exercise is just a little more difficult than Thumb Rolls, because the arms are held up a bit.

Benefits))

- ◉ Strengthens posture muscles, especially the scapular retractors.
- ◉ Improves shoulder function and posture.

Set It Up))

You will not need any special equipment. Some variations require a balloon or a balance disc and a chair with arms.

How to Do It))

The Start

- ◉ Sit tall with the back away from the chair. Hips can touch the chair, but the back should not. Shoulders are over hips, head retracted comfortably, and chin level. Feet should be flat on the floor, hip-width apart.
- ◉ Hold the arms out to the sides. Bend the elbows slightly and hold them close to the torso. Participants will resemble a big, tall-sitting *W*. Hands are a little lower than shoulder height, palms up. If money were placed on the palms of their hands, you could see it and it would not fall off.

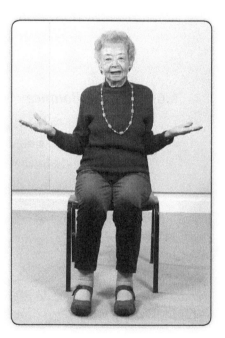

The Moves

- ◉ Inhale and sit tall.
- ◉ Exhale and pull the elbows back, squeezing the shoulder blades together.
- ◉ Hold each squeeze 2 to 3 seconds, while exhaling, and then relax.
- ◉ Repeat 6 times and progress to doing 12 times, as tolerated.
- ◉ Stretch the midback and do a few shoulder rolls when done.

Take It Further »

- Increase hold times.
- Gamble a little more with High Rollers. It's the same exercise but the elbows are held farther away from the torso, about 6 to 8 inches (12-17 centimeters). The new position is an elongated *W*.

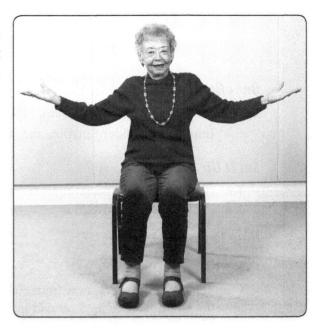

Give It More Balance »

- Sit closer to the edge of the chair.
- Place feet in a tandem position, heels lifted.
- Stand and Show Me the Money.
- Sit on a balance disc in a chair with arms.

Keep It Safe »

Cue participants to maintain the tall sit throughout. Do these gently at first.

Live It »

Participants should Show Me the Money and stand like a High Roller more often. It feels good and will improve midback posture.

KNEE LIFT, ABS IN

Knee Lift, Abs In can be done seated or standing. The goal is to draw in the abdominal wall with each knee lift, stabilizing the low back and core. The exercise looks similar to marching in place, only done in slow motion and with an emphasis on drawing abs in.

Benefits))

- ◉ Strengthens core muscles, especially the deeper abdominals.
- ◉ Improves step height and length.
- ◉ Increases core stability during gait.

Set It Up))

You will not need any special equipment. Chairs with arms would be best. Some variations require a balloon or a balance disc and a chair with arms.

How to Do It))

The Start

Participants sit all the way back in the chair. The hips and back should remain in contact with the chair during this activity. Place forearms on the arms of the chair for additional back support.

The Moves

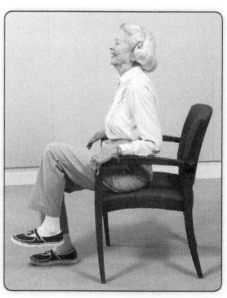

- ◉ Inhale, lift one knee toward chest and pull abdominals in toward chair.
  - The foot lifts about 6 inches (15 centimeters) off the floor.
  - Cue participants to pull their belly button toward the chair with each knee lift.
  - Each knee lift is held just long enough to feel the abdominal muscles brace the torso.
- ◉ Exhale as the knee is fully lowered; keep abdominals pulled in.
- ◉ Relax when foot is back on ground.
- ◉ Ask if they notice their low back pressing into the chair with each knee lift.
- ◉ Repeat with the same leg 4 times and build to 8 to 12 times, as tolerated; then do the other leg.
- ◉ Cue this exercise, "Knee lift, abs in. Knee lift, abs in."

Take It Further))

- ◉ Participants can recruit their abdominals better if they place one hand on their lower abdomen. This way, they will *feel* their abdominals draw in with each knee lift.
- ◉ Alternate legs with each repetition.
- ◉ Slow down the up and down motions.
- ◉ Lift knees higher, increasing difficulty.
- ◉ Sit away from the chair back (less back support).
- ◉ Sit with Genie Arms (arms crossed and lifted off the chest).

Give It More Balance))

- Add opposing head turns (e.g., lift right knee, look left; lift left knee, look right).
- Add opposing (reciprocal) arm swings.
- Add rhythm or music.
- Do Knee Lift, Abs In while wearing sunglasses or in a room with dim lighting.
- Do Knee Lift, Abs In seated on a balance disc in a chair with arms.
- Do Knee Lift, Abs In while standing (advanced). Stand beside the chair or a handrail for balance support. When standing, participants will notice how their hips tuck under just a bit with each knee lift (see the photo to the right). That feeling of hips tucking under the shoulders is ideal.

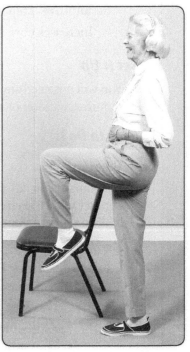

Keep It Safe))

Sitting all the way back in the chair with arms on the chair arms gives the most back support. If their chair has no arms, participants can place their hands on the sides of the chair, or on their thighs, to better support their back. Keep the torso as still and quiet as possible with each leg movement.

If done standing, be sure you have adequate balance support. Most participants will need to hold on to a chair on both sides of them with some needing another chair behind them as well. Some will be able to do this beside a handrail.

Live It))

Securing the abdominal wall while walking will improve core stability and balance.

WAIST WHITTLERS

Waist Whittlers challenges the oblique muscles on the sides of the torso. I call these muscles *sidewalls*. This activity challenges the positioning of the torso while the arms move.

Benefits))

- ◉ Challenges core muscles to stabilize against arm movement.
- ◉ Reinforces concepts of core stability and tall posture.
- ◉ Strengthens torso, especially the obliques.

Set It Up))

You will need one balloon or Slo Mo ball per person, plus a few extra. One variation requires a balance disc and a chair with arms.

How to Do It))

The Start

- ◉ Start with a tall sit (shoulders over hips, head retracted, chin level, feet flat on the floor). Lower abdominals are pulled in and up; ribs are lifted, lengthening the spine. Maintain this position throughout the exercise.
- ◉ Hold the balloon with both hands in front at waist height. Arms are almost straight, with elbows slightly bent.

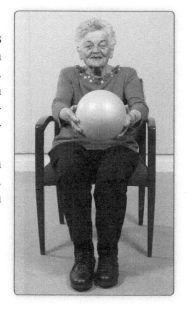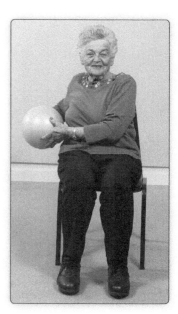

The Moves

Use the following cues.

- ◉ Keep the trunk tall and facing forward. You will be using only the arms to move the balloon from side to side.
- ◉ Pull the balloon back toward one hip. Both elbows will bend as you draw the balloon backward.
- ◉ Push the balloon forward again to the front position. Sit tall.
- ◉ Pull the balloon back toward the other hip. The trunk stays facing forward, only the arms should pull back.
- ◉ Push the balloon forward again to the front position. Sit tall.
- ◉ Keep moving the balloon from the right hip to the left without turning the torso.
- ◉ Repeat until you have moved balloon to both sides for six to eight repetitions on each side.
- ◉ Rest.
- ◉ Stretch *sidewalls* with gentle reach-ups when done. Try (Parentheticals) (page 80).

Take It Further))

- ⊙ Over time, build up to doing 8 to 15 repetitions on each side.
- ⊙ Push the balloon a little higher each time you return it to the center position.
- ⊙ Hold the balloon a little farther from the body.
- ⊙ Use a light weight, no more than 1 or 2 pounds (.5-1 kilogram), held with both hands.
- ⊙ Add a twist with Waist Whittlers With a Twist.
    - It's the same as Waist Whittlers, but as the arms pull to one side, the torso turns also.
    - Inhale and sit tall.
    - Exhale and turn the torso, arms, and balloon to one side.
    - Repeat to the other side.
    - Twists are not appropriate for people with osteoporosis.

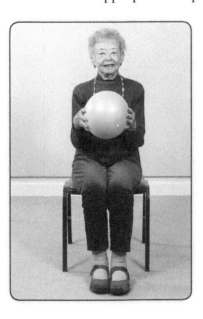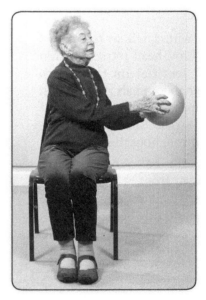

Give It More Balance))

- ⊙ Increase the speed of movement just a little.
- ⊙ Sit at the front of the chair.
- ⊙ Sit on a balance disc in a chair with arms.
- ⊙ Do Waist Whittlers standing in front of chair. For more variety try an off set foot pattern. When the right foot is forward, turn the balloon to the right. When the left foot is forward, turn the balloon to the left. Start with 6 Waist Whittlers to each side and progress to 12 repetitions.

Live It))

Movements like reaching to the sides are part of many everyday tasks. Core stability will make these moves easier on the back and safer.

PUSH-BACKS

This exercise strengthens and improves low back stability and the abdominals at once. Push-Backs are simply Tall Sits combined with pushing backward into a balloon, which provides resistance.

Benefits))

- Promotes core stability.
- Strengthens low back extensors and stabilizers.
- Strengthens abdominal muscles.

Set It Up))

You will need one balloon or Slo Mo ball for each participant, and a few extra. If you have a bigger budget, use Slo Mo balls. One variation uses a balance disc and a chair with arms.

How to Do It))

The Start

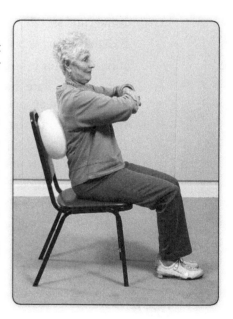

- Participants sit toward the edge of the chair. Feet are flat on the floor, shoulder-width apart. Shoulders are over hips, head pulled slightly back, and chin is level.
- Participants should place the balloon behind their back, between their back and the chair. The balloon should be at the small of the back for an easier exercise, and higher, between the shoulder blades, for more difficulty. Some participants may need assistance placing their balloon behind them.
- Once the balloon is in place, scoot back so the balloon is firmly held against the chair.
- Place the arms on the chest with the forearms crossed or for greater difficulty, use Genie Arms (as shown).

The Moves

Use the following cues.

- Inhale and sit tall.
- Exhale, draw shoulder blades together, and press back into the balloon.
- Keep the back tall and core braced.
- Hold 2 seconds. (Participants should notice that the abdominal muscles tighten and the low back is working, too.)
- Relax.
- Repeat six to eight times, as tolerated; progress to doing 12 repetitions.

Take It Further))

- Have your participants do Genie Arms. It is the same exercise except that participant will lift their crossed arms from the chest. Forearms are parallel to the floor. That's the Genie Arms look.
- Increase the number of repetitions or the hold time.
- Try combining Push-Backs with Whooh, Whoohh, Whooohhh! (see page 110).

Give It More Balance))

- Place the feet in tandem position, heels lifted.

Genie Arms With a Twist

This variation looks similar to a bear scratching its back against a tree. Participants brace their core muscles, then roll their shoulder blades over and around the balloon for the bear in the woods effect. They'll scratch their own back!

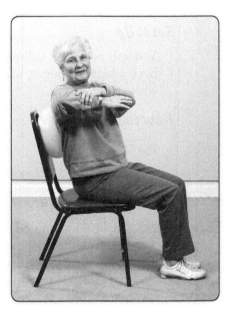

- Start out doing a Push-Back.
- Inhale and sit tall.
- Exhale and press back against balloon.
- Inhale and hold the breath.
- Exhale and rotate the trunk to the right (right shoulder blade will roll around the balloon).
- Inhale and rotate back to the center position.
- Repeat, but this time rotate to the left (left shoulder blade will roll around the balloon)
- Keep alternating until 6 repetitions are complete, build to doing 12 repetitions.
- Keep the spine tall and ribs lifted throughout.

Keep It Safe))

Remind participants to keep their core braced and their spine lengthened.

Live It))

Push-backs of any kind (basic, with Genie arms, or like bears in the woods) are great for low back stability.

CURL UP AND SIT TALL

This exercise has participants lift their trunk from a reclining position into the tall sitting position. Use it to develop abdominal and back strength.

Benefits))

- Strength training using a functional, everyday movement pattern.
- Strengthens torso, especially the abdominal wall.
- Encourages tall sitting.

Set It Up))

You will not need any special equipment.

How to Do It))

The Start

Participants sit about 4 inches (10 centimeters) from their chair back. Arms are crossed against the chest.

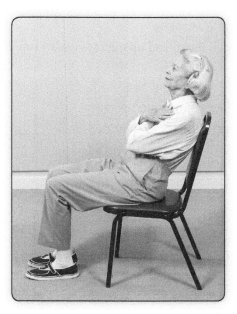 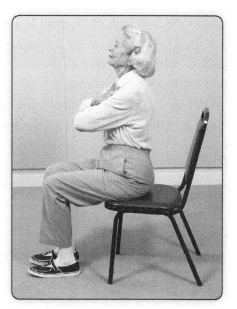

The Moves

Use the following cues.

- Roll your back toward the chair. See if you can tilt your hips back so that the low back touches the chair first, then the midback (see also Rock the Pelvis Backward, page 71). It looks like slouching.
- From this reclining position, breathe in and look up.
- As you exhale, lower the chin to the chest. Then use your abdominals to curl up and away from the chair. Lift your shoulders first to form the curl up.
- Curl up until shoulders are over the hips.
- Lengthen your spine into a tall sit as you finish the exercise.
- Think of lifting through your ribs upward into the tall sitting position.

- Hold the tall sit for 2 seconds.
- Relax and roll back to the slouched position.
- Use these cues:
  - Breathe in and look up.
  - Exhale, lower chin, curl up, and sit tall.
  - Repeat six times and progress to 12 to 15 repetitions, as tolerated.

Take It Further))

- Increase the length of time the tall sit is held.
- Lift elbows and make Genie arms as you bring yourself up to a tall sit.

Playground Swings

This great variation mimics swinging on a playground swing: When you're back, you lay back and your legs are extended. As you come forward, the legs get pulled under and you sit as tall as you can! With that picture in mind, tell them our modification is that only one leg will do the pumping action.

- Roll back on to the chair.
- Breathe in and look up. Extend one leg out straight.
- Exhale, curl up, and sit tall. Bring extended leg in and up into a knee lift (see Knee Lift, Abs In on page 121).
- Hold tall position 2 seconds.
- Relax, then repeat with other leg pumping your swing upward.
- Start with 3 repetitions per leg and progress to 12, as tolerated.

Keep It Safe))

These curl-up exercises should be avoided by participants with osteoporosis.

Live It))

Everything participants need to know for this exercise, they actually learned in kindergarten. The playground swing movement can make this activity feel joyous, and it works.

PURSE SNATCHER

This is called the Purse Snatcher because of how it looks and works. A balloon is held tightly under one arm, just like a woman would hold her purse tightly under her arm, so no one could come by and snatch it from her. The opposite arm is held up as if to signal a policeman for help. All this frivolity actually builds lateral core stability.

Benefits))

- ⊙ Improves posture and core stability.
- ⊙ Strengthens torso muscles, especially obliques and back extensors.

Set It Up))

You will need a small balloon or Slo Mo ball to play the role of the purse. One variation uses an agility disc and a chair with arms.

How to Do It))

The Start

- ⊙ Participants sit tall in the chair, feet on the floor, abdominals braced, ribs lifted, and shoulder blades back and down.
- ⊙ Place balloon purse under one upper arm.
- ⊙ Inhale and sit tall to prepare.

The Moves

Use the following cues.

- ⊙ Exhale and squeeze balloon moderately tightly under one arm, while reaching directly straight up with other arm.
- ⊙ Hold the squeeze for 2-3 seconds.
- ⊙ Relax between repetitions.
- ⊙ Repeat 4 times and progress to doing 8 per side.

Take It Further))

- ⊙ Wave for Help! The arm that is in the air makes small quick circles, like hailing a cab or calling for a policeman.
- ⊙ Do longer or bigger waves.

Give It More Balance))

- ⊙ Sit closer to the edge of the chair.
- ⊙ Sit with feet offset or in tandem.
- ⊙ Rest feet on a balloon when sitting in a chair with arms.
- ⊙ Lift crossed ankles off the floor when sitting tall.
- ⊙ Do Purse Snatcher standing.
- ⊙ Do Purse Snatcher walking.

POSTURE

Keep It Safe))

- ◉ Begin by gently squeezing the purse. Individuals with osteoporosis should be especially cautious about compressing a balloon to their ribs with great pressure.
- ◉ Some participants will not be able to lift the opposite arm. That is perfectly fine; just have them sit tall with each lateral compression. The activity will still benefit their core muscles.
- ◉ Nothing should hurt or cause any pain.

Live It))

Why not be imaginative with exercise? It can be fun and make a good exercise easy to remember. Keeping a purse close and standing or walking tall is a good functional exercise, too. Lateral core stability is good stuff.

BUDDHA'S PRAYER

The starting position looks similar to a meditating Buddha. The challenge is to keep the torso stable and braced while lifting the arms upward.

Benefits))

- Improves posture and core stability.
- Strengthens torso muscles, especially the back extensors.
- It's easy to remember because the name is fun.

Set It Up))

You will not need any special equipment. Some variations use a Thera-Band or a balloon on the floor.

How to Do It))

The Start

- Participants sit tall in the chair, feet on the floor, abdominals braced, ribs lifted, and shoulder blades back and down.
- They place their palms together, fingers pointing up, almost resting against the sternum (midchest).
- Lift forearms until parallel to the floor. This is the meditating Buddha look.
- Inhale to prepare.

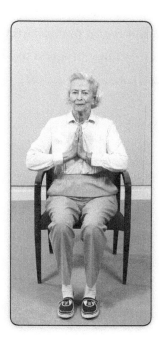 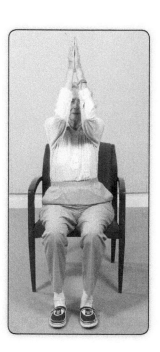

The Moves

Use the following cues.

- Exhale, begin moving the hands skyward and pressing the forearms toward each other.
- Keep the arms and hands close to the body throughout the lift. Movement is directly upward, not out.
- At the top of the movement, the hands are almost directly overhead.
- The eyes and face can follow the hands, if comfortable for the participant.
- Inhale in the up position.
- Exhale as you lower the hands.
- Repeat six to eight times, as tolerated.

POSTURE

Take It Further))

- ⊙ Use slightly longer holds at the top.
- ⊙ Increase the number of repetitions.
- ⊙ Good Mornings With a Thera-Band. It is this same exercise, but with a Thera-Band for extra resistance.
    - Place one end of a Thera-Band on the ground and secure it under both feet.
    - Clasp the other end of the band in both hands.
    - Bring the hands up under the chin, as if pulling covers up on a cold morning.
    - Sit with the hands together and the forearms parallel to the floor; this is the beginning position for Buddha's Prayer.
    - Inhale and lift the hands (and the band) upward until the arms are straight above. Lift the eyes and chin skyward, too, if possible.
    - Keep the abdominals pulled in; but let the ribs and shoulders lift.
    - Hold for a moment.
    - Exhale and return to the starting position.
    - Repeat 6-8 times; progress to 12 times, as tolerated.

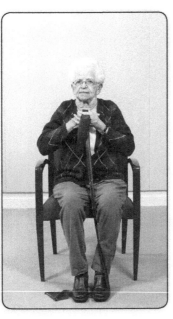 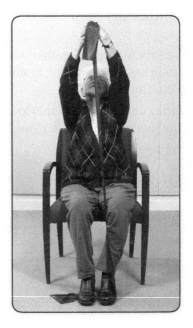

Give It More Balance))

- ⊙ Sit closer to the edge of the chair.
- ⊙ Sit with feet offset or in tandem.
- ⊙ Do Buddha's Prayer with feet on a balloon.

Keep It Safe))

Keep the arms close to the body throughout the exercise. They only need to lift as high as is comfortable for them. Keep the spine tall and stable. Nothing should hurt or cause any pain.

Live It))

Reaching up and looking up is much easier in slow motion and with core stability.

FORKLIFTS

Forklifts are recommended for people with osteoporosis, because they safely facilitate upright midback posture. This dual-action exercise strengthens the abdominal and midback muscles at the same time. Forklifts start out looking like a forklift but end up looking like the front loader on a dump truck. Picture how the front forks of a forklift scoop up a dumpster and lift it over the truck cab.

Benefits))

- ⊙ Improves midback posture, strength, and function.
- ⊙ Strengthens midback and trunk.

Set It Up))

You will not need any special equipment.

How to Do It))

The Start

- ⊙ Participants sit tall with their back away from the chair; the hips can touch the chair, but their back should not. Sit tall with abdominals braced, ribs lifted, shoulder blades back and down, and head retracted.
- ⊙ Arms start out close to their sides, then bend to 90 degrees with the forearms parallel to the floor, the palms facing up, and the figures sticking straight out.
- ⊙ Sit tall to prepare.
- ⊙ Do participants look like a forklift ready to pick up a pallet?

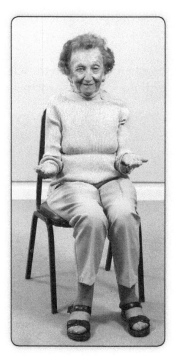 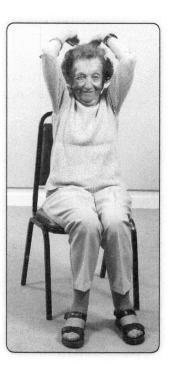

The Moves

Use the following cues.

- ⊙ Inhale and lift the elbows to about shoulder height. Keep a 90 degree bend in the arms.
- ⊙ If comfortable, continue rotating arms up and over the head, until the elbows are in line with the ears and the fingers point behind.
- ⊙ Keep the forearms parallel. (Participants tend to let forearms separate.)
- ⊙ Hold at top for 1 to 2 seconds.
- ⊙ Exhale and bring the arms back down. Relax.
- ⊙ Repeat 6 times and progress to doing 8 to 12 times, as tolerated.

POSTURE

Take It Further))

- ◉ Use slightly longer holds.
- ◉ Use more repetitions.
- ◉ Try it with Whooh, Whoohh, Whooohhhs! (see page 110).

Give It More Balance))

- ◉ Sit closer to the edge of the chair.
- ◉ Sit with feet offset or in tandem.
- ◉ Sit with feet offset or in tandem with lifted heels.
- ◉ Stand with feet in an offset position and a chair placed behind the participant.

Keep It Safe))

Cue frequently for participants to keep their forearms parallel to each other. That seems the hardest part for them to get right. Nothing should hurt. If it does, check their form and make sure they are keeping their abdominals pulled in before trying again. If pain persists, they should discontinue the activity.

Live It))

Participants can strengthen their core muscles effectively and may be able to reduce midback rounding with Forklifts. It's worth a try! Here's to better upright posture!

PUSH UP, PULL DOWN

The overhead passing movement pattern in this exercise is good for balance—reaching up directly overhead has a way of making a person feel very centered over their base of support. Passing the balloon overhead makes the movement between arms a reciprocal motion that is good for sequential coordination. It feels good and helps build core stability safely.

Benefits))

- ⊙ Enhances tall posture; facilitates length with strength.
- ⊙ Strengthens all core muscles, including the back extensors and abdominals.
- ⊙ Improves range of motion for the shoulders and scapulae.

Set It Up))

Have balloons or Slo Mo balls ready, one per person. Make sure they are a little soft; this makes them much easier to grasp. One variation uses light hand weights.

How to Do It))

The Start

- ⊙ Participants sit tall at the edge of the chair, with shoulders over hips, abdominals in, and head pulled back in line with shoulders.
- ⊙ They hold a balloon in the right hand and place it on the right shoulder.
- ⊙ They inhale to prepare.

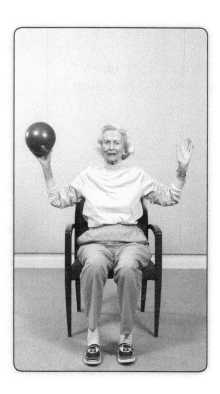
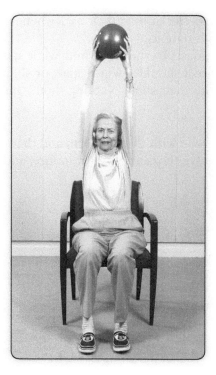
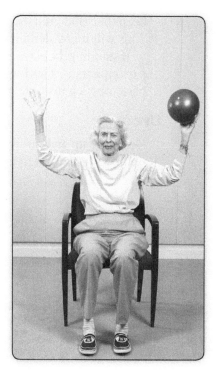

The Moves

Use the following cues.

- Exhale slowly and push the balloon up to a center point directly above the head.
- Use the arms, shoulders, and ribs to lift the balloon (Venus de Milo style arms, see page 63).
- Inhale and stay tall with the abdominals pulled in.
- At the top, reach up with the left hand to grasp the balloon.
- Pass the balloon to the left hand.
- Exhale and use the left hand to pull the balloon down toward the left shoulder.
- Repeat overhead passing for 8 to 10 passes, progressing to 20, as tolerated.

Take It Further))

- Increase the number of repetitions.
- Add a second set later in the class.
- Use very light weights, just 1 to 2 pounds (.5-1 kilogram).

Give It More Balance))

- Sit with tandem feet, heels lifted.
- Advanced: Perform while standing in front of a chair or with a walker.

Keep It Safe))

Many participants have rounded backs. If a participant cannot comfortably reach overhead, suggest they pass the balloon horizontally at chest level. Frequently cue them to keep their abdominals in to better support their back whenever their arms are overhead. This will increase their core stability.

If standing, be extra cautious. Overhead reaching while standing is a fall risk. Instruct participants to stand with feet shoulder-width apart or slightly wider, and have them place one leg in contact with their chair. Nothing should hurt.

Live It))

Reaching up and pulling down with the right arm and then the left becomes a gentle, undulating motion to improve thoracic range of motion and comfort.

THE UP AND UP

You can tell participants this activity is on the up and up. Really! The Up and Up uses concepts learned in Venus de Milo Arms (see page 63). It combines tall sitting and arm lifts to provide the torso with both strength and length. It's called *The Up and Up* because once they lift their arm up toward the ceiling, they then reach up a little farther.

Benefits 〉〉

- ◉ Improves torso function, flexibility, and strength.
- ◉ Strengthens back extensors and rib lifters.
- ◉ Improves shoulder flexibility and reaching skills.

Set It Up 〉〉

You will not need any special equipment. Some variations require light hand weights or a balance disc and a chair with arms.

How to Do It 〉〉

The Start

- ◉ Participants sit tall at the edge of the chair, heels under ankles, shoulders over hips, abdominals braced, ribs lifted, and head retracted.
- ◉ They begin sitting tall with the hands resting on the lap.

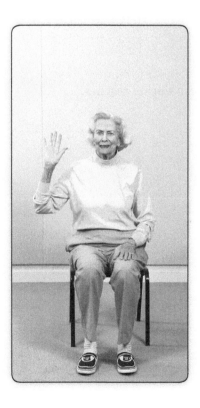
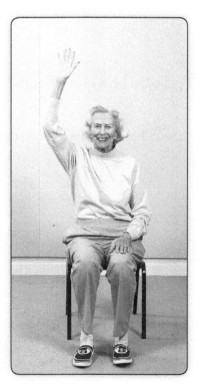
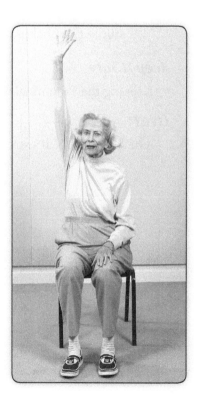

The Moves

Use the following cues.

- Lift the right arm up toward the ceiling, as far as is comfortable and, ideally, directly overhead.
- Reach a little higher by extending the ribs and shoulders (Venus de Milo arms).
- Return and relax.
- Sit tall again, lift the left arm toward the ceiling, and then reach higher.
- Remember there are two up phases; the second *up* phase is an extension through the shoulders and ribs.
- Repeat 6 to 8 times with each arm, and progress to 12 times, as tolerated.

Take It Further))

- Hold reaches a little longer.
- Encourage a little higher reach.
- Use a light weight, 1 or 2 pounds (.5-1 kilogram).

Give It More Balance))

- Sit closer to the edge of the chair.
- Use an offset foot position with heels lifted.
- Sit on a balance disc in a chair with arms.
- Do the The Up and Up standing up, with appropriate balance support (such as a sturdy chair behind).

Keep It Safe))

Keeping the abdominal wall pulled in better stabilizes the torso during reaches.

Live It))

The Up and Up! It's strength with length. That's good stuff!

POSTURE

BALLOON LIFTS

Balloon Lifts are a progression of The Up and Up. In this activity, both arms press a balloon upward.

Benefits))

- ⊙ Enhances torso and shoulder function, strength, and flexibility.
- ⊙ Strengthens especially the back extensors and abdominal wall.
- ⊙ Mimics everyday lifting and reaching skills.
- ⊙ Facilitates the concept of length with strength.

Set It Up))

Each participant will need a balloon, plus have a few extra on hand. Some variations use light-weight balls or hand weights.

How to Do It))

The Start

- ⊙ Participants sit comfortably with their back away from the chair, if possible. Hips can touch the chair , but the back should not. Abdominals are braced, shoulder blades back and down, chin level, and head retracted.
- ⊙ They hold the balloon in both hands, close to the body at waist level.
- ⊙ Inhale to prepare.

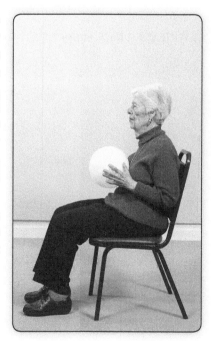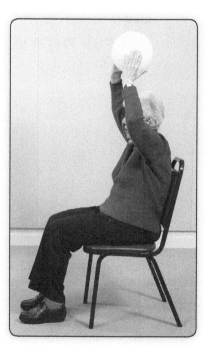

The Moves

Use the following cues.

- ⊙ Exhale, keep the balloon close to the body, and use both hands to push the balloon as far up and overhead as is comfortable. Allow the ribs to lift a little, too.
- ⊙ Can you push a little higher? (Allow participants to make that adjustment.)
- ⊙ Can you sit a little taller? (Allow participants to make that adjustment.)
- ⊙ Inhale and pull a little taller.
- ⊙ Exhale and lower the balloon to the starting position.
- ⊙ Repeat the lifts 4 times and progress to doing 12 times, as tolerated.

Take It Further))

- Use a lightweight ball (such as a soccer ball) instead of the balloon.
- Hold a single, 1- or 2-pound (.5- or 1-kilogram) weight with both hands instead of the balloon.

Give It More Balance))

- Sit closer to the edge of the chair.
- Sit on the edge of the chair with offset or tandem feet.
- Instead of pushing the balloon straight up, push it right and then left.

Keep It Safe))

Ideally, participants will keep balloons in line and above their shoulders as they lift and draw in their abdominal wall with each lift of the balloon. Many of your participants have bent-over backs. Keeping their abdominals in while reaching up will help support their back while they lift. Pushing balloons to right and left may not be appropriate for some individuals with osteoporosis. Nothing should hurt.

Live It))

Lifting both arms together with good back support is truly uplifting!

TAP AND CATCH A BALLOON

This activity is a progression that combines Push Up Think Thin (in chapter 6, page 209) and The Up and Up (see page 137). For a fun balance treat, Tap and Catch features a visual target (the balloon) and a coordinated activity (catching).

Benefits))

- Enhances torso and shoulder function and flexibility.
- Strengthens core muscles.
- Uses visual targets.
- Challenges eye–hand coordination.

Set It Up))

Each participant will need a balloon.

How to Do It))

The Start

- Participants sit tall at the back or edge of the chair (their choice), holding a balloon.
- Their shoulders should be over hips, abdominals in, and head pulled back in line with shoulders.

The Moves

Use the following cues.

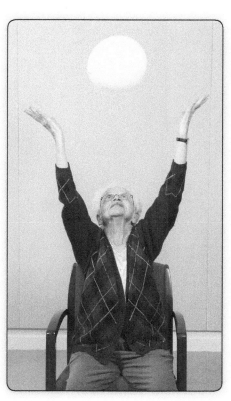

- Participant taps the balloon into the air, volleyball serve style, high enough above their head so that they must reach up to catch it.
- Quickly, pull in the abdominal wall, and extend both arms and the rib cage upward to reach and catch the balloon.
- Reach for the balloon with both hands while it is still overhead.
- Return to the starting position.
- Repeat the tap and catch 6 to 8 times and progress to doing 12 times, as tolerated.
- Pull in the abdominal wall each time when reaching up to catch the balloon.

Take It Further »

- Increase the number of repetitions.
- Tap the balloon a little higher to encourage a longer reach.

Give It More Balance »

- Sit at the edge of the chair with feet tandem and heels lifted.
- Tap the balloon to the left and right at varying tangents; 10, 11, 12, 1, and 2 o'clock spots, for example.
- Caution them to not lean out too far. The spots should be in the same plane as their body, not out in front of them.

Keep It Safe »

Pulling in the abdominal wall while reaching up and catching will help support their back and keep the exercise more comfortable. If they can't reach way up, then little taps and catches are fine. Nothing should hurt.

Live It »

Playing Tap and Catch is fun and promotes strength, length, and better balance.

This fun activity is one of the first to use rhythm and music. The song is actually a little too fast, but it works. They don't have to keep up with it to have fun and get some good exercise. Having participants sing along leads to audience participation and interaction. Some may even brag to their grandkids about doing this in your class.

Benefits))

- ◉ Uses music in a fun activity.
- ◉ Strengthens torso, especially the back extensors and abdominal wall.
- ◉ Improves torso and shoulder function and flexibility.

Set It Up))

If you have the equipment, cue up and have ready *YMCA* by the Village People. If your sound system can slow it down some that would be great, too.

How to Do It))

- ◉ Participants sit tall and look like a *W*: Arms out to their sides at shoulder height and elbows bent about 45 degrees. That's the W.
- ◉ Participants make an *A*. They sit tall and push both arms up to form an *A*, touching thumbs and fingers above the head.
- ◉ Tell them how great that looks, but you'd rather see a *Venus de Milo A*! They should lift high throughout their whole trunk and pull in abdominals. Coach them through it.
- ◉ Repeat *A & W*s 6 to 12 times, as tolerated.

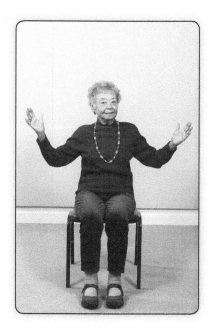 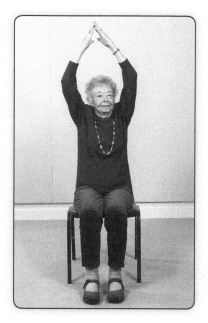

Take It Further »

⊙ Practice the letters for the *YMCA* song slowly and with good core stability.

- Have them form a *Y*.
- Have them form an *M*.
- Have them form a *C*.
- Then form a backward *C* (a mirror image, to work the other side).
- Then an *A* (they know that one already!)

⊙ Do the letters a little faster, cueing them frequently to keep the core stabilized.

Give It More Balance »

⊙ Once participants appear stable and comfortable with all the letters, introduce the *YMCA* song. Then play it with them and enjoy!

Keep It Safe »

Cue participants to keep abdominal wall braced while lifting ribs and arms. Do the movements and songs slowly for as long as they need.

Live It »

Everyone will have some fun at the YMCA! Thanks for playing!

POSTURE

6

Strength for a Purpose

Pretend for a moment you are an 85-year-old woman. You have been sedentary for many years. You may have developed complications from osteoporosis, arthritis, heart disease, and a hip replacement, and you may be taking several medications. You lack the strength and balance confidence you once took for granted. Getting around is difficult, and fear of falling influences almost every choice you make. Will you go out shopping? Spend holidays with the family? Take a walk and feed the ducks? Maybe those activities aren't options for you these days. The hustle and bustle of the crowds and the complications of uncertain terrains scare you.

Imagine a flight of stairs. At the top is a friend's door, a library, or a museum you love. Would you go up the stairs if you felt the effort or the risks were too great? It's not likely. Confidence, balance, and strength influence lifestyle decisions. Strength training that is oriented toward better balance and function can change a frail person's outlook on life. Purposeful strength training can restore a more satisfying lifestyle for participants, improving their balance, strength, and confidence.

This chapter focuses on strengthening the leg, back, arm, and chest muscles. ABLE Bodies exercises for core strength and stability were described in chapter 5. The exercises in this chapter are listed by muscle group and are presented from simple to more difficult. Seated exercises are first, followed by standing exercises, and then others, including some that involve moving. Where an exercise or activity bridges many muscle groups, the activity is included with the main group served.

Quick Reminder

As always, progress only as well tolerated by your participants. That means nothing hurts, they are willing and able to continue, and they show no signs of dizziness, nausea, excessive fatigue, and so on. Participants should be able to do the exercise using proper form before you add any difficulty. Review chapter 3 for more information on safe progression.

All activities in this chapter are available in PDF format! Visit www.HumanKinetics.com/ABLEBodiesBalanceTraining.

SEATED HEEL RAISES

Heel raises strengthen lower leg muscles, important for sway control. Stronger calf muscles can put a little extra oomph into the push-off phase of gait.

Benefits))

- Strengthens calf muscles (gastrocnemius and soleus).
- Enhances postural control for balance and gait.
- Allows participants to do a seated strength activity.

Set It Up))

You will not need any special equipment for this exercise. One progression has participants seated on a balance disc in a chair with arms.

How to Do It))

The Start

Participants start in the tall sitting position, with shoulders over hips, chin level, head retracted, and feet flat on the floor. Abs are pulled in and up slightly. The ribs are lifted and torso tall, lengthening the spine.

The Moves

Use the following cues.

- Lift both heels off the floor 3 to 5 inches (8-13 centimeters), as able. Balls of the feet should stay on the floor.
- Hold a moment.
- Return heels to the floor. Relax.
- Repeat 10 to 15 times, as tolerated.
- Stretch the calves when done (flex the ankle and turn the foot from side to side).

Take It Further))

- Lift both heels in stages.
  - Lift to balls of feet.
  - Lift to tip toes.
  - Push both heels forward so that they are almost over the toes and pressure is felt along the longitudinal axis of the foot.
  - Hold a moment and then return heels to the floor.
- Add a Thera-Band.
  - Place heels on the floor with toes up.
  - Place the middle part of Thera-Band under balls of feet. Hold the two ends in your hands. (Participants can adjust the resistance from here.)
  - Push the toes down against the band, toward the floor.

- Add additional weight to one leg.
  - Place both hands on one knee and lean the body forward to add weight to the heel raises of that leg.
  - Then add weight to other leg and do heel raises with that foot.

Give It More Balance 》

- Alternate heels; this will help improve agility and coordination.
- Slide to the front of the chair and maintain a tall sitting posture throughout the exercise.
- Sit on a balance disc (*only* if the chairs have arms).

SEATED TOE RAISES

Lifting the toes (flexing the foot) helps the feet clear the ground between steps. When the foot is not flexing between steps, a shuffling gait is apparent, and a toe that drags can cause a tripping hazard. Toe raises help prevent falls and improve gait.

Benefits))

- Strengthens muscles, especially the tibialis anterior muscle.
- Enhances postural control over swaying during standing.
- Improves foot action during gait.

Set It Up))

You will not need any equipment for this activity. One progression has participant seated on a balance disc in a chair with arms.

How to Do It))

The Start

Participants sit tall, with feet flat on the floor about hip-width apart, torso braced and tall, and spine lengthened.

The Moves

Use the following cues.

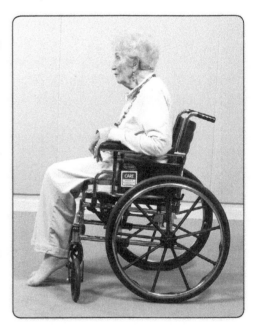

- Lift the toes of both feet off the ground (ankle and foot flexion).
- Hold a moment.
- Lower toes to the floor.
- Repeat 12 to 15 times, as tolerated.
- Stretch the shins when done (point and turn the foot and toes; do ankle circles).

Take It Further))

- Pull up more firmly.
- Hold the up position a bit longer.
- Add more weight to foot (place the heel of the other foot on the exercising foot).

Give It More Balance))

- Do alternating toe raises: Right, left, right, left. Alternating feet helps improve agility and coordination.
- Sit tall at the edge of the chair.
- Sit on a balance disc (*only* if the chairs have arms).

STRENGTH

DUCKS AND PIGEONS

Ducks and Pigeons is a variation of Seated Toe Raises.

Benefits))

⊙ Strengthens a broader range of ankle and lower-leg muscles than simple toe raises.

⊙ Allows participants to do strength work seated.

Set It Up))

You will not need any equipment for this activity, unless you choose to progress Duck Feet by adding resistance with a Thera-Band. Then each person would need a Thera-Band. One progression has participant seated on a balance disc in a chair with arms.

How to Do It))

The Start

Participants sit tall with feet flat on the floor, hip-width apart (same beginning position as Seated Toe Raises).

The Moves

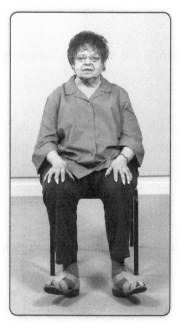
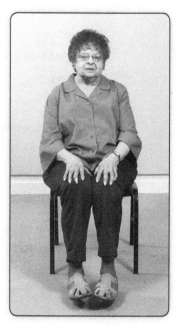

Use the following cues.

⊙ Keeping heels on the floor, lift the front of the foot as far as you are comfortably able. Hold a moment.

⊙ Turn the feet outward (duck feet).

⊙ Then turn them in (pigeon toes).

⊙ Lower the foot to the floor.

⊙ Repeat 8 to 12 times, as well tolerated.

⊙ Stretch the shins (point and turn the foot and toes; do ankle circles).

Take It Further))

⊙ Cue participants to make their ankles work harder. Tell them to pull up more firmly.

⊙ Do a few more repetitions, or increase hold times in the up position.

⊙ Use a Thera-Band to increase resistance for Duck Feet. Place band under both feet and hold ends in hands. Start with feet placed a few inches apart. Heels stay planted and forefeet move apart from each other.

Give It More Balance))

⊙ Sit at the edge of the chair.

⊙ Sit on a balance disc (*only* if the chairs have arms).

SEATED HEEL–TOE ROCKING

Proper heel–toe motion is essential for weight shifting during gait. During walking, weight transfers from the heel to the toe and then pushes off to the next foot. This heel–toe rocking exercise adds a sense of heel–toe motion to a seated foot exercise and an element of balance. Heel–Toe Rocking simply combines heel and toe raises.

Benefits))

- Mimics heel-to-toe weight transfer common in walking gait.
- Improves flexibility and circulation in the lower leg and ankle.
- Facilitates coordination for gait mechanics.
- Allows participants to experience Heel–Toe Rocking while seated.

Set It Up))

You will not need any special equipment for this exercise, unless you use the balance progression that suggests they place their feet on a balloon or balance disc. Then each participant would need a balloon or balance disc.

How to Do It))

The Start

Participants begin sitting tall, with feet flat on the floor, hip-width apart.

The Moves

Use the following cues.

- Heels up—press the toes down and lift the heels up until the foot rests on the ball.
- Toes up—press the heels down and lift the front of the foot up.
- Repeat 8 to 15 times.

Take It Further))

- Add more repetitions, up to 15.
- Pull up hard and press down firmly so the work is more difficult.
- Hold end positions longer.

Give It More Balance))

- ◉ Use opposing motions: Right toe up with left heel, then switch.
- ◉ Sit on the edge of the chair and work at maintaining Tall Sits during the activity.
- ◉ Place both feet on a balance disc and do Heel–Toe Rocking.
- ◉ Place both feet on a balloon. Allow the balloon to rock and roll under the feet, as legs move back and forth.

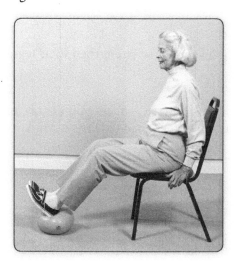 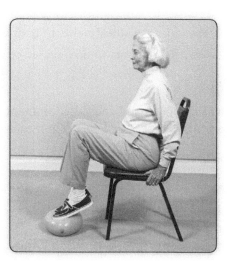

STRENGTH

HEEL DRAGS

This is an easy-to-learn, versatile exercise for strengthening hamstrings. Participants can change the difficulty simply by pressing harder against the floor or using a Thera-Band. Think of it as a seated hamstring curl.

Benefits))

- Strengthens hamstrings.
- Allows for easy adjustments to resistance.
- Allows participants to do a seated strength exercise to strengthen their legs.

Set It Up))

You will not need any special equipment for this exercise, unless you choose to add resistance with a Thera-Band. Then each participant will need a Thera-Band.

How to Do It))

The Start

- Participants sit tall at edge of their chair so that more of the hamstrings are off the chair.
- Feet are flat on the floor, hip-width apart.
- Participants place one foot forward of the other, still flat on the floor. The forward leg is almost extended.

The Moves

Use the following cues.

- Press the forward foot down into the floor to create resistance for the heel drag.
- Drag the foot backward until its toe is in line with the other heel, if able.
- Place the foot back out in front again and repeat the heel drag 8 to 12 times, as tolerated.
- Switch forward legs and repeat with the other leg.
- Stretch hamstrings when finished (seated Gentlemen's Bow).

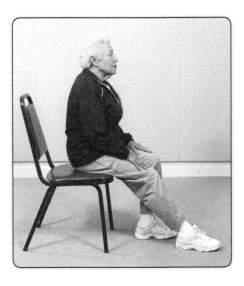 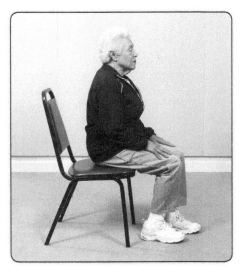

- ⊙ Add more repetitions, up to 15.
- ⊙ Cue participants to press more firmly against the floor to garner more resistance for the pullback phase.
- ⊙ Add difficulty with a Thera-Band using the following cues.
  - Run the middle part of the Thera-Band under both feet (hold the ends of the band in your lap to adjust resistance).
  - Push just one heel out of the looped band and hook it over the band. Place that heel on the floor.
  - Drag the hooked heel backward, as in Heel Drags, against the resistance. (The band adds extra resistance to the pull back phase.)
  - Maintain Tall Sit throughout activity.

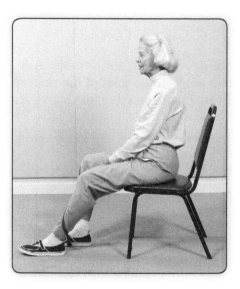 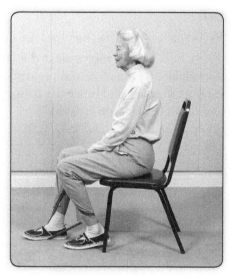

Keep It Safe))

In this exercise, participants begin seated at the front of their chair. To better support the back and torso in this position, ask them to place their arms on the chair arms and keep their core muscles braced.

CROSS-LEGGED KNEE EXTENSIONS

This simple exercise will help participants rise from chairs, climb stairs, and otherwise get on with their lives.

Benefits))

- Strengthens quadriceps and knee musculature.
- Helps reduce common types of knee pain.
- Allows participants to do a seated strength exercise to strengthen their legs.

Set It Up))

You will not need any special equipment for this exercise, unless you choose to add light ankle weights for some participants.

How to Do It))

The Start

- Participants sit all the way back in a chair.
- Their back should rest against the back of the chair and arms on the chair arms, if available. (If the chair has no arms, place arms on the sides of the chair to help support the back and brace the torso.) Abs are braced and shoulder blades are back and down. Ankles are crossed.

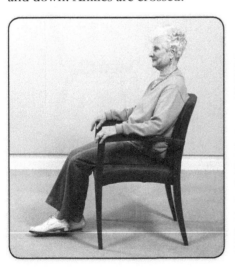 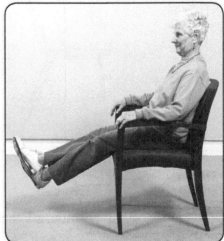

The Moves

Use the following cues.

- Lift legs upward until the knee of the lower leg is nearly straight.
- Raise the lower leg up to increase work.
- Hold a moment.
- Lower the legs.
- Repeat 8 to 15 times, as tolerated.
- Place the other ankle in top position and do same exercise with other leg 8 to 15 times, as tolerated.

Take It Further))

- ⊙ For greater difficulty, lengthen the time spent lifting and lowering the legs.
- ⊙ Cue participants to press down on the lower leg with their upper leg.
- ⊙ Use light ankle weights.

Give It More Balance))

As the legs come up, cue participants to pull their back away from the back of the chair, sit tall, and lengthen the spine. This will strengthen core muscles and require them to balance over their hips.

Keep It Safe))

Make sure participants sit all the way back in their chair with their hands on the chair arms or sides. This position keeps their back from feeling the weight of both legs lifting. If this exercise is too difficult for some, advise them to simply lift and extend one leg at a time.

SEATED LEG PRESS WITH A THERA-BAND

This exercise strengthens hip muscles, critical for getting out of chairs and walking up inclines or stairs. Strengthening hip extensors also plays a role in enabling upright posture.

Benefits 》

- Strengthens hip extensors.
- Uses Thera-Bands, which can be easily adjusted to increase or decrease difficulty.
- Allows participants to do this leg press seated.

Set It Up 》

You will need Thera-Bands or tubing for each participant.

How to Do It 》

The Start

- Participants sit all the way back in their chair and place a Thera-Band under one foot, like a stirrup. They should wrap the ends around their hands and hold the elbows to the torso.
- Lift the knee in the stirrup up toward the chest, bringing the forearms and hands toward the chest.
- They should keep their forearms and hands anchored to the chest throughout the exercise.

The Moves

Use the following cues.

- Press the foot and leg downward toward the floor (keep forearms and hands on the chest).
- Push down into the Thera-Band until that thigh touches the chair.
- Lift again.
- Repeat 8 to 15 times, as tolerated, with each leg.
- Stretch the hamstrings and gluteal muscles when finished (seated Gentlemen's Bow).

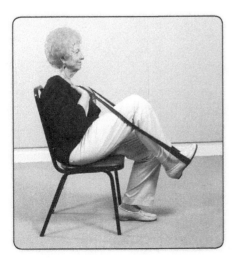 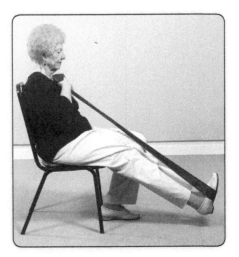

STRENGTH

Take It Further))

- Tighten up on the band (this shortens the length of the band and provides more resistance).
- Use a stronger band.
- Slow the speed of each push.

Keep It Safe))

Make sure participants sit all the way back in their chair. This position keeps their back from feeling the weight of their legs. Be sure to cue participants to keep their abs in on each lift.

STRENGTH

SEATED SIDE STEPS WITH A THERA-BAND

This exercise strengthens muscles important to side-to-side (lateral) stability. It may also help prevent falls, especially falls to the side, which are often the most devastating.

Benefits))

- Strengthens hip abductors.
- Allows participants to do seated strength training.

Set It Up))

You will need a Thera-Band for each participant.

How to Do It))

The Start

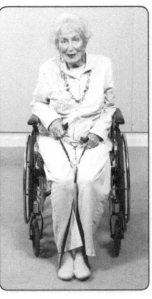
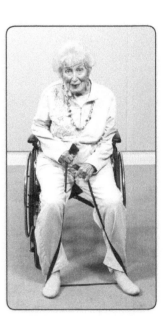

- Participants sit tall, as described earlier, knees bent 90 degrees and feet flat on the floor, hip-width apart.
- They place the middle part of the Thera-Band under both feet, bring the ends up between the knees, and hold the ends with the hands. The tightness, or resistance, of the band can be adjusted as appropriate during the exercise.

The Moves

Use the following cues.

- Without lifting the foot, slide one foot and leg out to the side, as far as is comfortable and against the resistance of the band. Continue to sit tall.
- Stop at the end point and hold a moment. Check that the knee is staying over the ankle.
- Slide the foot and leg back to the starting position.
- Repeat 6 to 12 times with each leg, as tolerated.
- Do the same with the other leg.
- Stretch the hip abductors when finished (cross one leg over the other and pull the knee gently toward the body).

STRENGTH

Take It Further ⟩⟩

- Get more resistance from the band by tightening up on the band. Or, use a stronger band.
- Increase repetitions to 15.
- Slow the pace or hold end positions a little longer.
- Press both legs out to opposing sides at the same time.

Give It More Balance ⟩⟩

Move closer to the front edge of chair and work at maintaining a braced, strong core.

Keep It Safe ⟩⟩

Participants should keep the sliding foot on the ground. They shouldn't lift it as it moves out to the side. Check that the foot travels directly under the knee throughout the exercise. (It shouldn't look like the Charleston dance step.) Check that participants are maintaining a good Tall Sit throughout the exercise.

STRENGTH

BALLOON KNEE SQUEEZES

Muscles of the inner thigh contribute to lateral stability and stability in gait. Better lateral stability is associated with reduced fall risk and improved knee function.

Benefits))

- ⊙ Strengthens hip adductors (inner thigh muscles).
- ⊙ Helps prevent falls, especially falls to the side.

Set It Up))

You will need a balloon or small Slo Mo ball for each participant.

How to Do It))

This exercise can be done either seated or standing.

Seated Position

- ⊙ Participants sit tall in a chair with feet closer together than the knees.
- ⊙ They place a balloon between the knees or thighs.

Use the following cues.

- ⊙ Squeeze the balloon tightly with the thighs. Make the balloon change its shape.
- ⊙ Sit taller.
- ⊙ Relax.
- ⊙ Repeat 6 to 15 times, as tolerated.

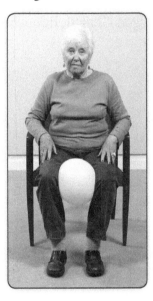
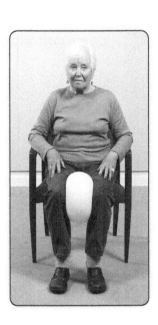

Standing Position

- ⊙ Stand with balance support as needed. Abs are braced, ribs lifted, hips tucked under shoulders, and head retracted.
- ⊙ Place the balloon between the thighs.
- ⊙ Squeeze the balloon with the thighs until it changes shape.
- ⊙ Relax.
- ⊙ Repeat 8 to 12 times, as tolerated.

Take It Further))

- ⊙ Do more repetitions, up to 15.
- ⊙ Hold the squeeze longer.
- ⊙ Squeeze harder.

ABLE Bodies Balance Training

Give It More Balance))

- Focus on maintaining ribs-lifted posture while squeezing.
- Sit at the edge of the chair.
- Sit at the edge of the chair with heels lifted.
- Add a single-arm lift and reach with each squeeze, as shown in this photo. Allow the ribs to lift upward with each reach.

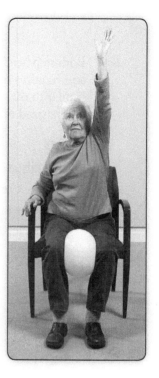

STRENGTH

MARCHING IN PLACE (SEATED)

Both step height and length are important aspects of gait. Marching exaggerates gait patterns and requires higher steps, which will facilitate longer strides. Seated Marching in Place is similar to the core exercise Knee Lift, Abs In. Keeping the abdominal muscles pulled in is emphasized in both activities, but this activity is done in a coordinated and faster pattern.

Benefits))

- Facilitates greater step height and length.
- Uses a reciprocal pattern similar to that of walking.
- Allows participants to sit, stand, or move to music.
- Adds an agility requirement to normal strength training.

Set It Up))

You will not need any special equipment for this exercise.

How to Do It))

The Start

- Participants sit all the way back in their chair, with forearms on arms of the chair to provide back support.
- They draw their abdominal wall toward the back of chair and brace core muscles.

The Moves

Use the following cues.

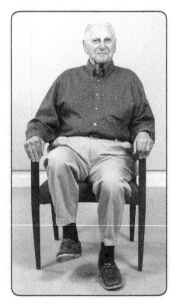

- Lift the right knee, keeping the core muscles stable; and then the left knee.
- Keep the back tall and abdominal wall pulled in toward the chair back.
- It's just like marching. Keep going!
- Try to maintain an even lift height and stepping pattern.
- Keep the core stable and still.
- Repeat until each knee has lifted 8 to 12 times, as tolerated.

Take It Further))

- Increase repetitions to 15, if well tolerated.
- Cue for higher knee lifts.
- Add Genie arms (tall sitting with arms folded across the chest).

STRENGTH

Give It More Balance))

- ◉ Move away from the back of the chair and maintain the tall sitting position. Have them keep their arms on the chair arms at first.
- ◉ Add reciprocal arm swings (right arm forward, left knee up; then left arm forward, right knee up).
- ◉ March to music. The music will help them coordinate movement patterns.
- ◉ Add arm swings to marching with music.

Keep It Safe))

Keeping the core muscles stable (abdominal muscles pulled toward the back of the chair and braced) and forearms on the chair arms will prevent back strain in the frailer adults.

STRENGTH

HEEL SIDE KICKS

These side kicks are similar to the Charleston dance. The upper leg stays in place while the lower leg kicks out to the side, allowing *internal hip rotation*. This activity can help correct the toe-out foot placement common in older adults.

Benefits))

- ⊙ Strengthens chronically weak internal hip rotators.
- ⊙ Allows participants to sit.
- ⊙ Helps to improve common stance and gait abnormalities.

Set It Up))

You will need Thera-Bands for each participant to add resistance.

How to Do It))

The Start

- ⊙ Participants sit tall at the edge of their chair, both feet flat on the floor, thighs parallel.
- ⊙ They can place their hands on the chair arms for better back support.

The Moves

Use the following cues.

- ⊙ Lift the right heel up and to the side. The lower leg moves like a clock hand moving from 6 o'clock to 4 o'clock. The upper leg rotates inward a bit, but should basically stay still and parallel to the other leg.
- ⊙ Return foot to the floor.
- ⊙ Repeat six to eight times, as tolerated.
- ⊙ Repeat with the other leg.

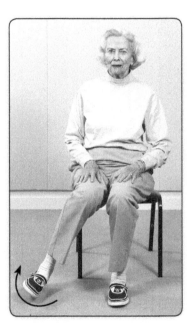

STRENGTH

Take It Further))

- ⊙ Increase repetitions or hold times.
- ⊙ Do Side Kicks With a Thera-Band.
    - Place a Thera-Band under both feet as if it were a stirrup.
    - Hold ends in hands.
    - Lift heels out to the side so the movement is resisted by the band.

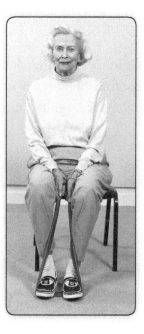 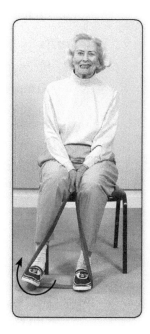

Keep it Safe))

Not everyone will be able to do this activity comfortably or well. To make it easier, participants can do it with the whole leg straight out. They simply turn the foot inward into pigeon toes, and the whole leg turns. Remember that nothing should hurt, and they should only do what is comfortable.

STRENGTH

KNEE CROSSES

This exercise strengthens the hip adductor muscles using a large, whole-body movement.

Benefits))

- ⊙ Strengthens inner thigh muscles.
- ⊙ Requires coordination of opposing sides of the upper and lower body.
- ⊙ Requires endurance, agility, and coordination.

Set It Up))

You will not need any special equipment for this exercise, unless you choose to add light resistance.

How to Do It))

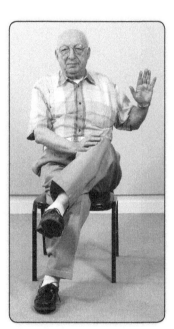

The Start

- ⊙ Participants sit all the way back in their chair to better support their back.
- ⊙ Cue them to lift their arms up to their sides, with elbows bent and hands up.

The Moves

Use the following cues.

- ⊙ Lift the left knee up and cross it over the midline of the body.
- ⊙ Bring the right arm and hand forward toward the left knee.
- ⊙ Touch the left knee with the right hand.
- ⊙ Pull the arm back to the beginning position and lower the leg back to the floor.
- ⊙ Repeat 6 to 12 times, as tolerated.
- ⊙ Repeat with the right leg and left arm and hand.
- ⊙ Stretch the inner-thighs when done (see Pull-Aparts on page 76).

Take It Further))

- ⊙ Increase repetitions to 15.
- ⊙ Cross and touch the knee to the opposite ankle (instead of to the knee).
- ⊙ Add a light ankle weight.

Give It More Balance))

Alternate legs, but make sure participants are core stable between each leg lift.

Keep It Safe))

Participants with recent hip surgeries should not do this exercise. Also, it's important for participants to sit all the way back in their chair for this exercise. Using the chair back for support protects the low back during leg lifts and torso twisting.

STRENGTH

TEETER-TOTTER CHAIR STANDS

Teeter-Totter Chair Stands build leg strength throughout the entire leg and are extremely functional. Being able to get up from a chair is vital for anyone with things to do and errands to run! Helping participants accomplish this everyday task is one of the best results of ABLE Bodies training. The physics of foot placement and momentum is the secret tool for easier get up and go power. Practice Teeter-Totter Chair Stands often and use them as a transition between seated and standing exercises.

Benefits ⟩⟩

- ⊙ Mimics an important activity of daily living.
- ⊙ Strengthens the entire leg.
- ⊙ Requires maintaining postural stability during a transition (sitting to standing).
- ⊙ Promotes everyday mobility.

Set It Up ⟩⟩

You will not need any special equipment for this exercise.

How to Do It ⟩⟩

The Start

- ⊙ Participants sit tall on the edge of their chair, feet hip-width apart and flat on the floor.
- ⊙ Heels should be pulled back, behind the knees.
- ⊙ Depending on the level of assistance required to get up, they can place their hands on the chair arms (easy), their knees (moderate), or their chest (difficult).

STRENGTH

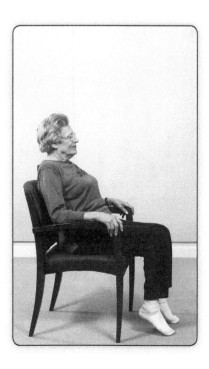 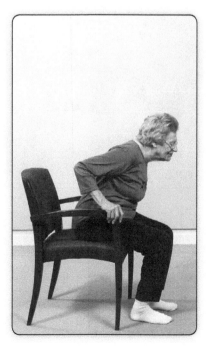 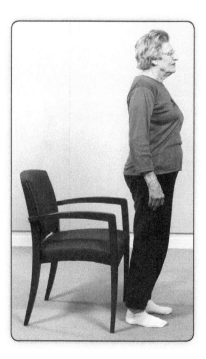

The Moves

Use the following cues.

- ◉ Lean back. Brace your core muscles and lift your heels.
- ◉ Then in one fell swoop, do the following.
    - Lean forward: tell them "Nose over knees."
    - Press down: Bring your weight forward and push it down into your feet.
    - Stand up: Quickly and firmly push up through the legs until standing.
    - The goal is to get the hips over the feet.

Take It Further))

One-Legged Chair Stand

- ◉ Beginning position is the same (edge of chair) but feet are offset. The back foot will be doing most of the work to stand up.
- ◉ Lean back, abs braced.
- ◉ Lift knee (leg that was pulled back).
- ◉ Lean forward and press down (cue them to stomp down as they lean forward).
- ◉ Stand up and balance yourself.

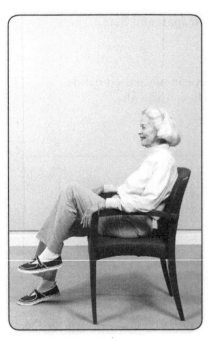 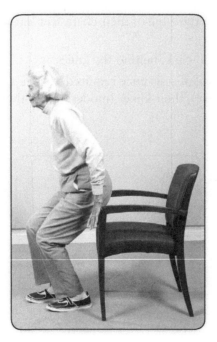 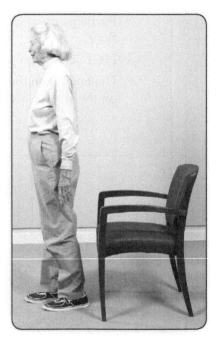

Use Thera-Band for added resistance

⊙ Place Thera-Band or tubing under both feet, with one end held in each hand.

⊙ Stand up; Thera-Band will resist the up movement. Adjust tightness of band to suit participant.

Keep It Safe))

Provide extra balance safety (a chair or handrail in front of them) and watch them closely the first two times. Remember that safely completing a Teeter-Totter Chair Stand will be a difficult task for many. Cue participants to maintain good posture (abs braced, ribs lifted) throughout. As they come to a stand, encourage them to push their hips forward to get themselves over their feet. Let them use their arms as needed. As they get stronger, they will gradually challenge themselves to use less arm strength. Staying close to the chair, or touching it lightly with a hand or leg, will help them to keep balanced and steady.

STRENGTH

STANDING HEEL RAISES

Heel raises are one of the most basic balance exercises. These heel raises incorporate more mindfulness on the part of participants. They are asked to notice the weight shifts and to rebalance in different positions. Strong calf muscles help control forward and backward swaying and add some extra oomph to the push-off phase of walking.

Benefits))

- ◉ Strengthens calf muscles (gastrocnemius and soleus).
- ◉ Teaches sway control.
- ◉ Adds elements of balance to basic heel raises.

Set It Up))

You will not need any special equipment for this exercise.

How to Do It))

The Start

- ◉ Participants should stand with good posture (feet parallel, soft knees, abs in, ribs lifted), behind a sturdy chair or beside a handrail.
- ◉ They place hands on balance support only as needed (both, one, tightly, lightly, hovered).
- ◉ Cue participants to distribute their body weight equally over both feet.

The Moves

Use the following cues.

- ◉ Shift your body weight forward to the front part of your feet. Can you feel your weight shift toward the balls of your feet? Good.
- ◉ Notice that your toes dig in a bit? Good.
- ◉ Find your balance in this position. Your weight is shifted forward but your heels stay on the ground. Hold your balance there for a moment to get steady in this position.
- ◉ Gradually lift your heels off the floor, slowly. Notice that your weight transfers onto the balls of the feet. Do you notice how the ball of the foot spreads out a bit to receive the weight?
- ◉ Hold this position for a moment. Get steady here.
- ◉ Let your knees soften. It will help. Do you notice how soft knees help? Good.
- ◉ Slowly lower heels to the floor with control.
- ◉ Shift your body weight back to the center of the foot (beginning position).
- ◉ Repeat 8 to 15 times, as tolerated.
    - Shift weight forward (heels stay down). Hold.
    - Lift heels, maintain balance, and keep knees soft.
    - Lower heels.
    - Shift weight backward.

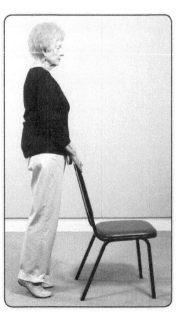

Take It Further))

- Use slightly longer holds in each position; just a second or two longer is adequate.
- Use an offset foot position to make one leg work harder.
    - One foot is forward, one back, shoulder-width apart.
    - Shift so that the body weight mostly is over the back foot.
    - Do a set of heel raises so that the back foot does most of the work.
    - Switch legs and repeat.

Give It More Balance))

Manipulate their footwork.

- Change the foot placement to wide apart or close together.
- Up and Hover: Lift heels, hold, and hover, maintaining balance.
- The Up and Up: Lift heels, then lift higher, hover, and lower.
- The Up and Step, Step: Lift heels, restabilize, take a few steps in place on the toes, rebalance, and then lower the heels.

Keep It Safe))

Let participants use as much balance support as they need. Participants should hold on with either one hand or both; tightly or lightly; or hover their hands just above the support.

SHALLOW SQUATS

Strengthens the whole leg in a movement pattern that is used when rising from a chair.

Benefits))

- Strengthens hip and knee extensors.
- Uses an everyday movement pattern as a leg-strengthening activity.
- Requires postural stability for balance maintenance.

Set It Up))

You will not need any special equipment for this exercise.

How to Do It))

The Start

- Participants stand with tall posture in front of a sturdy chair.
- Their feet are parallel and shoulder-width apart. Abs are braced.
- They can increase balance support by touching the front of the chair with their legs or finger tips.

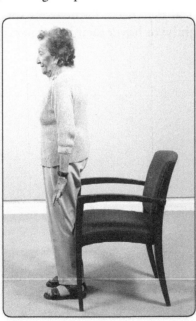 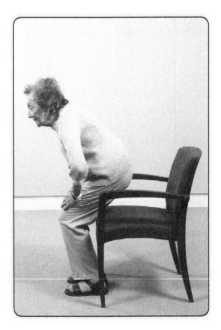

The Moves

Use the following cues.

- Bend the knees and hips; the goal is to lower the hips over the chair. It should look like you're about to sit down. A quarter to half of the way down is a reasonable shallow squat.
- If done correctly, the knees will stay over the ankles throughout the squat.
- Stand tall again, pushing the hips forward and up.
- Repeat 8 to 12 times, as tolerated.

Take It Further))

- ◉ Increase the repetitions, up to 15, if able.
- ◉ Hold a moment in the lowered position.
- ◉ Encourage a deeper squat.
- ◉ Use an offset foot position, with feet shoulder-width apart. This position will make the back leg work harder. Instruct participants that their back leg should stay in contact with the chair for better balance.

Give It More Balance))

- ◉ Focus on standing tall and feeling balanced at top of each rise or repetition.
- ◉ Lift one arm upward, directly overhead (if possible) with each squat.

Keep It Safe))

It's common for participants to squat in a way that puts their knees forward instead of their hips back. The correct way is hips back over the chair. Do not do these squats if participants are unable to do them correctly. If participants experience any hip, back, or knee pain, check their form. If pain persists, discontinue the exercise.

STRENGTH

MARCHING IN PLACE (STANDING)

This progression of seated marching strengthens the hip flexors. The movement pattern is specific to walking and helps participants initiate, practice, and complete safe weight transfers.

Benefits))

⊙ Simulates coordination and timing for leg action while walking.

⊙ Improves step height and length.

⊙ Requires core stability during leg movement.

Set It Up))

You may need some additional chairs for this activity. Additional balance support is often needed.

How to Do It))

The Start

Participants should stand with good posture (soft knees, abs in, ribs lifted) and adequate balance support. Here are some examples of balance support for Marching in Place. Place each participant:

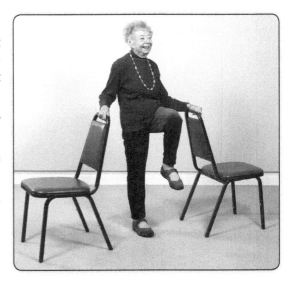

⊙ Between two sturdy chairs with another chair or wall behind them

⊙ With a wall to their back and one chair beside them

⊙ In a corner with two walls for balance support, perhaps a chair or walker in front of them

⊙ With hands on a railing or counter

The Moves

⊙ Have them begin marching in place.

⊙ Cue participants to keep their abs braced, ribs lifted, and their gaze on the horizon (a visual aid helps maintain balance).

⊙ Frequently cue them to keep their upright braced posture and to draw their abs in with each knee lift. Ask them if they notice how that helps them to keep their balance.

⊙ Continue marching slowly and deliberately for 15-30 seconds, as well tolerated.

⊙ Rest for a while, and then repeat if desired

Take It Further))

⊙ Longer march, up to a minute or two

⊙ Higher knees

⊙ Slightly faster marching

STRENGTH

Give It More Balance))

- ◉ Lessen the balance support.
  - - They can use a lighter hold on handrail or chair.
  - - They can use one hand instead of both to hold onto balance support.
- ◉ Add one arm swing (with the free arm).
- ◉ Add music. Use a slower melody, especially at first.
- ◉ Add reciprocal arm swings with or without music *only* if participants are comfortable letting go of their support. Arm swings are very difficult for frail participants.
- ◉ Dim the lights.

Keep It Safe))

Watch participants carefully. Marching is hard work and involves one-legged standing, if only for a brief time. Provide as much balance support as needed for each participant to feel comfortable and safe. After finishing, use Farmer's Stretch to stretch the hip flexors.

STRENGTH

STANDING HAMSTRING CURLS

This exercise strengthens the hamstrings and requires good standing balance.

Benefits))

- ⊙ Strengthens hamstrings.
- ⊙ Requires successful weight shifting.
- ⊙ Improves one-legged balance.
- ⊙ Builds kinesthetic awareness.

Set It Up))

You may choose to add light ankle weights for some participants.

How to Do It))

The Start

Participants stand tall behind a sturdy chair or other suitable support with knees soft and feet parallel.

The Moves

Use the following cues.

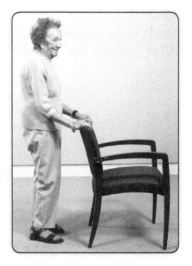
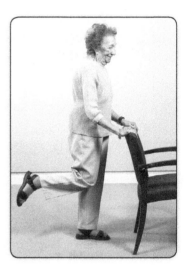

- ⊙ Keeping the fronts of the knees and thighs parallel (side by side), shift your weight to one leg and lift the other heel up toward the buttocks.
- ⊙ Lower the heel so the foot is back beside the other.
- ⊙ Repeat 8 to 12 times, as tolerated.
- ⊙ Repeat with the other leg.
- ⊙ Stretch the hamstrings when you're done. (Gentleman's Bow works great for this).

Take It Further))

- ⊙ Increase the repetitions to 15, as able.
- ⊙ Lift and lower more slowly.
- ⊙ Add light ankle weights.

Give It More Balance))

- ⊙ Have participants notice how the weight transfer feels when they change legs.
- ⊙ Reduce their balance support: Suggest that they use only a light touch on their chair or walker.

Keep It Safe))

Make certain they are keeping their knees and thighs aligned and parallel. Most will tend to lift their knee forward, breaking the frontal plane; this is a different exercise (hip flexors are used instead of hamstrings). You want them to lift their heel back, toward the buttocks. If proper form is difficult for them, have them place the working foot beyond the support foot before lifting the heel.

HEEL-TOUCH FORWARD, TOE-TOUCH BACK

This is a progression of heel–toe strength work, and it requires more balance control than easier versions. The leg swinging from front to back is a balance perturbation that participants will learn to manage as they practice this activity. Arm swings are a natural addition.

Benefits))

- ◉ Requires postural stability during limb movement and weight shifting.
- ◉ Enhances elements of gait, including leg swings and heel–toe motion.

Set It Up))

You will not need any special equipment for this exercise.

How to Do It))

The Start

- ◉ Provide participants with adequate balance support. Start with a balance support on both sides, such as standing with a walker or between two chairs. Participants with better balance can use a single balance support.
- ◉ Participants stand with good posture, feet shoulder-width apart, knees soft.

The Moves

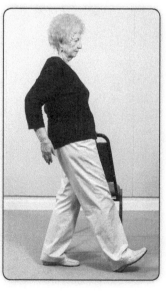 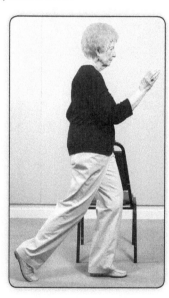

- ◉ Participants shift weight to the left leg.
- ◉ They place the right heel out in front on the ground.
- ◉ They allow the left knee to bend as the forward foot lands. Cue this movement with "Heel."
- ◉ They swing the leg behind so that the toes touch down behind. Cue this movement with "Toe."
- ◉ On your cue: "Heel," the leg swings forward; "Toe," the leg swings backward; and so on.
- ◉ Repeat 8 to 12 times, as tolerated. Heel, pause, toe, pause, heel, pause, toe, pause, etc. (think Step and Stop on page 237).
- ◉ Use a deliberate pace that allows them to maintain their balance with each foot placement.
- ◉ Repeat with the other leg.

Take It Further))

- ◉ Increase repetitions.
- ◉ Increase speed or shorten pause times between heel and toe.
- ◉ Cue more bend from the supporting leg.

Give It More Balance))

- Ask participants to focus on how the leg swings affect their balance.
- Use fewer balance supports.
- Change legs more frequently. Always bring the feet back together before switching.
- Add a single-arm swing (hold the balance support with the other hand).
- Add swings with both arms.
- Use music or counting to set a rhythm.
- Place hands on the hips.

Keep It Safe))

This activity takes a fair amount of balance. If participants find that placing the toe behind them is too difficult, have them place the foot beside the other instead of back. Cue it as "Heel, together. Heel, together." As with many activities, developing a rhythm will make it easier, too.

PENDULUM LEGS

Strong hip abductors are important for side-to-side stability, and the ability to make quick transitions may prevent falls to the side. This exercise for hip abductors teaches participants to successfully do repetitive lateral weight transitions.

Benefits))

- Strengthens hip abductors.
- Enhances balance awareness during lateral weight transitions.
- Uses reciprocal, sequential motion between lower and upper body.

Set It Up))

You will not need any special equipment for this exercise, unless you choose to use light ankle weights for some participants.

How to Do It))

The Start

- Participants stand tall behind their sturdy chair or other appropriate balance support (facing a handrail or using their walker).
- Both hands should be placed on balance support to start (tightly or lightly).
- Abs are braced, shoulder blades back and down, feet shoulder-width apart and parallel, and knees soft.

The Moves

Use the following cues.

- Keeping the core stable and as still as possible, lift the right leg up to the side.
- The lift just needs to be a few inches; 4 to 6 inches (10-15 centimeters) is adequate.
- Bring the legs back together for just a moment.
- Lift the other leg as soon as the other comes down—just like a pendulum. The transition in the center is just for a moment.
- It will help participants if you cue them to allow knees to soften just a bit between weight transfers. (It kind of feels like a little bounce, a quick "down, up" in between opposing leg lifts.)

Take It Further))

- Do slightly higher lifts to the side.
- Use light ankle weights.

Give It More Balance))

- Cue participants to *really notice* the feeling of each weight transfer. Noticing this feeling enhances their kinesthetic learning.
- Reduce balance support just a bit. Hands hover over the back of the chair, for example.

STRENGTH

- Add opposing arm lifts.
    - As the right leg lifts to the side, lift the left arm up and directly overhead (it looks like the arm movement used in the classic jumping jack, but with only one arm).
    - Switch sides and lift the left leg to the side and the right arm overhead.
    - Repeat for 8 to 12 repetitions, switching sides each time.
    - Arms should be lifted overhead, not out to the side. Have them try it both ways—they will learn more and learn it better with their own bodies. Sampling an activity in two ways is great inside/out learning! Participants should notice that their balance is better with arms overhead instead of out to the side.

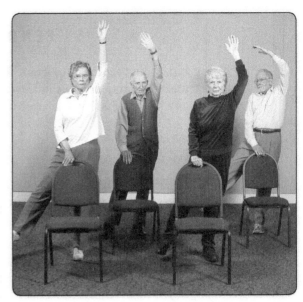

- Do the activity on a soft carpet or lawn.
- Stand on an easy balance pad, if available and if you can supervise personally.

Keep It Safe))

For the greatest balance stability, cue participants to keep their torso quiet, tall, and still. Comment on how core stability steadies the body against limb movements. Allow them to use balance support as needed for them to feel safe. The following changes will make this activity easier:

- Participants can lightly touch their foot out to the side, instead of lifting the leg up.
- Participants can perform multiple repetitions on one side, and then switch sides instead of alternating each time.

SIDE STEPS WALKING

Sidestepping adds a little maneuverability to an everyday skill. A side step with a bit of a knee bend actually turns this activity into a modified side lunge. Side stepping will strengthen hip abduction and reduce fall risk.

Benefits))

- ◉ Combines strength, balance, and mobility.
- ◉ Builds lateral stability by strengthening hip abductors and adductors.
- ◉ Practices lateral stepping for improved agility.

Set It Up))

You will not need any special equipment for this exercise, unless you choose to use light ankle weights for some participants. Tubing with ankle cuffs should be used only in one-on-one training.

How to Do It))

The Start

Participants stand tall with appropriate balance support. This exercise is done moving, so a handrail, counter, or row of sturdy chair backs will work best. Good balance support can also involve holding hands with each other. Pairs of participants can face each other and hold each other's hands or forearms (see Waltzing Matildas on page 320).

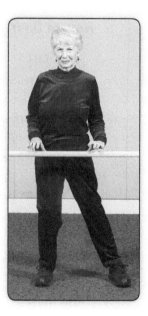

The Moves

Use the following cues.

- ◉ Step six to eight times to the right.
- ◉ Step six to eight times to the left.
- ◉ Rest.
- ◉ Repeat once or twice.

Take It Further))

- ◉ Take wider steps.
- ◉ Add big knee bends to each step. Cue participants to bend and straighten the receiving knee with each step.
- ◉ If you are working with individual clients, use tubing to add resistance and more balance challenge.

Give It More Balance))

- ◉ Reduce balance supports.
- ◉ Cue participants to place their hands on their hips. Supervise them closely.
- ◉ Add music to provide rhythm. Waltzes are great for this.

STANDING HEEL-TOE ROCKING

Heel–Toe Rocking is a great addition to other activities. It mimics the heel-to-toe pattern used in gaits and is similar to some common balance challenges (getting something from a top shelf, for example). The balance challenge for them is to feel and control this kind of rocking and rhythmical motion.

Benefits))

- Strengthens the entire lower leg.
- Requires upper body awareness and control.
- Provides a difficult balance challenge.

Set It Up))

You will not need any special equipment for this exercise.

How to Do It))

The Start

- Participants should stand tall with feet offset, shoulder-width apart, and the knees soft.
- Ask them to hold onto a walker or a handrail, or stand between two sturdy chairs for support as needed.
- Before starting, have participants practice the two individual parts of this activity:
  - Rolling forward onto the balls of their feet and back down.
  - Pulling up their toes (forefoot, actually) a few times. Have them do the front foot first, then the back foot, and then both. Cue them to hold on to their balance support firmly. This is a tough balance challenge.

This practice time gives them a chance to experience how combining the two moves will work for them.

The Moves

Use the following cues.

- With feet in offset position, begin a rocking motion:
  - Rock forward up onto the balls of the feet.
  - Balance just a moment in this position.
  - Lower the heels.
  - Rock backward just a bit so weight on the heels is enough that they can lift their forefoot.
  - At first, just lift one forefoot, then the other.
  - Gradually progress to lifting both forefeet.
- Repeat the full rocking motion 8 to 12 times, as tolerated.

Give It More Balance))

- Position the feet parallel, hip-width apart. This narrows the base of support. Do heel–toe rocking in this position.
- Cue participants to gaze ahead, not down. A horizon-level visual target helps them maintain balance.
- Encourage them to notice how the rocking motion feels.
- As they improve at this rocking activity, suggest that they lessen their balance support. They can hold onto the chair lightly, instead of tightly, for example.
- Add an overhead arm lift at the top of each heel lift.
- Dim the lights, just enough to make them a little unnerved; but still able to see. Reducing visual input gets them to focus more on somatic and vestibular sensations.

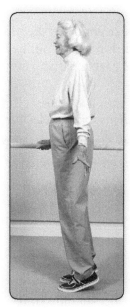 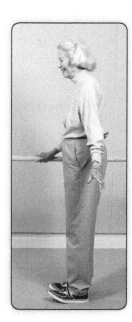

Keep It Safe))

Unless your group is quite capable, rocking backward should be done individually, with your personal supervision at first. They can take turns with you at their side or holding their hands. Keeping their back close to a wall is another way to make this activity safer. Rocking backward onto the heels is especially difficult and can be unnerving at first. Don't insist they do this part, if they are uncomfortable or look very rocky doing it. Allow them to use as much balance support as they feel they need.

Participants tend to bend at the waist and drop their hips back when you ask them to rock backward. Cue them to maintain upright posture and keep their hips over their ankles throughout.

KNEE LIFT, TOUCH BACK, AND SQUEEZE

This exercise strengthens the hip extensor on the back side of the hip (gluteals) while stretching the hip flexors on the front of the hip—a very efficient way to train. Strong hip extensors enable participants to climb stairs and hills.

Benefits))

- ◉ Strengthens hip muscles for everyday tasks.
- ◉ Practices elements of balance and gait (one-legged standing, leg swings).
- ◉ Provides temporary relief of sciatic pain for some participants.

Set It Up))

You will not need any special equipment for this exercise.

How to Do It))

The Start

- ◉ Participants should stand beside a handrail or chair. Standing beside the chair allows room for the leg-swing motion
- ◉ Cue particpants to stand tall with good posture (abs braced, knees soft, shoulder blades back and down, ribs lifted).

The Moves

Use the following cues.

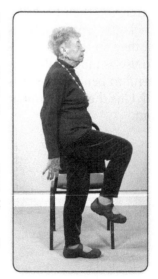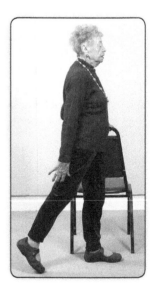

- ◉ Lift one knee upward (toward the chest) until you feel a stretch in the back of the leg (across the gluteal area).
- ◉ Lower the knee and begin to extend the leg out behind until your toes touch down on the ground behind you and you feel a stretch in the hip flexors.
- ◉ Tighten the gluteal muscles (buttocks).
  - Hold the position a moment. (Toes will still be on the ground behind them; the knee will be almost straight.)
  - Keep the supporting knee soft with a slight flexion.
- ◉ Start with 6 repetitions and build to 10, with each leg.

Take It Further))

- ◉ Increase repetitions until 15 can be done successively.
- ◉ Hold the tightened position longer.

Give It More Balance))

- Lean slightly forward, and instead of touching the toe down behind, lift rear leg up a few inches and tighten gluteals.
- Hold lifted position a little longer.

Keep It Safe))

Make sure participants have adequate balance support while lifting their knee and swinging their leg back. Some may experience back pain when placing the leg behind them. Suggest that they lean forward a bit and keep their abdominals tight. If pain persists, discontinue.

STRENGTH

MODIFIED LUNGES

Lunges work the whole leg in ways that enhance both balance and gait and they are extremely versatile. Lunges can be modified for a variety of abilities and goals and can be done in just about any direction. This activity is a basic beginning lunge that emphasizes the quadriceps.

Benefits))

⊙ Strengthens all major leg muscles.

⊙ Provides greater balance challenge through a narrow base of support.

Set It Up))

You will not need any special equipment for this exercise.

How to Do It))

The Start

⊙ Participants stand with good posture and appropriate balance support. They should stand behind their chair with both hands on the chair back. Get them in an offset foot position.

⊙ One foot immediately behind the chair and flat on the floor (keeping the front knee right behind the chair will help them keep that knee over the front ankle during the lunge.)

⊙ The other foot should take a big step (or scoot) back, as far as they comfortably can.

⊙ Maintain a shoulder-width stance. Keep both feet aligned parallel to each other and straight (the tendency is to turn the back foot out).

⊙ Lift the heel of the back foot off the floor.

⊙ Feet are now parallel and straight, shoulder-width apart, one forward, one back.

⊙ Both knees are slightly bent. This is the ready position. (Whew!)

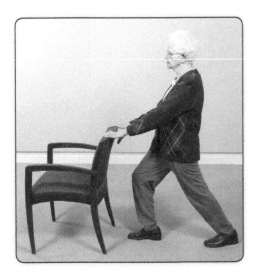 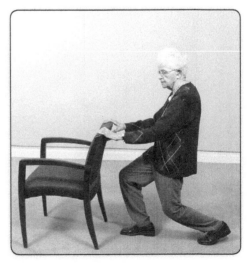

The Moves

Use the following cues.

- Cue them that this move looks like a curtsy. It's a dipping or dunking kind of motion.
- That is, bend both knees to lower the upper body 5 to 7 inches (10 to 15 centimeters).
- Keep the torso upright, braced, quiet, and centered between both legs.
- Cue them not to lunge forward; but straight down, keeping the torso upright.
- Cue them also to keep the front knee aligned over the front ankle.
- Repeat 6 times with each leg and build up to being able to do 10 to 12 repetitions.

Take It Further))

- Increase repetitions until participants can do 15 successively with each leg.
- Do lunges more slowly.
- Add a hold, or even a small bounce, in the down position.
- Increase the lunge depth, but only if participants can maintain good form (the front knee over the arch of the front foot).

Give It More Balance))

- Add an arm lift to each dip. If the right leg is forward, lift the left arm up and overhead with each dip down.
- Switch legs more often. Work up to doing alternate legs. This is difficult, so give plenty of time for participants to make the switch and get set up to safely do the next lunge. Monitor them for form and safety.
- Lunge to standing position. Do this with your personal supervision, first. Instead of standing behind their balance support, participants stand beside a handrail or their chair. They do a shallow lunge. After the lunge, challenge them to pull back up to a standing position using mainly the front leg. This requires both strength and balance.

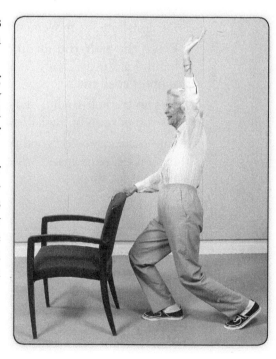

Keep It Safe))

Watch participants' form carefully. They will tend to lean and lunge forward and to push the forward knee out past the toes. If they are unable to correct this, or if they experience pain, stop or modify the exercise.

HEEL RAISES AND ROCKING ON A HALF-ROUND

A half-round is a foam column cut in half to create a flat and a round side. Generally these are about 3 feet (1 meter) long. When heel raises are done, the balls of the feet are on the half-round side and the flat side is down. These heel raises are more difficult because greater range of motion is available. When the flat side is up, heel–toe rocking motions are easier. Heel–toe rocking improves ankle flexibility and foot motions for gait. Using a half-round is fun for participants, partly I think, because it is something new. At first they will think, "There's no way I can do that!" But then they do. This activity requires one-on-one supervision, especially at first.

Benefits))

- Strengthens calves while incorporating elements of balance, gait, and flexibility.
- Requires balancing on the balls of feet.
- Adds something new to heel–toe raises and rocking.

Set It Up))

Eventually you'll need enough half-rounds for all participants. (Three-foot [1-meter] half-rounds can be cut in half to make two half-rounds.) But to start, you need only the one because you'll have to supervise participants closely. Class members can take turns.

How to Do It))

The Start

- Demonstrate the movements for the class before having them try it.
- Place the half-round on the floor, flat side down, beside a handrail or behind a sturdy chair. At least one hand should be in contact with balance support at all times.
- Get on the half-round. Stand with legs shoulder-width apart, balls of the feet on the top portion of the half-round. Heels hang off the back.
- Cue participants for good posture. Hips and shoulders should be aligned above the ankles (participants will tend to drop their hips backward; cue them to push the hips forward).

The Moves

Use the following cues.

- Lift the heels so they're level with the top of the half-round.
- Lift the heels a little higher so they're above the half-round.
- Try to balance and hold the position a moment.
- Slowly lower the heels below the level of the half-round so that the heels almost touch the ground and you feel your calves stretching.

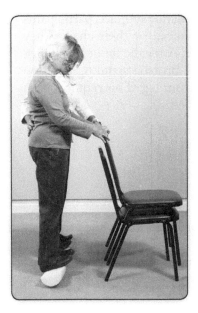
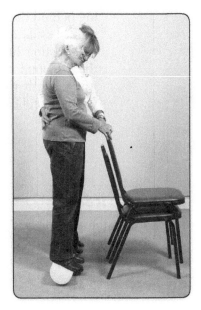

STRENGTH

- Are your hips still aligned directly over your ankles? Or did you bend at the hip? Make the needed correction.
- Lift and lower the heels for 6 repetitions and then build to doing 12 repetitions, as tolerated.

Take It Further ⟩⟩

- Increase repetitions until 15 can be done successively.
- Hold the up or the down position longer.

Give It More Balance ⟩⟩

Have participants do heel–toe rocking on the half-round.

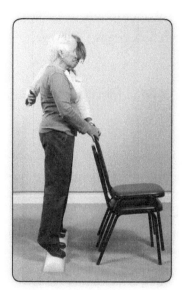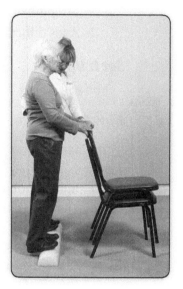

- Turn the half-round over so the flat side is up.
- Carefully help participants get on the half-round.
- Once they are on, cue them for tall posture. No bending at hips, please.
- Commence heel–toe rocking. Drop the heels back and feel that stretch; press the toes forward and down for a heel raise.
- Repeat 6 to 15 times, as tolerated.
- Remind them to keep their hips over their ankles throughout.

Keep It Safe ⟩⟩

Do these only with your personal supervision at first. Let participants decide for themselves if they want to try this one. Always provide a handrail or the back of a sturdy chair for balance support. If your chair backs are too short for a good support, or if you have tall participants, you can stack two chairs together; just be sure the chairs remain stable.

SIDE STEPS WITH A THERA-BAND

This is almost the same exercise as Side Step Walking, except a Thera-Band provides additional resistance and participants only take one step each direction so they can stay in front of their chair for balance safety. This can be a tricky one to teach safely, so follow the instructions carefully.

Benefits))

- ◉ Strengthens hip abductors.
- ◉ Adds difficulty to Side Steps Walking.

Set It Up))

You will need a Thera-Band for each participant.

How to Do It))

The Start

- ◉ Participants begin sitting down. Have them put the middle of the Thera-Band under both feet, stirrup style. They will hold the two ends on the outside of their knees, one end in each hand.
- ◉ Ask them to stand up carefully while holding the ends of the bands. They can also keep the heel of their hand on the chair to give them help and balance.
- ◉ Once they are up and comfortable, ask them to move back a bit until they feel their legs touch their chair. Let them know that touching the chair with their legs is a balance aid that will help them feel more stable.
- ◉ Then have them step sideways toward one edge of the chair. Tell them that the width of their chair will be their stepping width. They will be stepping side to side in front of their chair.
- ◉ Tell them that the chair is their back up balance safety plan—a place to sit should they lose their balance or get tired.
- ◉ Cue them to stand tall: Knees soft, abs braced, ribs lifted, and shoulder blades back and down. Now they're ready to begin stepping.

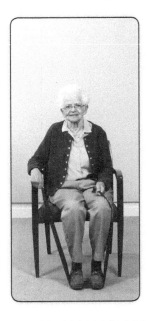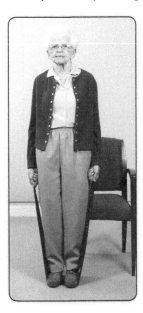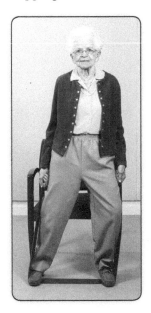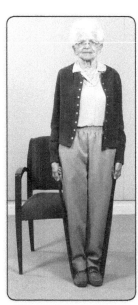

The Moves

Start from one edge of the chair and side step to the other. Then bring the other foot beside the first. The band will provide resistance. Use the following cues.

- Step, together, step from edge to edge of the chair.
- Touch your chair with your legs. (Remind participants of this throughout the exercise so they always keep the chair behind them.)
- Do 8 to 15 side steps in each direction.
- Stand directly in front of your chair when finished, again with your legs touching it.
- Let go of the band; just let it drop onto the floor.
- Touch your chair, so you know where it is.
- Now you can sit down.
- Once you're seated and rested, pick up the band from the floor.

Take It Further))

- Add a knee bend to each side step. As they step to the side, the stepping leg will bend and then straighten. Cue them, "Bend and straighten."
- Tighten the band for greater resistance by flexing the arms at the elbows with each side step. Effectively it's a bicep curl done with a side step.

Give It More Balance))

If participants are well supervised, they can move away from the chair. While side stepping, they should keep their back to a wall for safety. Have them start with just a few steps in one direction, perhaps four to eight in each direction. Personally supervise this activity.

Keep It Safe))

Follow the directions for getting up and back down carefully. Watch that participants stay in front of the chair, just in case they lose their balance. Remind them to touch their chairs periodically and to sit if they need to. This activity should not be done with any participants who use walkers or canes since it requires both hands to hold the Thera-Band. Participants who cannot do this activity standing can do the seated version (see Seated Side Steps With a Thera-Band on page 158).

CLOCK STEPPING

Daily living happens in all directions. Falls can also happen in any direction. Hence, multidirectional stepping and lunges are valuable for maintaining everyday balance. Clock Stepping involves a series of lunges to various points of an imagined clock. Lunge size, depth, and hand position can all be varied to suit various goals and abilities.

Benefits »

- ◉ Strengthens the whole leg (especially the abductors) in functional movement patterns.
- ◉ Requires balance recovery from multiple directions.
- ◉ Combines with upper body movement for greater balance challenge.
- ◉ Uses a familiar icon (a clock) as a visual tool.
- ◉ Requires thinking and memory.

Set It Up »

You will not have to have any special equipment for this exercise. When training just one person, you can use agility discs as the numbers on a clock. Their job will be to step to the number you indicate. How clock stepping works best: You will be calling out easy positions first. Easiest numbers are on the top half of the clock. Repeat each position two to four times in a row, before moving on to a new number. It's best to do just one leg at a time. Call out each number for one leg. Then have them move to the other side of the chair and you call out each number for the other leg. Eventually you will call out numbers randomly with no return to center between the numbers. After that you can add arm reaching along with the stepping.

How to Do It »

The Start

- ◉ Participants stand tall at the right side or back of their chair, hips in line with chair back. Their left leg and arm are next to the chair. They should keep their left hand on the chair back for balance safety.
- ◉ Have participants imagine they are standing at the center of a big clock. Can they picture these times: 9 o'clock? 1 o'clock? 5 o'clock? Dinner time? Nap time? TV news time?

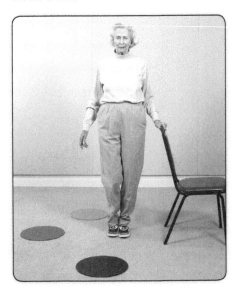 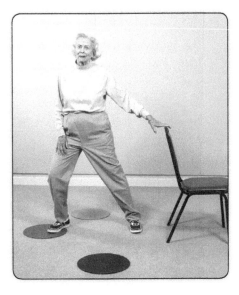

The Moves

- ◉ Call out these types of cues:
    - Step the right leg out to the 9 o'clock position.
    - Don't just touch it with your right foot; actually transfer your weight to that foot. Let your knee bend some as it takes on your body weight. Good job!
    - Now return to center position: Push! Push with that leg to bring it back to the center of the imaginary clock.
- ◉ Repeat this first position three or four times until participants are comfortable with that lateral lunge.
- ◉ Next, work on 12 o'clock the same way.
- ◉ Then work on 6 o'clock (stepping backward).
- ◉ Expand from there.
- ◉ Have participants walk around to the other side of their chair. Talk about clock positions they will use on this side.
- ◉ Work on lunges out to 3 o'clock first.(The upper half of the clock is sideways and forward stepping; the lower half is backward stepping, which is more of a balance challenge.)
- ◉ Participants will step to clock time, and then push on that leg to bring it back to the center of the imaginary clock.
- ◉ Ask if they felt the lift they got from the push (it's like floating back to center).
- ◉ Work on lunges to 1 o'clock and 5 o'clock, repeating each hour a few times until they are comfortable with it.

Take It Further))

- ◉ Do more repetitions to each hour on the clock.
- ◉ Use greater knee bending and weight transfers when stepping to each point on the clock.
- ◉ Include movements that go from the top of the clock to the bottom without returning to center.

Give It More Balance))

- ◉ Change numbers more quickly.
- ◉ Vary the timing or speed of your calls.
- ◉ Vary the spacing between hours (imagine the clock is much bigger).
- ◉ Add opposite-arm reaching past the stepping knee with each step to facilitate counter-rotation.
    - They need to be comfortable without both hands on the chair and supervised closely.
    - When reaching sideways (1 o'clock through 4 o'clock and 7 o'clock through 11 o'clock), they should reach with the opposite hand.
- ◉ Play Rock Around the Clock. Lunge to noon, 1, 2, 3, 4, 5, 6, and back up; then repeat without returning to the center. Repeat once or twice and then do the other side.
- ◉ For able participants, use diagonal movements or call numbers from either side of the clock.

- Add dual tasks. Mix up the names of the positions to make them think and react. What time do they take their first medicines? What time is their local news? What's their youngest grandchild's age? When is their nap time? How many letters are in their name?
- Dim the lights.

Keep It Safe))

Watch your group closely and pace the movements so everyone can keep up and feel safe. Don't be too quick or wild—you're not trying to tie-up their legs or play Twister. The goal is to practice and master everyday transitions. Keep participants close to their chair or handrail for balance safety.

AROUND THE WORLD

While balancing on one leg, participants will move the other forward, to the side, and backward, strengthening the muscle groups that surround the hip. It's a series of straight-legged leg lifts in multiple directions, done standing.

Benefits))

- Improves one-legged balance.
- Strengthens both legs.
- Requires maintenance of balance on one leg while the other limb is in motion.

Set It Up))

You will not need any special equipment for this exercise.

How to Do It))

The Start

- Participants stand tall with soft knees beside a chair or railing.
- Explain that they will be doing a series of straight-legged leg lifts.
- The directions will be forward, side, across, and backward.
- Each lift needs to be only about 6 to 12 inches (15-30 centimeters) high.
- The knee of the supporting leg should stay soft.

The Moves

Use the following cues.

- Place the right leg out in front and set it on its heel, foot flexed. Do six to eight straight-legged leg lifts to the front (strengthens quadriceps and hip flexors).
- Return to the beginning standing position.
- Lift the right leg out to the side. Do six to eight leg lifts (strengthens hip abductors).
- Return to beginning standing position.
- Lift the right leg forward again and then cross it over in front of the left foot. Lead with your heel. Do six to eight of these leg lifts (strengthens hip adductors on inner thigh).
- Return to beginning standing position.
- Lean forward a bit, using a handrail or chair for support. Lift the right leg behind. Do six to eight lifts to the back (strengthens hip extensors, gluteal muscles).
- Repeat sequence using the left leg.

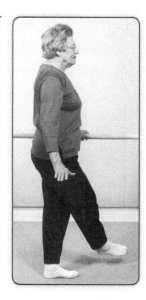

Take It Further))

- Increase the number of lifts in each direction.
- Slow down (adds difficulty and requires more balance).
- Take out rest stops between positions.

Give It More Balance))

- Do the activity on a carpeted floor.
- Stand on a step placed by a handrail, if you can supervise personally.
- Stand on an easy balance pad, if you can supervise personally.

Keep It Safe))

The short, little lifts tend to be small balance perturbations. Provide the necessary balance support so participants feel safe standing on one leg while moving the other. They should always keep the supporting knee soft.

STRENGTH

FRONT STEP-UPS

Stairs are almost always hard work for older adults. Some can no longer do stairs at all. Strengthening the leg muscles and teaching participants how they can more easily do the stepping-up motion will help restore some of their lost abilities. This exercise also provides balance practice for this common, everyday kind of transition and should carry over to other activities.

Benefits))

- ◉ Practices an important everyday activity (stepping up and down stairs and curbs).
- ◉ Develops skill and confidence to stay active in the community.
- ◉ Requires postural control of momentum.
- ◉ Front Step-Ups strengthen primarily hamstrings and hip extensors.
- ◉ Side Step-Ups strengthen the hip abductors and adductors and quadriceps.

Set It Up))

Unless you plan to take turns, which is a great idea, each participant will need a small step, no higher than 4 inches (10 centimeters) tall to start. Ahead of time place the step beside a handrail or inside a walker with the brakes on for good balance support. Demonstrate first and then walk participants through the procedure so everyone is familiar with the sequence. The first few times have participants take turns with you beside them to provide individual help.

How to Do It))

The Start

- ◉ Participants should stand tall facing the step, one hand on the handrail or both hands on the walker's side rails.
- ◉ They place one foot on the step. Suggest that they start with their strongest leg.

The Moves

- ◉ Cue participants to lean forward toward the stair and then step up. It's kind of one movement. Ask them if they notice how leaning forward toward the step helps get their center of gravity over the stair, making it easier to get up there. Momentum helps too. You might remind them that it's similar to Teeter-Totter Chair Stands. That is, it's one motion: Lean toward the step and when the knee is aligned over the foot on the stair, they push into the stair and step up. At the top, they may need to stop their momentum. Use these cues:

  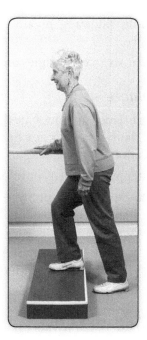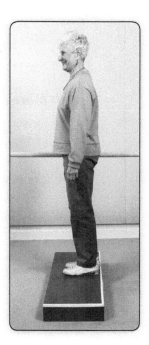

  - Place your foot on the step.
  - Lean toward the step until you feel your weight pushing through your knee and down onto your foot.
  - Pressing through the heel of the stair foot, lift your body upward and forward onto the step.

- Bring the other foot up onto the step and balance yourself there (stop the forward momentum).
- Step back down carefully, holding rail or walker. Balance again and get ready for the next step up.
- Start with just 4 to 6 step ups and progress to doing 6 to 10 step ups over time, with each leg, as tolerated.

Take It Further))

- Increase the number of repetitions with each foot.
- Slow down the movement.
- Use a bigger step, such as 6 inches (15 centimeters).
- Do Side Step-Ups. Side Step-Ups use the same techniques as Front Step-Ups, but participants step up onto the stair from standing parallel to the stair. It's a side step to a stair.

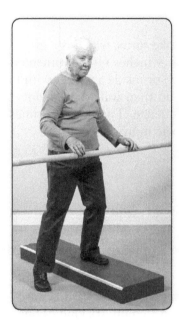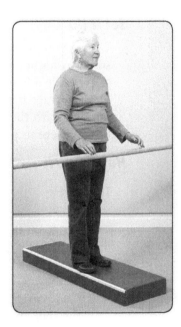

  - Place the foot on the step parallel to the edge of the step (be sure they leave room for the other foot to join it).
  - Lean over the step a bit to transfer body weight and align the knee over the ankle.
  - Step up sideways; regain balance.
  - Repeat six to eight times and progress to doing sets of 8 to 12; change legs.

Give It More Balance))

- Lessen the balance support. Cue them to hold onto their support lightly, not tightly, or maybe their hand can just hover over the support to be used only if needed. They can choose the challenge.
- Try new stepping patterns onto the step, with appropriate balance support.
  - Wide-Stepping Front Step-Ups: Right foot steps up wide to right; then left foot steps up wide to left. When coming back down, the feet come back together. Cue as wide, wide, narrow, narrow.
  - Side Step Up and Over: Step up with the right foot, then left. Step off to the other side with the right foot, then left.

Keep It Safe))

Always demonstrate first. Provide balance support. Be willing to hold their hands. Stress the importance of leaning toward the placed foot and using some momentum. The momentum gained from the forward lean makes stepping up much easier.

ROWS WITH CHECK-MARK FEET AND A THERA-BAND

This one gets its name from the position of the feet, which are placed out in front of the knees, toes up. The feet and lower legs look like a check mark.

Benefits))

- ⊚ Strengthens muscles of the midback.
- ⊚ Encourages and reinforces tall sitting.
- ⊚ Allows participants to strengthen back muscles while remaining seated.
- ⊚ Feels great!

Set It Up))

Each participant will need a Thera-Band for this exercise.

How to Do It))

The Start

- ⊚ Participants Tall Sit at the edge of their chair.
- ⊚ They place their heels on the ground beyond the knees and lift their forefeet off the ground so only the heels are touching the ground. (Feet and lower leg will form a check mark.)
- ⊚ Place the middle section of the Thera-Band on the floor under the feet, stirrup style.
- ⊚ Wrap the ends of the band around the hands until the band is tight when the hands are on their lap, near the knees. Hold hands in the thumbs up position.
- ⊚ Participants inhale to prepare and pull their trunk up into a Tall Sit position (abs braced, ribs lifted, head retracted, shoulder blades back and down, shoulders over hips).

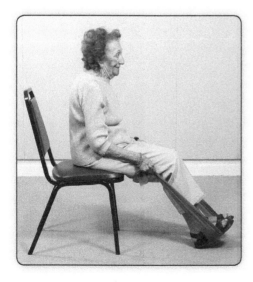 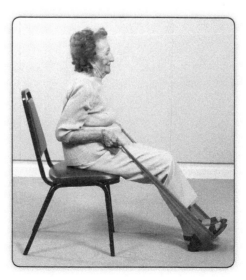

STRENGTH

The Moves))

Use the following cues.

- ⊙ Exhale and pull the band backward in a rowing motion.
- ⊙ Pull the band far enough back that the elbows end up behind the torso.
- ⊙ Pull yourself into a slightly taller sit. Hold that position a moment.
- ⊙ Inhale and return to the starting position.
- ⊙ Repeat 8 to 15 times, as tolerated.

Take It Further))

- ⊙ Tighten up on the bands or use a heavier band with more resistance.
- ⊙ Do slower repetitions.
- ⊙ Hold the end point longer.

Give It More Balance))

- ⊙ Pull the arms back alternately.
- ⊙ Place heels on a balance disc.
- ⊙ Dim the lights.
- ⊙ Participants close their eyes (*only* if the chairs have arms).
- ⊙ Sit on a balance disc (*only* if the chairs have arms).
- ⊙ Sit on a balance disc, alternate arms, and close eyes (*only* if the chairs have arms).

Keep It Safe))

Participants should keep their heels on the ground at all times. Most will tend to lean back whenever they pull the band backward. To prevent backward leaning, simply remind them to keep their shoulders over their hips and core stabilized.

STRENGTH

COPS AND ROBBERS

This exercise uses the hand and arm position that a robber wants when he commands, "Stick 'em up!" Cops and Robbers enhances participant posture and adds a nice chest and shoulder stretch to each repetition as an added bonus.

Benefits))

- ⊙ Strengthens upper and midback and posterior deltoids.
- ⊙ Facilitates external shoulder rotation and stretches the chest.
- ⊙ Reduces thoracic rounding of the spine.

Set It Up))

You will not need any special equipment for this exercise, unless you elect to use light hand weights for some participants.

How to Do It))

The Start

- ⊙ Participants sit tall, with abs in, ribs lifted, spine lengthened, head retracted, and shoulder blades back and down.
- ⊙ Lift both arms straight out in front of shoulders at shoulder height.

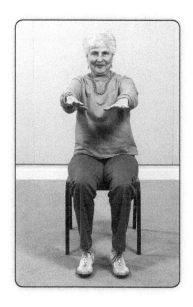 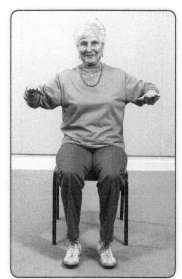 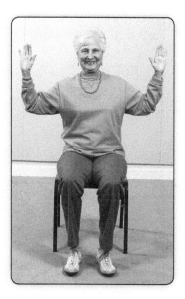

The Moves

Use the following cues.

- ⊙ Pull both arms back until elbows are in line with the torso. Keep forearms at same level as the upper arms. Squeeze shoulder blades toward each other.
- ⊙ Rotate your forearms upward so that your hands move skyward. This is the "stick 'em up" Cops and Robbers part of the movement.
- ⊙ You should feel the muscles in your back and shoulders tighten as they do the work of lifting your forearms. Can you? Good.

- Can you feel your core muscles tighten, too? Perfect.
- Lower the forearms back to level position and then back out to the starting position. The out position stretches the shoulder-blade retractors. Can they feel that?
- Repeat 6 to 12 times, as tolerated.

Take It Further))

- Slow the movements down.
- Squeeze the shoulder blades together each time you pull arms back from the forward (starting) position.
- Lift forearms up into the up positions each time with a little more oomph!

Give It More Balance))

- Sit at the edge of the chair.
- Sit at the edge of the chair with feet tandem and heels lifted.
- Stand to do this exercise.
- Sit on a balance disc in a chair with arms.

Keep It Safe))

Nothing should hurt their shoulders or back. Many older adults with shoulder problems may be unable to do this exercise successfully. See if they can do shoulder rotation a different way: suggest they keep their upper arms by their sides and then rotate just their forearms out to the side. The forearms would stay parallel to the floor. Encourage tall sitting throughout.

STRAIGHT-AHEAD LAT PULL-DOWN

Straight-Ahead Lat Pull-Downs are easier than overhead lat pull-downs. They strengthen the mid- and low back, and they also develop arm strength.

Benefits))

- ◉ Strengthens low and midback muscles.
- ◉ Incorporates tall sitting into a classic strength exercise.
- ◉ Aids everyday tasks, such as opening doors or carrying objects.

Set It Up))

Each participant will need a Thera-Band for this exercise.

How to Do It))

The Start

- ◉ Participants sit tall with their back away from the chair back, shoulders over hips, abs in, and ribs lifted.
- ◉ Hold the middle part of Thera-Band out in front at shoulder height. Participants can wrap the band around the palms of their hands; it's easier for those with arthritic hands. Arms are straight and hands are about shoulder-width apart.

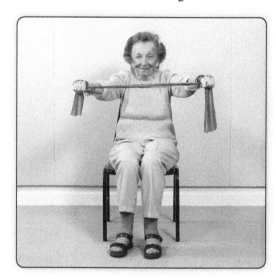 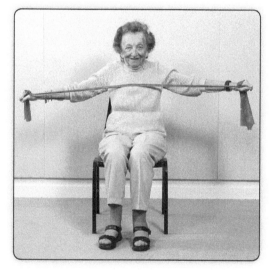

The Moves

- ◉ Participants pull their straight arms back, until they are laying the band across the chest and have greatly increased the distance between the two hands.
- ◉ At the end point, hands are out wide to the sides. The band touches the chest at the collarbone.
- ◉ Hold a moment.
- ◉ Repeat 8 to 15 times, as tolerated.

STRENGTH

Take It Further ⟩⟩

- ⊙ Increase repetitions, up to 15 repetitions.
- ⊙ Tighten up on the band or use a band with greater resistance.
- ⊙ Slow the motion down.
- ⊙ Hold the end point a little longer.

Give It More Balance ⟩⟩

- ⊙ Sit at the edge of the chair.
- ⊙ Sit at the edge of the chair with feet offset and heels lifted.
- ⊙ Cross the ankles and hold the feet up, just off the ground.
- ⊙ Sit on a balance disc (*only* if the chairs have arms).
- ⊙ Close eyes (*only* if chairs have arms).

Keep It Safe ⟩⟩

Encourage participants to maintain tall sitting throughout in order to maintain core stability. Do not combine closed eyes with sitting on a balance disc unless you are training one on one.

BALLOON LAP PRESS-DOWNS

The form for this activity encourages tall sitting while strengthening the low back and triceps. Strong low back muscles help maintain upright posture and reduce common kinds of back pain. Triceps are the arm muscles that participants often use to get out of chairs.

Benefits))

- ⊙ Strengthens back and arms.
- ⊙ Incorporates tall sitting into a strength exercise.
- ⊙ Aids many activities of daily living.

Set It Up))

Each participant will need a Balloon or a Slo Mo type of ball for this exercise.

How to Do It))

The Start

- ⊙ Participants place a balloon (or soft, medium-sized ball) in their lap, near the knees. This distance is to help ensure that the arms are almost straight.
- ⊙ They place their palms on the balloon and lift the fingers away from the balloon.
- ⊙ Inhale to prepare and pull the torso up into the ABLE Bodies Tall Sit position.

The Moves

Use the following cues.

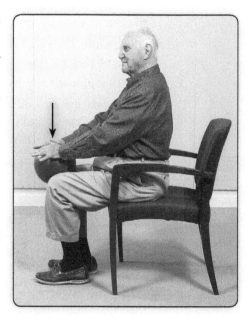

- ⊙ Exhale and press down on the balloon through the palms of your hands, using arm and back strength.
- ⊙ Hold the press 1 to 2 seconds while maintaining the Tall Sit.
- ⊙ Can you feel the low back and arms doing the work?
- ⊙ Relax.
- ⊙ Repeat 8 to 12 times, as tolerated.

Take It Further))

- ⊙ Press harder or longer.
- ⊙ Move the balloon farther away in the lap. The arms will be straighter.

Give It More Balance))

- ⊙ Place feet in tandem position with heels lifted.
- ⊙ Cross the ankles and hold the feet just off the ground while pressing.

Keep It Safe))

Keep the abs braced, ribs lifted, and shoulder blades back and down throughout.

BOWS AND ARROWS

This is one of my favorites. I like how the chest is stretched while the back is strengthened—it's a great combination! When done correctly, participants will look like archers aiming at their target and pulling back their bow string. Talk about targeted exercise!

Benefits))

- Strengthens upper and midback; especially those important shoulder blade retractors.
- Enhances posture and uses tall sitting posture and core stability.
- Incorporates head turns to enhance neck flexibility.
- Allows participants to do the exercise either seated or standing.

Set It Up))

Each participant will need a Thera-Band for this exercise.

How to Do It))

The Start

- Participants Tall Sit toward the front of their chair. Abs are in and spine is lifted.
- They hang the middle part of a Thera-Band over one hand (between the thumb and four fingers).
- Hold that arm out to the side, straight and at shoulder height.
- Turn their head to look down the length of the arm pointed to the side. Cue participants to pretend they are aiming a bow, looking down their arm at their target.
- Meanwhile, the other hand takes hold of the hanging part of band about 8 inches (20 centimeters) down from the other hand.
- Lift that elbow away from the chest.
- Now participants look like archers ready to pull back the bow. The head is turned toward the target and they are looking down their extended arm. The back hand is holding the Thera-Band taut as it would be on a bow string. Participants are ready.

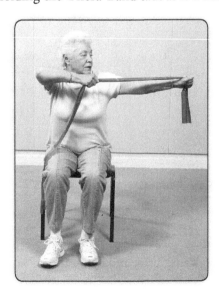
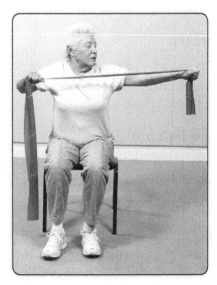

STRENGTH

The Moves

Use the following cues.

- Draw the pretend bowstring back and across the chest. Your hand will slide across your chest from forward shoulder to back shoulder. The shoulder blade of the pulling arm will pull toward the spine.
- Can you feel your shoulder blade slide in next to your spine? I think it feels like parallel parking for the shoulder blade!
- Repeat 8 to 12 times, as tolerated, with each arm.
- Repeat with the other arm.

Take It Further))

- Tighten up on the Thera-Band or use a band with greater resistance.
- Increase repetitions to 15.
- Slow the movement and hold the end point longer.

Give It More Balance))

- Sit with feet tandem and heels lifted.
- Stand in front of a chair, feet parallel. The back of one leg should touch the front of the chair.

Keep It Safe))

Cue participants to maintain tall sitting posture throughout. Nothing should hurt.

STRENGTH

OVERHEAD LAT PULL-DOWN

This is a progression of the Straight-Ahead Lat Pull-Down. Everything is the same except that the starting position is with hands overhead, which is more difficult.

Benefits))

- Strengthens mid- and low back muscles.
- Incorporates tall sitting into a back strength exercise.
- Aids everyday tasks such as reaching up, opening doors, or carrying objects.

Set It Up))

Each participant will need a Thera-Band for this exercise.

How to Do It))

The Start

- Participants sit tall with their back away from the chair back, shoulders over hips, abs braced, and ribs lifted.
- They hold the middle part of the Thera-Band overhead. Participants can wrap the band around their palms; it's easier for those with arthritic hands. Arms are straight and hands should be wider than shoulder-width.

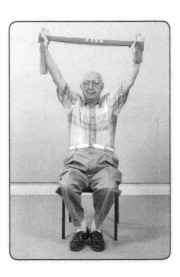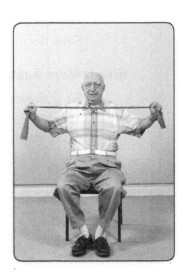

The Moves

Use the following cues.

- Pull both arms down and out to the sides, bringing the band across the chest and greatly increasing the distance between the hands.
- At the end point, the hands are out wide to the sides. The band touches the chest at the collarbone.
- Hold a moment.
- Repeat 8 to 12 times, as tolerated.

Take It Further))

- Increase repetitions to 15.
- Tighten up on the band or use a band with greater resistance.
- Slow the motion down and hold the end point a little longer.

Give It More Balance))

- Sit at the edge of the chair.
- Sit at the edge of the chair with feet offset and heels lifted.
- Cross the ankles and hold the feet just off the ground.

Keep It Safe))

Cue participants to keep their ribs lifted and abs in. Remind them that they can do the straight-ahead version if it's more comfortable for them.

PUSH UP AND THINK THIN WITH A BALLOON

I could have named this activity *Suck It In*, to be more descriptive; but it didn't sound as nice. Either way, it's about drawing in the core muscles to support overhead reaching.

Benefits))

- Challenges and strengthens core muscles.
- Strengthens back extensors.
- Helps with the everyday skill of reaching overhead.

Set It Up))

You will need one balloon per participant. Optionally, you may choose to add a light-weight medicine ball or a balance disc for some participants.

How to Do It))

The Start

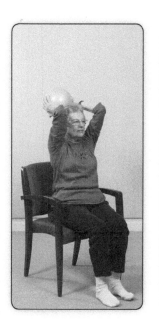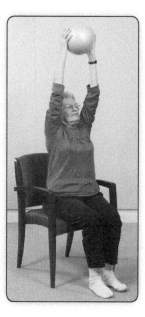

- Participants sit tall in their chair with hips touching the chair back for extra support.
- They lift balloon to just overhead, almost touching the head. Elbows are bent.
- Inhale and sit tall to prepare.

The Moves

Use the following cues.

- Exhale and extend both arms to push your balloon directly upward, a little farther overhead.
- Inhale again and draw in the abdominal wall tightly.
- Exhale and push the balloon a litle higher (extend the arms and torso a little more).
- Keep your abs tight, but allow your torso to extend.
- Take your time.
- Do only 4 to 6 repetitions to start and progress to being able to do 6 to 12.

Take It Further))

- Increase the number of lifts.
- Move slowly and encourage more height.
- Use a lightweight ball.

STRENGTH

Give It More Balance))

- Sit closer to the edge of the chair.
- Sit on the edge of the chair with offset or tandem feet.
- Place feet on a balance disc.
- For private training, try sitting on a balance disc, but be careful!

Keep It Safe))

Drawing abs in while lifting tall will do wonders for keeping this exercise comfortable because the back is better supported. Nothing should hurt.

ONE-ARM BANDITS

If participants magically turned into slot machines, their torso would be the big box and their arms would be the levers. There are many versions of this exercise, all of which involve keeping the torso stable while one arm does the stipulated movement. Let's play slot machines and pull a few levers!

Benefits))

- Facilitates a steady, stable torso.
- Strengthens shoulders, arms, core, and low and midback muscles.
- Uses Thera-Band to add appropriate resistance.

Set It Up))

Each participant will need a Thera-Band for this exercise.

How to Do It))

The Start

- Participants sit tall at the edge of their chair, with abs braced and ribs lifted.
- They hold a Thera-Band between their hands, about shoulder-width apart. It may be most comfortable to wrap the bands around the palms of the hands. This is especially nice for participants with arthritis.

The Moves

- Position 1: Both arms are out straight and in front of the shoulders. Use the following cues.
  - Pull back the left arm, keeping it as straight as a lever.
  - Repeat 8 to 15 times, as tolerated.
  - Rest; then do the other arm.

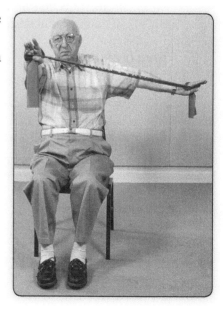

STRENGTH

- Position 2: Move both arms to the right and lower them toward the lap. This position will allow for a diagonal line of pull.
  - Pull the left arm diagonally upward and to the opposite side. Ending point depends on them, but aim for out to the side and above the shoulder.
  - Do 8 to 15 times, as tolerated.
  - Rest and do the other arm, pulling from left to right.

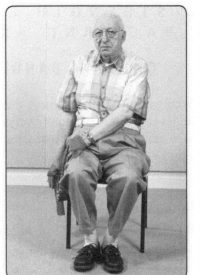 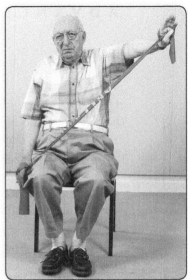

- Position 3: Hold arms overhead, as is comfortable.
  - One arm stays up while the other pulls down to the side.
  - Do 8 to 15 repetitions, as tolerated.
  - Rest and then do the other arm.

Take It Further))

- Move through each repetition more slowly and hold the end position longer.
- One-Arm Bandits With a Twist: Do position 1 in a way that allows the torso to turn in the direction of the pulling arm. Remind participants to keep their back tall and abdominal wall braced throughout the exercise.

Give It More Balance))

- Sit closer to the edge of the chair.
- Can be done standing. Position 1 is the easiest, so try it first.

Keep It Safe))

Throughout, it is important that they keep their core muscles braced. Spend a few weeks working on each variation before moving on to a new position.

STRENGTH

DRIVE ME UP THE WALL

This activity is basically reaching an arm up the wall. It's similar to the daily activity of retrieving items from overhead places. The extension can be felt the whole length of the body.

Benefits))

- Develops core stability during reaching-up activities.
- Improves posture.
- Strengthens back extensors.
- Uses standing position to promote real-life balance while standing and reaching.

Set It Up))

You will not need any special equipment for this exercise. But you do need a suitable wall or corner space for your participants to use.

How to Do It))

The Start

Use the following cues.

- Stand tall, facing the wall.
- Place the feet in an offset position shoulder-width apart. The right foot is forward with the toe touching the wall.
- Place both hands on the wall at shoulder height.
- Lean toward the wall so that most of your body weight is over the front foot.
- Brace the torso and inhale to prepare.

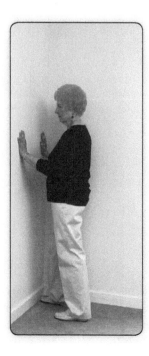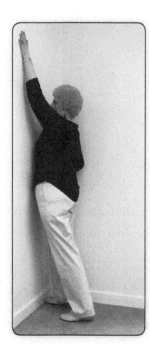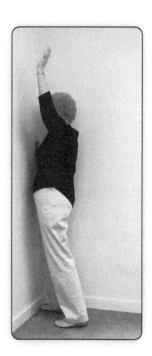

The Moves

Essentially the move is one arm will be pushing up the wall, then pulling back and being lowered to the shoulder. It's like one arm drawing a big oval circle and trying to push out the top of the oval as far as they can.

- Exhale and slide the left hand up the wall as far as comfortably possible.
- Hold that spot a moment while you inhale.
- Exhale and push that hand up a little farther. Allow the ribs to lift this time, but keep the abs braced.
- Hold steady a moment again as you exhale and stay lengthened.
- When you're ready, pull the arm off the wall; you'll shift some of your weight to the back foot.
- Lower the arm to shoulder height and place it back on the wall.
- Repeat six to eight times, as tolerated.
- Change feet so the left foot is forward and right arm moves up the wall six to eight times, if tolerable.

Take It Further))

- Increase repetitions.
- Use a very light wrist weight on the reaching arm; .5 to 1 pound (.25-.5 kilogram) is enough.
- Try Drive Me With a Twist:
    - Each time the arm is pulled off the wall, allow the torso, shoulders, and head to rotate to the same side as that arm, as shown in the photo.
    - Cue participants to pull the left arm off the wall and look left.
- Reverse starting foot position, so that the forward foot is on the same side as the lifting arm.

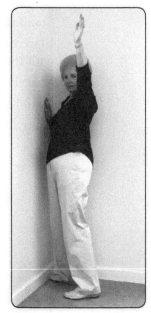

Give It More Balance))

- Stand on a plush carpet or firm balance pad with feet offset.
- Roll a small Slo Mo–type ball up the wall.

Keep It Safe))

Reaching up and pulling an arm back can be a fall risk, so be careful. Using an offset foot position will reduce the risk. Keeping one hand on the wall also steadies their balance. Remind them to take their time and to feel steady before they pull their hands off the wall. Cue them to keep the torso as braced as possible while moving arms upward. Advise them to be careful when adding the *twist* option. They should stop if the activity feels unsafe or painful or makes them dizzy.

FLAG SALUTES

The starting position of this exercise looks as if you are about to say the Pledge of Allegiance; hence the name *Flag Salutes*. It consists of bending and straightening the arm against the resistance provided by a Thera-Band.

Benefits))

- ◉ Strengthens triceps to assist with chair stands.
- ◉ Mimics movement pattern of arms during a chair stand (function-based exercise).
- ◉ Allows participants to sit, stand, or move.
- ◉ Can be done with participants seated, standing, or moving.

Set It Up))

Each participant will need a Thera-Band. One progression has participant seated on a balance disc in a chair with arms.

How to Do It))

The Start

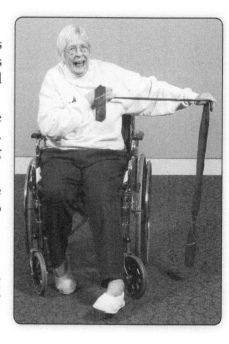

- ◉ Participants sit tall, with feet flat on floor, shoulders over hips, chin level, head retracted, abs braced, ribs lifted, spine lengthened, and shoulder blades back and down.
- ◉ They drape the middle of the Thera-Band over the right hand and place the right hand on the left shoulder. This is the part where they look as if they'll be saying the Pledge of Allegiance.
- ◉ They grasp the dangling portion of the band with the left hand and lift the left elbow away from their torso and to the side.

The Moves

- ◉ Participants extend the left arm out and to the side, straightening the elbow. It's simply elbow flexion and extension, done in a backward and sideward direction.
- ◉ Repeat 8 to 12 times, as tolerated.
- ◉ Repeat with the other arm.
- ◉ Stretch the triceps when finished.

STRENGTH

Take It Further 》

- ⊙ Increase repetitions to 15.
- ⊙ Add a second set after resting.
- ⊙ Tighten up on the band, double it, or use a band with a stronger resistance.

Give It More Balance 》

- ⊙ Sit at the edge of the chair, with feet in tandem position and heels lifted.
- ⊙ Sit on a balance disc (*only* if the chairs have arms).
- ⊙ Stand tall, with one leg touching the chair (to steady balance).

Keep It Safe 》

Maintain a tall sitting or tall standing posture, throughout.

A&W CHEST PRESSES

These are called *A&Ws* because the arms form an *A* and a *W* while doing the chest presses.

Benefits))

- Strengthens arms, chest, and shoulders.
- Strengthens core stabilizers.
- Incorporates tall sitting to enhance form and posture.
- Allows participants to choose sitting or standing.

Set It Up))

Each participant will need a Thera-Band for this exercise. One progression has participant seated on a balance disc in a chair with arms.

How to Do It))

The Start

- Participants run a Thera-Band behind their back and arms, just below the shoulder blades. They hold one end of the band in each hand, with hands next to the chest and elbows behind the chest.
- They sit tall and lift their elbows away from the torso so arms are parallel with floor and hold their hands palms down. This is the *W*.

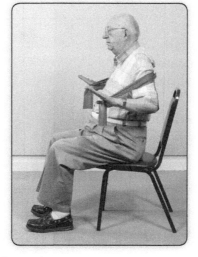 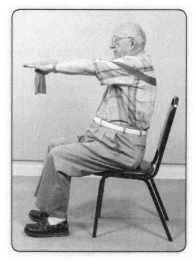

The Moves

Use the following cues.

- Press the arms straight out until the thumbs touch. This is the *A* position.
- Pull the arms back again to the *W* position.
- Repeat 8 to 12 times, as tolerated.

Take It Further))

- Increase repetitions until 15 can be done successively.
- Tighten up on the bands or use a stronger resistance band.
- Hold the *A* position longer.

Give It More Balance))

- Sit closer to the edge of the chair, feet tandem, heels lifted.
- Do seated on a balance disc (*only* if the chairs have arms).
- Stand, with one leg touching the chair.

Keep It Safe))

Make sure bands are across the back and not the neck. If this is tough for some to do, have them run the band under their arms instead of over.

BALLOON-SQUEEZE CHEST PRESSES

It's always good to have several choices for each type of equipment. Here is a good activity to use your balloons in your repertoire. It's especially valuable because the push and pull motion strengthens the involved muscles throughout a broad range of motion.

Benefits))

- ◉ Strengthens chest and shoulders.
- ◉ Enhances core strength.
- ◉ Can be done with participants seated or standing.

Set It Up))

Each participant will need a balloon or a soft, medium-sized ball, such as a Slo Mo ball. One progression has participants seated on a balance disc in a chair with arms.

How to Do It))

The Start

- ◉ Participants sit tall and hold the balloon between the palms of both hands at about chest level.
- ◉ They lift the elbows out to the sides.

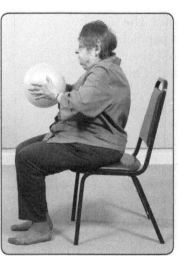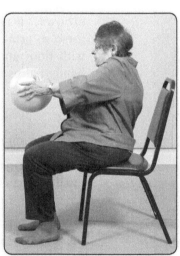

The Moves

Use the following cues.

- ◉ Squeeze the balloon tightly between the palms of your hands.
- ◉ Keep squeezing and begin to push your arms away from the chest about 6 inches (12 centimeters), and then draw them back in toward the chest.
- ◉ Relax the squeeze. That's one repetition.
- ◉ Repeat 8 to 12 times, as tolerated.

Take It Further))

- ◉ Increase repetitions until 15 can be done successively.
- ◉ Press harder against the balloon.
- ◉ Change the angle of the push: Push balloon a little to the left for one rep and to the right the next rep.
- ◉ Change the height of the movement. Keep balloon lower, or go from low to high.

Give It More Balance))

- ◉ Sit at the edge of the chair, with feet tandem.
- ◉ Sit on a balance disc (*only* if the chairs have arms).
- ◉ Do while standing.

Keep It Safe))

Cue them frequently about sitting tall and keeping core braced. All reps should be done slowly.

STRENGTH

RIGHT CROSS, LEFT CROSS
AND RIGHT HOOK, LEFT HOOK

These are fun and effective variations of the basic chest press. Crosses are a diagonal movement pattern, which is efficient training as two planes of motion are used. Hooks are punching movements done low to high and involve more core muscles than a standard chest press.

Benefits))

- Enhances everyday activities such as pushing or lifting.
- Facilitates core stabilization for arm movement.
- Provides a fun and familiar activity with easy-to-teach movements.
- One of the few exercises done quickly to garner power.

Set It Up))

Each participant will need a Thera-Band for this exercise.

How to Do It))

The Start

- Participants sit or stand tall and run a Thera-Band behind the back, just under the shoulder blades.
- They hold the ends of the bands in their hands.

The Moves

Crosses

Use the following cues.

- Lift the arms away from the torso and hold them parallel to floor.
- Extend the right arm across and out to the left, across the body at shoulder height. (The right hand should end up in front of the left shoulder.)
- Do it slowly at first to learn proper form, then quickly. Boom! That's your Right Cross!
- Return to the starting position.
- Do same diagonal pattern with the left arm. Slowly at first to learn proper form, then quickly. Boom! That's your Left Cross!
- Keep alternating, completing 8 to 15 repetitions with each arm.

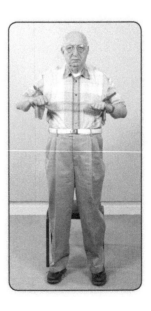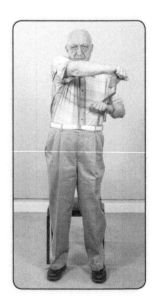

Hooks

Use the following cues.

- Anchor the Thera-Band around the back, lower than for crosses (more toward the waist). Or, sit on your band, with it under your hips.
- Hold your bent arms close to the torso to start.
- Draw the right arm back so that the hand is at the hip. (You are preparing to throw this punch from the hip, upwards and diagonally.)
- Keeping the elbow bent, bring the right hand up and to a point left of center and in front of you. Notice that this is a hooking punch pattern; that means that the arm stays bent throughout. Imagine that this hook shot is a glancing blow off an opponent's chin. Now do it quickly. Boom! This is your right hook.

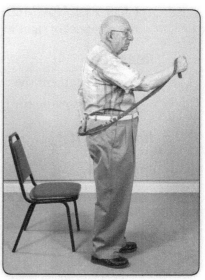

- Return to the beginning position, and then push the left hand up and to the right of the center point in front of you. Slowly for form and then quickly for fun. This is your left hook.
- Alternate arms until each arm has thrown 8 to 15 hook shots.

Take It Further 》》

- Tighten up on the band or use one with stronger resistance.
- Increase the speed and power of the punches.

Give It More Balance 》》

- Sit at the edge of the chair.
- Allow the trunk to twist with each hook shot (keep abs braced).
- Try it standing in front of a chair, feet offset. One leg should stay in contact with the chair.

Keep It Safe 》》

Maintain tall, stabilized posture for the best results and back comfort. Keep arms below shoulders for all of these activities.

CHAIR PUSH-UPS

This is a tough one but a good one. It will definitely help participants get out of chairs. I commonly assign this one to participants who cannot do a full chair stand. That is, while the rest of the class is doing Teeter-Totter Chair Stands, they'd be doing Teeter-Totter Chair Push Ups. Much of the movement is similar. They lean back, lean forward, and then instead of standing up they do the Chair Push-Up. It is very functional.

Benefits))

- ◉ Strengthens the triceps.
- ◉ Helps participants get out of chairs with greater ease and control.

How to Do It))

The Start

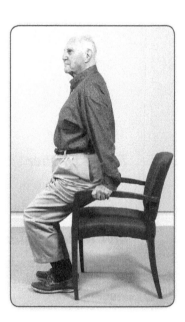

- ◉ Participants sit at the edge of their chair with feet pulled back behind the knees, hip-width apart and flat on the floor.
- ◉ They place their arms on the chair arms, with elbows pointing directly backward.
- ◉ They should get a firm grip on the chair arms so they are prepared to push up through the palms of their hands.

The Moves

Use the following cues.

- ◉ Lean back, bracing the abdominal wall.
- ◉ Lean forward, keeping the back tall and stable.
- ◉ Push up from the chair until the arms are straight and the hips are lifted off the chair. (Hands stay on the chair.)
- ◉ Then use your arm strength to lower yourself back to the chair, with control (don't just plop back down).
- ◉ The legs can assist, if needed.
- ◉ Do just one or two repetitions to start, and then rest. Then try a few more. Build up to doing six to eight reps.

Take It Further))

- Add a few more repetitions.
- Lower more slowly.
- Do a second set.

Keep It Safe))

This is a difficult one that requires the strength to lift most of their body weight off the chair. Build repetitions slowly. Like ABLE Bodies' chair stands, foot placement (feet behind knees) and momentum (leaning back then forward) will make this exercise easier to do successfully. Cue them to lower themselves back down to their chair with control; not to just plop back down.

WALL PUSH-UPS AND WALL PUSH-OFFS

Push-ups are a classic exercise. They have many beneficial effects, including enhanced core strength. Doing push-ups on a wall is an easier variation that many frail participants should be able to do.

Set It Up))

You will need appropriate wall space for this activity. You will not need any special equipment for this exercise.

Benefits))

- Strengthens torso, chest, back, and arms in one fell swoop.
- Combines both strength and balance work.

How to Do It))

The Start

- Participants stand tall 18-30 inches (46-76 centimeters) from a wall, feet shoulder-width apart.
- Both hands are on the wall, a little lower than shoulder height.
- Core muscles are braced.

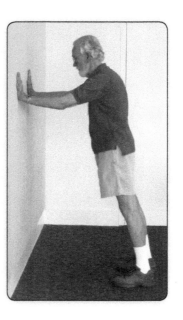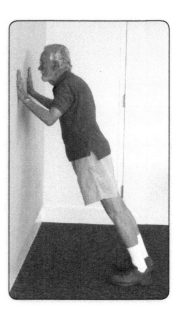

The Moves

Use the following cues for wall push-ups.

- Lower the chest toward the wall until your nose almost touches the wall.
    - Participants will tend to bend forward at hips; try to prevent that.
    - Cue them to keep the abs braced and back straight.
    - Have them think about keeping their ears, shoulders, hips, and ankles all in a line, like ducks in a row.
- Push back up to straight-arm (beginning) position.
- Repeat six to eight times and build to doing 8 to 12 reps.

Take It Further))

- Hold the down position for 5-15 seconds.
- Do Wall Push-Ups slower.
- Increase repetitions to 15, as well tolerated.
- Use more of a lean. That is, place the feet farther from the wall to start. The further back the feet are, the more difficult the push-up becomes.

Give It More Balance))

Have your participants do Wall Push-Offs. Use the following cues.

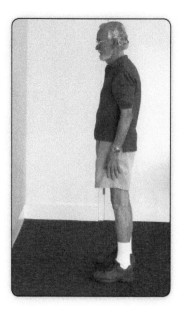

- ⊚ Lower yourself to the wall (as in Wall Push-Ups).
- ⊚ Then give a quick push to push yourself off the wall and back over your feet.
- ⊚ Regain your balance.
- ⊚ Place your hands back on the wall.
- ⊚ Repeat: Lower down, then "Push!" back to standing position.
- ⊚ Repeat the push-off 8 to 12 times.

Keep It Safe))

Nothing should hurt. And participants should feel safe and comfortable doing the activity. Master the push-up before trying the push-off. For both activities, core stability and maintaining ear, shoulder, hip, and ankle alignment is crucial.

STRENGTH

7

Balance and Mobility

This chapter is probably why you bought this book. There are more than 70 activities here for you to use and enjoy, and I hope that you're excited to start and your participants will love the new ideas as well. Everybody loves pulling out the balance toys! They make balance class feel more like recess than exercise class. I think you'll find the ABLE Bodies progressive way of teaching balance to be conservative, intuitive, and supported by exercise science literature, including ACSM best practices position statements (Mazzeo et al., 1998; Nelson et al., 2007).

Chapter 7 is divided into subsections that reflect the main balance system they are intended to target: somatosensory, vision, vestibular, and motor coordination. In reality, many activities will overlap into other categories or subsections, just as in real life everyday tasks engage more than one balance system. But for the most part I have tried to place each activity in its most specific subsection. For the specific needs of one client, you can use activities by subsection to create appropriate challenges for that one client or you can select your activities from a variety of subsections to provide a more multicomponent program that will likely be more beneficial when working with groups.

Let's review a few caveats before we begin. By this point, you should recognize the value of first preparing participants for this chapter. Participants need a solid foundation for balance training, including flexibility, posture, core stability, and strength. For any balance activities beyond beginning levels, participants will need to be able to stand on their own comfortably and follow your instructions. Standing on their own includes standing with some balance support, such as a walker, sturdy chair, or handrail. The second safety principle worth repeating is the arm's-length rule. If participants are more than an arm's length from their balance support, they need a spotter (i.e., you) by their side. And finally, whenever the balance toys are out, keep close control of your classes, have them take turns, hold their hands, and be careful.

Quick Reminder

As always, progress these challenges only as well tolerated by participants, meaning nothing should hurt, they are willing and able to continue, and they show no signs of dizziness, nausea, excessive fatigue, and so on. Also, participants should be able to demonstrate proper form before adding any difficulty.

Practice the activities before you present them. Choose only activities that you feel comfortable teaching. Pick activities that you believe your clients will both enjoy and be able to do successfully. If you're unsure an activity will fit your class, it's probably best to wait.

All activities in this chapter are available in PDF format! Visit www.HumanKinetics.com/ABLEBodiesBalanceTraining.

BALANCE

THE BALL GAME

This is a fun, easy game that's a great introduction to balance and somatosensory learning. This kind of learning is where you learn about your world from the inside out; from sensory systems inside your body. I call it inside-out learning! Anyone can play this ball game. Participants will learn about their somatosensory system in a fun and interactive way. (The somatosensory system is made up of sense receptors inside the body that help you learn about the world around you.) You will be teaching your participants to listen to their body.

Benefits))

- ⊙ Requires participants to listen to their body and recall former learning experiences in a fun and easy activity.
- ⊙ Explores light touch, pressure, and recognizing shapes (proprioceptive learning).
- ⊙ Increases self-awareness, self appreciation, and interest in learning more.

Set It Up))

- ⊙ You'll need balls of various sizes, shapes (footballs, Wiffle balls, playground balls), textures (tennis balls, golf balls, Hacky Sacks, Wiffle balls), densities (grapefruits, baseballs, foam balls, light medicine balls), and even smells (oranges, grapefruits). Have a few items that clearly are not balls (fuzzy dice, barbell). Check out the local dollar stores for these items.
- ⊙ Keep the balls hidden; do not bring them out until participants have their eyes closed.
- ⊙ Ideally, provide enough balls for everyone to have one. Alternatively, a few volunteers can use a smaller number of various balls. The audience will enjoy watching them guess and learn.

How to Do It))

- ⊙ Participants should be seated comfortably.
- ⊙ Begin the activity with a few hand stretches:
  - Flex and extend the fingers (make a fist; make a starfish).
  - Each finger takes a bow by touching its thumb and then extending again into a starfish.
  - Play the piano with the fingers (curl fingers up and out at knuckles).
  - Do a few wrist circles.
- ⊙ Ask participants (or volunteers if there aren't enough balls for everyone) to close their eyes (or you can use blindfolds). This is a guessing game! They should keep them closed until told to open them.
- ⊙ Hand out one object to each participant.

- They will be "looking" for sensory clues with their fingers. First they will feel the texture of the ball.
- Use a light, soft touch of your fingers to learn about the texture.
    - Is it bumpy? Fuzzy? Smooth?
    - Does it have lines? Does it have any holes in it?
    - Does the texture tell you anything about the ball?

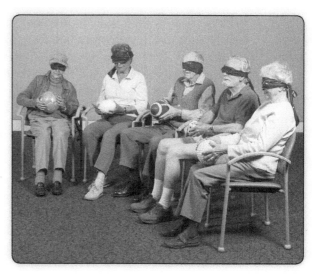

- Squeeze the ball (firm touch).
    - Is it firm or soft?
    - What about squeezing the ball? Does that tell you anything?
    - Thump it. What sound does it make?
    - What does the thump say about the ball?
- What shape is the ball?
    - Is it big? Small?
    - Does anyone have a ball that is not round?
    - How can you tell the shape without looking?
- Are there other sensory clues?
    - Does the ball have a smell?
    - Is it heavy or light?
    - If the ball is heavy, how does the body know that?
    - Do participants notice how weight is felt because it pulls on the arm muscles?

By now, people will have a pretty good idea of what object they're holding. When you call out their ball, have them raise their hand but still keep their eyes closed.

- Who has a tennis ball?
- Who has a golf ball?
- Whose ball is not actually a ball at all?
- Call out all the balls. Participants raise their hand when they hear their object named.
- Now they can open their eyes. Congratulate them on good guesses!
- Ask them how they knew all of this without sight.

They may say they just could tell, and you can discuss how that's learning from past experiences and knowledge. But probably most interesting to them will be that they used their somatic senses for light touch, firm touch, pressure, and position to learn about the shape, weight, and size of the object. They also may have been able to use smell and sounds for more clues. All of these sensory clues combined with past experience and knowledge helped them gather information about the objects.

Discuss how their body figured out the shape of their ball without sight. The answer is that kinesthetic receptors line each joint and communicate the position of the joint to the brain. If the positions of the fingers describe a round object, that's what the joint receptors tell the brain. And then we know the object we hold is round. Similarly, other somatic receptors tell us if the ball is fuzzy or smooth, firm or soft. Still others in our muscle cells tell our brains something about how much an object weighs; we feel the pull on a muscle.

Live It))

Participants will better appreciate the body and all of its sensory devices. Without using vision, the body can still perceive the environment. Density, texture, position, shape, smell, and weight all provide important sensory information about the world around us. These sensory clues combine with past experience and knowledge to help the body coordinate a great deal of information from which to draw a conclusion or form a plan.

COMING TO YOUR SENSES

Smell, touch, and recognition again combine to learn about the environment. Coming to Your Senses is a fun, easy, and inexpensive activity in which almost anyone can participate and do well. Participants will remember this activity every time they use hand lotion, at least for a while. It will boost their appreciation of their amazing body and help build balance confidence. Participants will need to pay attention to senses other than sight to learn about hand lotions.

Benefits)))

- ◉ Encourages listening to the body (proprioceptive learning).
- ◉ Engages senses of touch, pressure, temperature, and smell.
- ◉ Encourages recall and recognition.

Set It Up)))

Bring to class three or four scented hand lotions with easy-to-identify one-scent fragrances; also pick one unscented lotion. Do not let participants see the bottles or the lotion; sometimes seeing the color of lotion will give away its scent.

How to Do It)))

Begin the activity with a brief discussion about smells. What smells do they remember from childhood? Fresh bread? Hay? Farm smells? Mom's perfume or Dad's cologne? (I remember the smell of my mom's scarf and her leather purse.) If participants smelled these scents again, they'd still probably recognize them accurately and immediately, even all these years later. Of all the senses, smell has the most accurate and long-term memory.

- ◉ Participants should be comfortably seated. Tell them you'll be giving them lotions to rub into their hands. If they have an aversion to scents, they may wish to sit out this activity.
- ◉ Tell them that this activity is about learning without eyes. Ask them to please close their eyes and keep them closed until the end. It won't take long.
- ◉ Give each participant a small dollop of lotion. Mix up the scents from person to person. Remind them to keep their eyes closed.
- ◉ As participants rub the lotion into their hands, use the following cues.
  - Feel the coolness of the lotion (temperature sensation).
  - Feel its softness and how it glides across the skin.
  - Feel how the skin moves, too (light touch receptors).
  - Feel the length of each finger and the hardness of the fingernails (light touch, texture, and pressure).
  - Feel how one hand can feel the other hand. Notice the pressure of the touch.
  - Notice the depth and the curve of your palm.
- ◉ Now, concentrate on the fragrance. Ask participants to bring their hands to their nose and take a deep, slow breath. Do they recognize the fragrance?
  - One by one, call out the names of the fragrances you have used for class. Participants can raise their hand when they recognize theirs.

- Does anyone have an unscented fragrance? They may. Remember, one lotion was unscented.
- Allow that some participants won't guess right. That's okay, it's the effort to explore with their senses that's important.
- Participants open their eyes. Did they enjoy coming to their senses? The sensory exploration of their hands?

Keep It Safe))

Perfumes bother some people or can cause allergic reactions. Ask all participants whether fragrances bother them. If anyone is sensitive to the smell of scented lotions, do not do this activity in their presence. Additionally, many older adults no longer have a keen sense of smell. People who have no sense of smell can still enjoy the other wonderful sensations of touch and coolness. Before you begin the activity, let participants know you plan to use these fragrances. They can opt out for any reason.

Live It))

The senses of the body are enjoyable and informative. This is a chance to explore somatic sensations. The human body is amazing!

OVER THE MOON—BASIC STRETCH

Large exercise balls can be intimidating for older adults. You want participants to like these balls because they may be using more of them in the future. Here is a wonderful activity to introduce them to the ball. It's a simple back stretch that feels great. The roll of the ball provides the kinesthetic stimulus, a slight change in balance and back support.

Benefits))

- Provides a positive, early, and easy ball experience for participants.
- Stretches the low back and sides.
- Participants have a ball!

Set It Up))

Round up as many exercise balls as possible; But you'll need at least one. Participants can take turns—this activity goes quickly.

How to Do It))

Demonstrate the movement for participants.

The Start

- Participants sit tall on the edge of their chair, knees as wide as comfortably possible, abs in, and shoulder blades back and down.
- Place hands on the ball.
- Take a deep breath and sit tall to prepare.

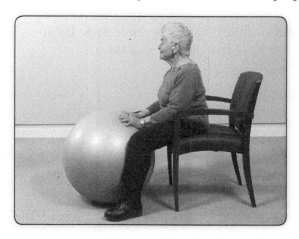 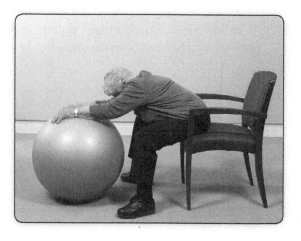

The Moves

- Keeping hands placed where they lay, exhale fully and roll the ball forward.
- Use these cues:
  - Keep your back tall and straight. The forward lean should happen at the hip, not through the spine. (Hip flexion, not spinal.)
  - Keep your hands where you originally placed them on the ball. As you roll the ball away from you, the ball stretches you.
  - At the end of the forward roll, lower your head and relax a few moments (10-15 seconds, if tolerable) while your back is gently stretching.
  - Do you feel a nice stretch across the low back and shoulders?
  - Can you feel how the arc of the ball helps the stretch?
- Roll the ball back and sit tall again. Repeat, if desired.

Roll Ball to the Side

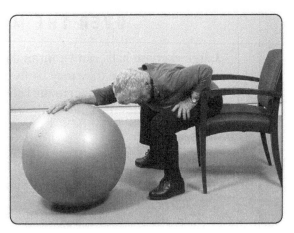

- Place just one hand on the ball. Use the other hand for back support; put it on your chair or opposite knee.
- Inhale deeply and sit tall to prepare.
- Exhale and roll the ball to the side to stretch the opposite sides and shoulders.
- Inhale and roll the ball back to the center and sit tall again.
- Exhale and roll the ball out to the other side.
- Lean from the hip; allow the shoulders and sides to extend and stretch (think Venus de Milo arms for added stretch).
- Hold each gentle side stretch 10 to 15 seconds—relax and enjoy the stretch.
- Roll back to center and sit tall.

Keep It Safe)))

Nothing should hurt. Show and discuss the difference between hinging at the hip joint and spinal bending—they want hip hinge, not back rounding. Also, because this activity involves forward leaning, support for the back must be provided. The ball provides back support because participants are resting part of their weight on the ball. When moving to the side, keep one hand on the opposite leg for additional back support.

Live It)))

The ball takes on body weight as participants lean forward, and its big round shape helps stretch a tight back. Participants should be Over the Moon about using the ball!

OVER THE MOON—ROCK FORWARD, STAND UP

Getting out of a chair is difficult for many participants. This intermediate activity uses the ease of rolling a stability ball to initiate the momentum that helps a person rock forward and then stand up from a chair. The ball provides both movement initiation and balance support. The sensation of rolling forward and up provides a unique somatic learning experience.

Benefits))

- ⊚ Mimics the forward and up sensation of getting up from a chair or doing one of our Teeter-Totter Chair Stands.
- ⊚ Facilitates kinesthetic awareness and learning.

Set It Up))

Provide at least a small variety of stability balls. Bigger balls work best. It is easy to share the balls because the activity goes quickly.

How to Do It))

The goal is simply for each participant to experience a short little ride with the ball, forward and up. First, demonstrate and discuss how the activity looks. Then pick a volunteer to try it first so the others can see. Then invite them to try it.

The Start

- ⊚ Participants sit on the edge of their chair, legs wide apart.
- ⊚ Place the ball in front of them.
- ⊚ They sit tall and place their hands on the ball. They are to keep their hands on the ball until just before they are ready to stand up.
- ⊚ Remind them to keep their hands where they started.

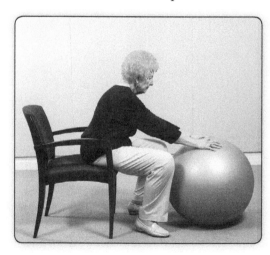 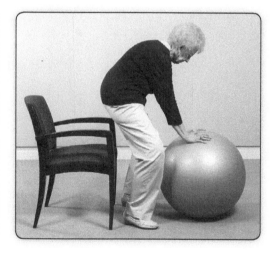

The Moves

- ⊚ Cue them that this will be done in one continuous movement. They will roll the ball forward and then stand up. The forward momentum of the first part of the roll will bring their hips up off the chair and over their feet. Then, when their hips are over their feet, it is easier for them to stand upright. When they are ready, have them give the first part of the sequence a try. Roll the ball forward until their hips rock up and off of the chair. Let them try it a few times first; then ask these kinds of questions:

BALANCE

- Do you notice a point during the roll where your hips start to leave the chair?
- Did the momentum help?
- Is it a bit similar to a chair stand?

⊙ They return to the beginning position and repeat the movement, but this time, they roll forward and then stand all the way up. Ask these questions.

- Did getting your hips over your feet make it easier to stand up?
- Did the momentum help?
- Did it surprise them how easily they rose from their chair?

Keep It Safe 》

Not everyone will figure out this movement successfully. Some won't be able to get the *rise* out of rolling forward, and others may feel unbalanced rolling away from the edge of their chair. And it is possible to lose balance coming to a standing position. So stay close to your participant. Let participants decide for themselves what they are willing to do.

Live It 》

Stability balls are great. Over the Moon and up to standing is such a nice experience!

STEP AND STOP

This activity has been one of the most helpful for my clients. It involves breaking down a series of stepping movements into fewer pieces. Before participants move to any other position, they steady themselves and then continue when they're ready. Later you can apply this concept to many mobility activities. It works great!

Benefits))

- ◉ Facilitates somatic learning (listening to the body's sense of balance).
- ◉ Teaches a technique that is helpful for transitions.

How to Do It))

The Start

- ◉ Participants stand in front of a wall with a chair beside them, or they stand in a corner with a chair or walker in front of them. It is fine for them to keep their hands on a balance support for this activity.
- ◉ Place a line 12 to 18 inches (30 to 40 centimeters) in front of them. You can use tape, chalk, a ruler or yardstick, or a design on the floor. The line is their visual target for where they will be tapping their foot.

The Moves

- ◉ Do a few Step and Stops without the stops.
  - Participants tap one foot on the line, and bring it back beside the other foot.
  - Tap the other foot on the line.
  - Did they notice any instability going back and forth? (probably) Did one leg do better than the other? (it's common)
- ◉ Now do a few Step and Stops with each foot a few times.
  - This time, they tap one foot out and leave it there, momentarily, until they're comfortable, steady, and ready to pull the foot back. Cue with different words for regaining their balance between steps: Steady, rebalance, hesitate, hold, get steady and ready, step and stop.
  - Continue, using each leg a few times. Tap the line (stop and steady), back (steady), tap (balance), back (hold), tap (rebalance), back (stop); step, stop, step, stop.
  - Rebalance, or steady themselves with change in foot position. Step and stop, step and stop. The little hesitations help steady balance.
- ◉ Begin alternating feet.
  - Right tap, stop; back, stop. Left tap, stop; back, stop.
  - Start with just 2 taps (1 right,1 left) and progress to doing 8 taps (4 right, 4 left).
  - Use the same kinds of cues and a slow, doable but deliberate cadence: Step, stop, back, stop; step, stop, back, stop; and so on.
- ◉ Cue participants to *feel* their bodies' transitions from left to right and to notice the sensations of weighting and un-weighting.
  - How does it feel to change legs? Do they notice one leg must be unweighted to move the other and then their weight must shift back?

- Are they keeping their knees soft? (they should) Does it help? (yes)
- Is their core stable? (yes) Are the shoulders staying over the hips? (yes , they should be)

Give It More Balance))

- ◉ Count a cadence out loud for them in sets of four, then eight. You can also have the participants count the cadence out loud.
- ◉ Play appropriate music.
  - For slower music, try "Tennessee Waltz."
  - A little faster music could be "Blueberry Hill."
  - Progress to doing a whole song's worth. Vary the stepping patterns.
- ◉ Advanced: Have them do this with hands on their hips.
- ◉ Have them tap their foot on a short step instead of a line. The added height of a small step is a much bigger balance challenge.

Keep it Safe))

- ◉ Make sure participants have ample balance support; wall or corner behind, railing beside or a walker in front.
- ◉ Take time to work through the progressions: One leg at a time, before alternating legs. Start with just two taps on the line. An even cadence will help.
- ◉ Practice frequently. It is a skill that takes time and practice.

Live It))

Smooth stepping transitions can be tricky, icky tasks for participants. Mastering them with a tool that really helps, like Step and Stop, can boost their confidence and keep them more active.

B A L A N C E

BELLY BUTTON TRAINING

Belly buttons are very cool. Centering the activity on them makes it a little more fun and memorable. The goal is to create an understanding of how participants' center of gravity affects their balance. The preactivity discussion will help them understand the concept intellectually as well as kinesthetically. All of this makes belly buttons easy, fun, and practical to use in balance training.

Benefits))

- ⊙ Introduces center of gravity and builds sensory awareness of it.
- ⊙ Works well with many other ABLE Bodies activities.
- ⊙ Offers practical applications in everyday tasks.

Set It Up))

For most of these versions, each person will need a Thera-Band knotted at one end. A long scarf or heavy string may work also. If you have it, tie a golf ball or heavy object in the knot so the cord will hang straighter and work better as a plumb line. Participants will hold it in their hand as a plumb line between their belly button and the floor. The line and where it hits the ground provides a visual marker of where their center of gravity meets the ground.

How to Do It))

Start with a discussion about how each person's belly button is approximately their balance point, or center of gravity. That is, if they were a spinning top, or if they did a million cartwheels, their limbs would spin through the air around their center, their balance point—their belly button! The belly button marks their center of gravity.

Then you might begin with a review of an earlier activity such as Anchors A-Sway, if you've done that one with your participants. The review will link previous information with this new information and expand their understanding. In Anchors A-Sway, participants discovered that the farther they leaned forward, the more likely it became that they'd need to take a step or risk toppling over. Demonstrate this for them. As you lean further and further forward, it is your center of gravity (belly button) that moves closer and closer to the edge of your base of support (your feet). At a certain point, you need to take a step. Explain and demonstrate that if their center point (their belly button) moves beyond their base of support (their feet), they too must take a step or topple forward. They have reached their tipping point. Encourage a few to try this tipping point exercise.

The Start

Hand each participant the knotted Thera-Bands you have ready and ask them to stand in front of their chair or with other balance support, as needed.

The Moves

Belly Stands

- ⊙ Participants' feet are shoulder-width apart, equally weighted; torso is braced.
- ⊙ Shoulders are over hips, abs are in, and head is retracted.
- ⊙ Weight should be equal over both feet.
- ⊙ Participants hold one end of the band against their belly button and adjust the length so the other end barely touches the floor.

- Ask the following:
    - Can you feel your weight evenly distributed over both feet?
    - Where is your belly button in relationship to your feet? (Between.)
    - If you drew a straight line down from your belly to the floor, where would it land? (Between.)
    - Observe where your band touches the ground. (Because their weight is equally distributed over both feet, the band should touch the floor right between their feet).
    - Now, look down. Is that where the band is touching the floor?
    - It is? Perfect! That's as it should be. It means that your center of gravity is centered over and between your feet.

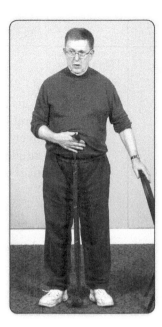

Belly Weight Shifts to One Side

In this activity, participants practice shifting their weight from one foot to the other. Where their Thera-Band touches the floor will change with their sways. The object of the lesson is to explore these changes. The band will follow the movement of their belly. As they shift their weight to the right, the band will move toward the right foot, and vice versa. The first goal is for them to notice the effect of weight shifts on the movement of the band and to get a sense that the band marks the plumb line position of their center of gravity over the ground. A secondary goal is to help participants understand how centering their belly button over their supporting leg is necessary for eventually standing on one leg successfully.

- Without changing how they are standing (weight equal on both feet), participants try to lift one foot off the ground. (It should not be possible.)
- What, no luck? What happened?
- Let them try again. Remember, no weight shifting or leaning!
- It's just not possible to lift one foot with their weight still on it. To lift one leg, they must first remove the weight from it. The question is how to do that without losing their balance.
- Using their belly button hand, participants will drag the belly button to the right. That means shift the whole torso—head, neck, and trunk. Don't lean or tip the box, just move it directly sideways and over the right foot. (Participants should be standing upright with weight over the right leg.)

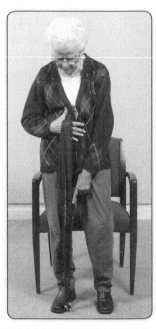

    - Which foot feels your weight now? (Right)
    - Which foot is unweighted? (Left)
    - Look down and notice where your Thera-Band is touching the floor. (Inside of right foot)
    - It should have moved over, too. It should be touching the inside of the right foot. The plumb line reflects the change in position of your center of gravity to the right.

BALANCE

- Participants return their belly button to the center position.
  - Drag the belly button left. The whole torso moves left (head, neck, trunk).
  - No leaning! Shift the whole torso, like it's one big box.
  - Is the band touching the inside of the left foot? It should be!
- Participants return their belly button to the center position.
- Repeat sways several times. Watch how band moves along the ground, side to side, with the weight shifts.
- Be sure they are moving the whole torso left or right, and not just leaning or tilting the upper body.

Belly Weight Shifts to a One-Legged Stand

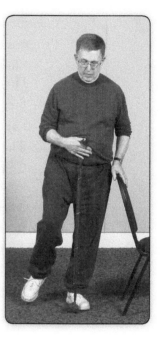

- Participants begin in a tall posture, as before—feet shoulder-width apart, torso stable, and knees soft. (Soft knees will help them maintain balance when shifting weight over one leg.)
- Drag the belly button right. Move the whole torso over.
  - Check your band. Is it showing that your belly button is over the left foot?
  - Do you notice that your right foot is *unweighted*?
  - Move your right foot slowly up and in front of the other foot; keep the abs in and body tall. Now the left leg is almost in line with the right. Carefully lift the right foot off the ground, bringing the knee in close to you.
  - Wow! You're standing on one leg.
  - Put the foot back down to the side.
  - Did the belly button shifting help prepare you for the move?
  - Was it much easier to hold the up position with the left foot in front, as opposed to beside it?
  - Why do you think this worked better? (More of the body weight is aligned over the base of support than when the foot is held to the side.)
- Have participants do the same in the other direction. Participants shift or drag their belly button so it's over the left foot.
  - Lift the right foot, bringing the knee right and up toward the body. Balance a moment on one leg, again.
  - Can they notice how knee placement affects balance? It's a good time to stress "knee lift, abs in" posture.
- Repeat these brief one-legged stands until they become easier.
- Increase difficulty by having participants maintain balance longer on one leg.

Belly Steps

This is an intermediate activity of moderate difficulty. Belly Steps progress the knee-lifted, single-leg stance into a forward step. The goal is to get participants to step forward with their foot and their belly button, together. You want them to feel the sensation of moving their belly button forward and over the stepping foot. This will make subsequent stepping motions easier.

- ◉ Participants shift their weight over the right foot, lift the left knee, and come into a single-leg stand.
- ◉ Repeat to the left.
- ◉ Continue repeating until participants show ability and confidence.
- ◉ Progress to taking a step.
    - Shift weight to the right leg and lift the left knee. Hold a moment.
    - Step forward with the left foot as shown.
    - Land heel and then toe.
    - The belly button moves, too—it follows the foot.
    - Commit to the step. That means let the belly follow the left foot forward.
    - Then bring the other foot beside it.
- ◉ Repeat a few times with each leg.
    - As the right foot steps, follow it with the belly button.
    - Land heel and then toe.
    - Bring the other foot beside it.
    - Ask, do you notice how the belly button helps initiate and then complete the step?

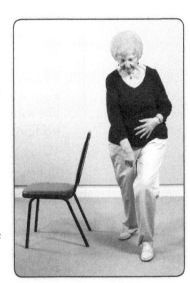

Belly Lunges

This is an intermediate activity of moderate difficulty. Lunge steps are bigger steps than normal and carry the person a longer distance. Participants should take turns doing this activity under your supervision.

- ◉ Put down two lines of masking tape to form a *V* that is 6 to 10 feet (2-3 meters) long. The lines should be only 6 inches (15 centimeters) apart at the narrow end and 3 feet (1 meter) apart at the other end. Participants will practice crossing over the two lines at ever-widening spots using the techniques from Belly Steps. That means the belly button will move forward with the stepping leg for each step across the *V*. The ever-widening lines will soon require that they use a lunge step to cross.
- ◉ One participant at a time will stand at the lines at a point they think they can cross safely. You should stand beside them and model the activity the first few times.

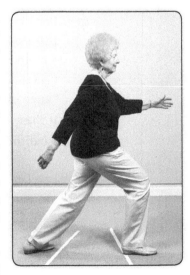

- Here are some cues to use as participants cross:
  - Make a plan and spot where you want your foot to land.
  - Weight shift to one leg.
  - Big knee lift with the other leg.
  - Step that foot out and across to the chosen spot. Move your foot, belly, and torso.
  - Land heel–toe and bring the other foot beside it. Stop there.
  - Did you make it? Did getting your belly out there help? Good job!
  - Belly Lunges are awesome. Turn around and do it again!
  - See how far up the *V* you can go.
  - Practice really improves this skill and reinforces the utility of the concept.

Belly-Ups

This is a difficult activity because it requires participants to climb stairs. Start by using one step placed near a handrail and spot them personally. Later you can progress to a short staircase with handrails. To step up each stair, participants place their whole foot on the stair and then move their weight (their belly button) over the ankle that is up. This moves their center of gravity forward and makes it easier to lift themselves up the stair.

- Participants step up and move the belly (torso) forward.
- They push through the up heel to lift their weight over that step.
- Bring the other leg forward and step up to the next step.
- Belly up and lift up to the next stair.
- Keep going for 8 to 12 steps, until they reach the top of the stairs, or until they tire.

Keep It Safe))

For the greatest balance safety, have participants take turns during most of these activities. Let participants choose what kinds of challenges they are willing to try.

Live It))

Participants should move belly and body together. Where the belly button goes, so goes the body. To be in balance, the center of gravity needs to be over the base of support.

BALANCE

BALL ON THE WALL

Ball on the Wall, which mimics a squat, is an advanced exercise that strengthens the whole leg in everyday ways. Balloons or balls create the need for wobble control by core muscles, facilitate upright posture, and provide kinesthetic sensation.

Benefits))

- ⊙ Adds more balance and kinesthetic work to the common squat.
- ⊙ Builds leg strength.
- ⊙ Increases core strength and awareness.

Set It Up))

You will need stability balls, Slo Mo balls, or balloons, and a clear, safe space along a wall or in a corner.

How to Do It))

The Start

- ⊙ Participants stand with their back to a wall or a corner. Place the stability ball behind them in the small of their back. Smaller balloons or balls can be placed at shoulder blade level.
- ⊙ Tell participants to press their back against the ball. Use these cues.
    - Can you feel your stomach tighten? Good, now brace your abdominal wall.
    - Draw your shoulder blades back and down.
    - Press your back into the ball and keep that position.
    - Inhale to prepare.

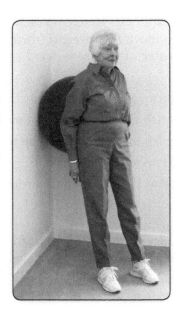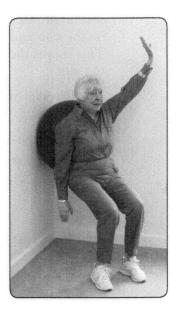

The Moves

- ⊙ Keeping pressure on the ball, participants exhale and lower themselves into a shallow squat.
- ⊙ Check their position:
    - Knees over ankles—don't let them move forward over or past the toes.
    - If the knees go past the toes, step out a little farther from the wall for the next squat.
    - Are shoulders level?
    - Is the core braced?
- ⊙ Come up again.
- ⊙ Repeat 8 to 15 times, as able.

BALANCE

Give It More Balance))

- Add arm lifts: With each squat, lift one arm up, reaching overhead.
- Lift one heel: Lifting one heel makes the heel-down leg do most of the work and requires more balance control.

Take It Further))

Have your participants do Ball on the Wall With a Twist. This activity is advanced and requires closer spotting. It's simply a ball squat with torso rotation added. Cue the torso rotation as rolling one shoulder blade onto the ball with each descent, coming back to the middle position on ascent. Practice the rolling motion before adding the squat. Cue participants also to keep the core muscles braced. The exercise looks like a bear in the woods scratching his back on a tree (stability ball).

- Stand with your back against the ball.
- Both feet are flat, core muscles are braced, and forearms are crossed on the chest.
- Inhale to prepare.
- Exhale. Push the back against the ball and maintain this pressure throughout the squat.
- Slide down the wall, turning the torso, arms, head, and neck to one side with each squat.
- Lead with the arms to help pull the torso into the greatest rotation that is comfortable.
- The torso rotation should look like a spool of thread turning on its bobbin. There is no bending of the back; just rotation.

Keep It Safe))

I think that this activity should be done one person at a time or in private training sessions. Putting the ball in a corner makes it safer because the ball will stay in place better and because corners provide two-sided balance support. If you decide to try the twisted version, teach the rotation first without the squat. Supervise closely until the participant is comfortable.

Live It))

With Ball on the Wall, 10 squats a day will keep the walker away!

BALANCE

TAI CHI

I am neither a certified nor a registered tai chi instructor. But for the past few years I have been working with Drs. Fay Horak and Laurie King at Oregon Health and Science University's (OHSU) Neurological Sciences Institute (NSI) to develop exercises for Parkinson's disease (PD). The program, called HELP PD, has made some remarkable differences already in our subjects. The one-hour workout consists of 10-minute segments of six familiar physical activities; Tai chi is one of those activity blocks. Recently I have begun using some of the tai chi poses with music. Using music with tai chi is not officially sanctioned by any tai chi expert; but then again, I am not officially sanctioned myself. Putting music to basic tai chi has helped my clients master the weight shifting and mind–body awareness that is true tai chi.

Benefits »

- Practices slow weight shifts intrinsically cued.
- Encourages mind–body awareness and inside-out (kinesthetic) learning.
- Offers movements that can be done in multiple directions.

Set It Up »

You will need to learn three movements on your own. They are all simple movements, but it is beyond the scope of this book to teach you how to do them. Please consult other books or tai chi instructors if you need help.

- Prayer Wheel
- Tai Chi Cat Walk
- Cloud Hands

Prayer Wheels are weight shifts done in place, Tai Chi Cat Walk is forward walking, and Cloud Hands is sideward walking. When you are teaching these, at least initially, teach them without the hand movements. Emphasize slow, mindful weight shifts, deep even breaths, and upright posture (shoulders over hips, head over shoulders). Tai chi text describes the upper body as "riding a horse." The weight shifts are not a rocking, up and down vertical movement, but a transfer along a horizontal plane, from one foot to the other.

How to Do It »

Prayer Wheel

- Feet offset, shoulder-width apart, one forward, one back.
- Shift body weight from rear foot to forward foot, slowly, maintaining shoulders over hips.
- Add hands moving in the shape of a large wheel.
- Pretend hands are holding a 12-inch (25-centimeter) ball between the palms of the hands. Move the ball in a big wheel, between hips and shoulders, extending arms fully out in front, at hip level, then back towards the body at shoulder height and then back down to the hips.
- Add breathing cues:
  - Exhale out to mid point of wheel; inhale back.
  - Equal breaths for each turn of the wheel.
- Slow moves, upright posture throughout.
- Repeat 10 times, then change feet and perform 10 more prayer wheels.

ABLE Bodies Balance Training

Tai Chi Cat Walk

Tai Chi Cat Walk starts where Prayer Wheel leaves off. It takes the forward weight shift and turns it into a step, hence walking forward begins. To do the cat walk participants shift backward and turn the front foot out to 45 degrees. Then as they shift forward again, the rear foot is brought forward to take a step, landing heel-toe. Once the foot is landed, body weight shifts forward, then back again and the cycle repeats. Hand movements play a role, too, but they can be added later. When the movements are basically learned, but maybe not quite correct, try adding music. My favorite is Patti Page's *Tennessee Waltz*. It's slow and methodical; the weight shifts and foot turns just happen.

- Shift forward.
- Shift back, turn the forward foot out.
- Travel (that's how I cue it, anyway. It means lift their back foot and bring it forward). During the traveling section, cue them to notice how their body weight needs to align over the supporting leg for them to stay balanced while the other foot travels to its forward spot and lands heel-toe.
- New foot lands, very lightly, heel then toe.
- Shift forward.
- Shift back, etc.

Cloud Hands

This activity encourages slow sideways walking. The imagery is that they are walking on a bank of clouds, trying not to fall through. When ready, try the first few stanzas of Henry Mancini's *Pink Panther*. The music there has that perfect, sneaking quietly across a room feel to it.

- Transfer their weight from their left to right foot.
- Cue them to stand with most of their weight on their left foot. They should push hard enough into their left foot that they feel the ground pushing back at that left foot.
- Slowly they release that push and they will feel their body weight transfer from the bottom of the left foot, up their leg, across their pelvis, and down the length of their right leg until they feel the right foot pushing against the ground.
- Staying upright, lift the left foot slowly up and move it to the left.
- Place left heel then toe on the ground on the inside of that foot.
- Shift body weight to it, as foot rolls to its middle.
- Begin transferring body weight to left foot, when it is fully weighted bring the right foot beside it, in toe-heel fashion.
- Repeat 10 times in each direction.

Keep It Safe))

Keep each participant near a balance support. They will need it, especially for the walking movements, where they are on one foot for brief moments between weight transfers. For groups, long rows of chairs work great. Spread out long rows of chairs and put 2-3 people on each row. Then they simply move along with the chair backs acting as a handrail.

Live It))

Tai chi does a great job nurturing body awareness, deep breathing, slow mindful weight shift, body mapping, and upright posture throughout. Balance is felt all through each weight transfer. The magic of adding music is a great example of how music has a way of helping coordinate complicated patterns, making them easier, and making them happen with the whole body. It is a real smile maker!

ABLE Bodies Balance Training

BALANCE

STANDING WEIGHT SHIFTS

Coaching awareness of body weight and movement while practicing weight shifts helps to improve balance. Multiple patterns of weight shifting make this exercise very effective.

Benefits))

- ⊚ Practices postural control during weight shifts.
- ⊚ Facilitates kinesthetic learning, listening to their body. I call it inside/out learning.
- ⊚ Provides a good and very practical early standing balance activity.

Set It Up))

You will not need any special equipment for this exercise.

How to Do It))

The Start

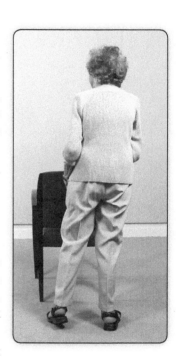

- ⊚ Participants stand behind a sturdy chair with good upright posture and with feet shoulder-width apart or slightly wider.
- ⊚ They place both hands on the chair; tightly, lightly, or hovered, as able. Some participants may be comfortable with only one hand on the chair. To start, be conservative and cue both hands on the chair.
- ⊚ Participants begin with their body weight equally distributed over both feet, with proper upright posture.

The Moves

Use the following cues.

- ⊚ Shift your weight toward the right foot then back to center, three to six times. Don't lean with the upper body, rather shift the whole, tall torso over the desired foot. Borrowing an expression from tai chi, the shift is like riding a horse, no leaning, the trunk just shifts to the side. Body stays upright.
- ⊚ Do three to six shifts to the left. Again, don't lean; instead, shift the whole upper body.
- ⊚ Change the foot position to a wider stance. Repeat the shifting, but add knee bends to the leg receiving the body weight. Do these weight shifts three to six times. Again, no leaning and keep the torso tall.
- ⊚ Change the foot position to an offset stance. Shift the weight forward and bend the front knee. Shift back and bend the back (receiving) knee. Repeat three to six times.
- ⊚ Change to an offset stance with the other foot in front and repeat the sequence.

Take It Further))

- ⊚ Hold each weight shift longer.
- ⊚ Widen the foot placement.

BALANCE

Give It More Balance))

- ⊙ Cue participants to lift the heel of the foot that is being *unweighted*. This will make each weight shift more complete.
- ⊙ Add arm reaches to the weight shifts to further increase the weight shifting effects.
  - Shift to the right, reach to the right with the left arm; and vice versa.
  - Ask if they notice how reaching up tends to re-center their balance.

Keep It Safe))

Keep participants near their support chair, with one arm available to grab it, if needed. Remind them that they can hold the chair tightly, lightly, or just hover their hands over it. Participants should use whatever balance support makes them comfortable.

EYES ON THE PRIZE

Eyes on the Prize refers to the value of visual targets. The prize is their visual target. This activity teaches participants to use a visual target at horizon level to guide their path, keeping their eyes on the prize.

Benefits))

- Allows participants to experience visual targets.
- Improves lateral stability.
- Requires participants to pay attention to their sense of balance.

Set It Up))

Put down a line (or two or three) using your widest tape (0.5 to 2.0 inches [1.0 to 5.0 centimeters]). At one or both ends, place visual targets at horizon level, such as a prize they'll win or pictures of beautiful vacation spots, tasty food treats, or favorite celebrities for participants to focus on.

How to Do It))

Start by discussing a little about visual targets: Where you place your gaze guides your path when moving. When people learn to drive, for example, they are taught to look far ahead at the middle of the road. When skiers learn to ski through the forest, they quickly learn to avoid the trees by looking at the paths between the trees—not at the trees. It's a lesson quickly learned. Where the eyes focus is where the body follows. Why not use this innate visual sense when training for balance? Visual targets also make the footwork of balance more automatic.

Let participants know that they will be invited to walk this line several times. Demonstrate for the participants how you want them to walk down the line with good posture, soft knees, and above all, eyes on the prize. Then have participants walk the line, one at a time. Their goal is to keep on the path as much as possible. On the first pass, let them work it out themselves a little at a time. Ask them

- Where are you looking when you walk? (Most look down at the line.)
- What might you remember about looking down from previous lessons? (See Parts of the Whole on page 92; looking down moves their center of balance closer to their toes, so they were less centered over their feet.

Now it's time to walk the line again. During this next pass, suggest they keep their gaze on the horizon. They can look down occasionally as needed, but ask them to try their best to keep their gaze on the horizon. For those who are still uncomfortable looking at the horizon, try to convince them to sweep their vision at least a little farther up the line with each subsequent path.

- Once participants start across the line, get them to lift their gaze to the horizon.
- During subsequent passes across the line, use these cues.
  - Abs are braced, ribs lifted, and shoulder blades back and down.
  - Keep your eyes on the prize; it will help direct your path.
  - Can you notice how this helps with gait and balance? Is it a little easier?
  - Try walking a little faster. Do you notice you can walk faster more easily? (It's true.)
  - Experts say that a visual target makes balance more automatic. Would you agree?

BALANCE

Give It More Balance))

- ⦿ Add some music to give their steps a rhythm.
- ⦿ Add arm swings to give it more challenge.
- ⦿ Have participants sing, recite a poem, or count by 3s as they walk.
- ⦿ Dim the lights or have them wear sunglasses.
- ⦿ Have participants use a visual target while trying to stand still on the tandem line. This is very difficult (static balance is trickier than moving balance), but it's interesting for them to try. Provide ample balance support.
- ⦿ Try Follow the Light; it's with the vestibular activities on page 257.

ABLE Bodies Balance Training

BALANCE

TIGHT TANDEM WALKING ON A LINE OR BEAM

A tight tandem walk is one in which the heel of one foot is placed directly in front of and touching the toe of the other. This activity is one of the most difficult in the program. It's tough but not impossible. Because of the narrow base of support, it takes both good balance and leg strength. Plan to work with one person at a time.

You might use this activity as a test in week 2 (when even two steps on a line are difficult) and then again in week 16 to measure improvements. The changes will be remarkable, with all they have learned. These kinds of changes build confidence, and can help prevent falls to the side. Self-efficacy experts say that nothing builds confidence like achieving something that has been difficult in the past.

Benefits))

- Strengthens hip abductors and adductors for reduced fall risk.
- Practices dynamic balance over a narrow base of support.
- Uses visual targets.
- Requires cognitive skills; participants practice making and executing their plan.
- Builds confidence.

Set It Up))

Put down a 12-foot (3.5-meter) line beside a handrail. Alternatively, perhaps there is a line in the carpet that you can use; just make sure balance support is nearby. There's no shame in everyone using a walker at first. It will be that much easier to learn the foot work. This activity should be done with just one person at a time, with yourself nearby. You might lock forearms with them or hold both hands the first few times. You will be walking backward in front of them. It also helps if you hold their hands up a bit and out to the side.

How to Do It))

The ultimate task is to walk heel-touches-toe style down the line. Describe and model a tandem step. Participants can do an easier pattern, if they like, by having their feet land farther apart. The goal is that it just needs to be challenging. Consider reminding them of ABLE Bodies tools they've learned previously. They may think of some themselves. That would be better. Then let them make their own plan about how they will walk this challenging line.

- Remind participants of similar activities you've already done successfully with them, such as The Straight and Narrow, Eyes on the Prize, and Holiday Lines (see Walk the Line).
- They should plan for a stabilized torso, aligned posture, and soft knees.
- They should look ahead using a visual target at horizon level or at least look 8 feet (2.5 meters) ahead.
- They might hold their arms out to the sides (if comfortable).
- With each step they will be moving their torso forward toward the new supporting leg—belly button walking. Cue them to be aware of each transition.
- They should find a pace that works for them. A little faster is generally easier.
- Rhythm adds symmetry and cadence.
- My, oh my, look at all the tools they have to help them do great! (Really!)

Get Started))

For the first few passes, just get the hang of it. Focus on one or two tools at a time from the previous list. Little by little, participants will do better. They will keep improving one step at a time. Soon they'll have done far better than they ever would have thought.

Give It More Balance))

- ⊙ Have participants sing, recite a poem, or do simple math problems as they walk.
- ⊙ Have them carry a mug filled with water. No spilling!
- ⊙ Dim the lights or have them wear sunglasses.
- ⊙ Use a flashlight to get their gaze farther ahead.
- ⊙ Have them walk on a poly beam. Participants should feel comfortable with the beam and willing to try. Many won't want to try until they see a friend do it. Let them know their trusty walker is welcome as they cross the beam. Only let them try the challenges that they're 90 percent sure they can do. Encourage them to use as much balance support as they want. Support and praise their choices.

Keep It Safe))

Adequate balance support may be a challenge. Tight tandem walking could be difficult for almost anyone. Always provide plenty of balance support, including walkers. Consider having participants share walkers if you need extras. Make sure you only send one participant across at a time, and be there yourself to hold hands, catch a misstep, inspire, and give cues. Participants should make a plan before they start; that is, recall ideas that will help them, and then do the best they can. This and the other Walk the Line activities (see page 312) should be fun and used occasionally for special days. Participants seem to really like the single line and balance beam kinds of challenges; but they do require extra supervision.

Live It))

What will be your participants' chosen path? Visual targeting really helps with all kinds of line challenges. Practice at line challenges improves their balance over a narrow base of support and will strengthen muscles related to lateral balance. These attributes may help prevent devastating falls to the side, so practice, practice, practice. Use the tools! Participants should keep soft knees; use a stable, upright posture; use visual targets; find a rhythm; feel each transition; and glue each foot to the ground (figuratively, of course) when crossing a beam or line.

OPPOSING CIRCLES AND HIGH FIVES

Walking against the flow of others creates balance challenges. The little bumps and jostles (perturbations) common in crowds can be frightening and the constant every-which-way flow of moving people can be dizzying for vestibular systems. The following progressive challenges are safe, fun ways to practice crowded walking situations. These two could easily be visual or vestibular. They are both normally fairly easy for most groups.

Benefits))

- Helps build confidence for walking in crowds.
- Incorporates visual targets.
- Practices common vestibular challenges.
- Promotes fun social interaction.

Set It Up))

You will need a large, safe area for several people. Clear the area of any obstacles or hazards. Plan the route your participants will use ahead of time.

How to Do It))

Explain the activity and let participants know that some of them may get a little dizzy. Explain that if they do, they should stop and sit down or let you know and you will help them. Participants who use walkers can use them during this activity.

Opposing Circles

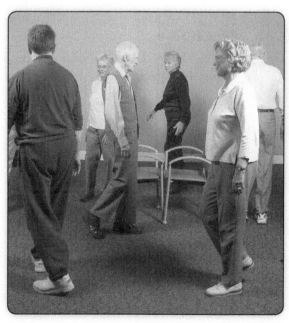

- Divide participants into two groups. Have them form an outer circle and an inner circle.
- One circle of participants walks counter-clockwise while the other walks clock-wise.
- Observe all participants. Ask if anyone is uneasy or dizzy and look for signs that they may be.
- If all is going well, have the class slow down and then change directions.
- After a little while, switch inner and outer circles and go again.
- Encourage participants to move the circles close enough to each other to occasionally bump shoulders with the inner circle. Just little bumps, though!
- Ask them to pay attention to the visual sensations they get walking in opposite directions from others.

BALANCE

High Fives

Use the same double opposing circles, but this time, cue participants to stabilize their torso and give each other high fives as they pass.

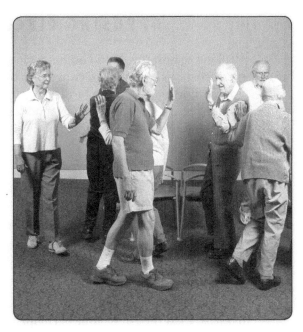

- Participants should be cautious at first and go easy on each other. Little bumps.
- Here are some cues to use:
    - Your visual target is the other person's hand. Watch it until you high five it.
    - Spot your target. Watch the hand, hit it, and then go to the next hand.
- Change circles and directions. Do it once more.

Give It More Balance))

Do allemande hands around the circle! This variation is an advanced challenge because of the weaving passes participants make as they allemande around the circles. The hands of the oncoming person become the next visual target. (See Allemande Left on page 311 for more details.)

Keep It Safe))

Take things slow. Vestibular dysfunction is common in older adults. Watch participants closely, especially at first, for signs of dizziness.

Live It))

Fitness can't fix vestibular dysfunction, but practicing problem moves will help participants predict and manage the challenges better. This practice will also help them walk in crowds and survive the little inevitable bumps that happen.

FOLLOW THE LIGHT

It's hard not to like a flashlight. It doesn't matter if you are 4 or 84 years old; if someone hands you a flashlight, you turn it on, flash it around, and light up a few things. It's just fun. Follow the Light uses flashlights to enhance visual skills for improved mobility. In Walk the Line (see page 312) and other activities, participants are taught to keep their eyes on the horizon (or at least a few feet farther ahead). Horizon-level visual targets help participants walk more upright and maintain their path and momentum.

Benefits))

- Uses visual targets in a fun way with flashlights.
- Improves posture, gait, and balance.
- Engages other senses (darkness heightens the attention paid to vestibular and somatic senses).
- Links previous learning to a new activity.

Set It Up))

You will need one flashlight per person, ideally; or at least four or five so participants can go in groups (check at your local discount store). You will need a clear, unobstructed area; and the ability to dim the lights. You can also tape down four to six lines (optional). They should be perpendicular to one end of the space and about 8 feet (2.5 meters) long and 4 feet (1.3 meter) apart.

How to Do It))

- Announce you will be dimming the lights for this activity, but not so much that the room will be completely dark. Give participants the chance to opt out if they prefer.
- Pass out flashlights. Participants should test them to see how they work.
- With the room lights still bright, line up small groups of four to six at one end of the room. The rest of the group stays seated and watches.
- Have the group turn on their flashlights.
- Dim lights enough so that the flashlight's beam will be bright.

Stand Normally

- Participants should stand normally and point the flashlight where they normally look at the ground when they walk.
- Ask them to note where they shone the light.
- Those with the least balance will likely be pointing the flashlights just in front of their feet.

Bring Out the Bent Over Posture

- Remind participants of the Bent Over Posture activity (see page 103). They are to pretend they're 98 years old, very frail, and bent over.
- Give them a moment to assume the position. Try these cues:
  - Stand with your knees and back bent and your head tilted down, looking down.
  - Do you notice your weight shift toward your toes? (Remind participants of Parts of the Whole.)
  - Shine your light at the spot on the floor where you suspect a bent over person is seeing the floor.

- ⊚ Participants now get to take years off their life.
  - Stand Tall with your head retracted and chin level, looking more directly ahead.
  - Can you feel a difference in how weight is distributed over your feet? (It moves toward the heels.)
  - Shine the light to where you're looking now.
  - Assume a bent over posture again.
  - Do you feel the difference? Do you see the difference?
  - Compare to where you normally see the ground.
  - Which feels more balanced? (Tall posture and level chin, right?)
- ⊚ Discover where they are looking now that they have improved their posture.
- ⊚ You want participants to feel a difference between looking ahead and looking down. If they feel more balanced while looking ahead, they will be more willing to look ahead while walking.
- ⊚ Discuss how not only posture and balance point change with bent over posture, but also visual perception; that is, where they see the ground also changes. If our bent over person was walking, he'd be looking down. The up tall person would be looking out ahead.

Follow the Light
- ⊚ Participants shine the flashlight beam back to where it was when they stood normally (normal standing posture).
- ⊚ Now they shine the light out about 6 to 8 feet (2-2.5 meters) farther ahead than normal.
- ⊚ Participants assume ABLE Bodies tall posture (shoulders over hips, head retracted, chin level, core braced, knees soft). Then they begin to walk toward the beam of light.
- ⊚ As they begin to walk, use the following cues.
  - Keep your light 6 to 8 feet (2-2.5 meters) ahead of you.
  - Follow the light.
  - You want to be looking farther ahead than you normally do.
  - Keep your focus ahead. Notice your posture. How do you feel?
  - Walk the full length of the room, turn, and stop at the end.
  - How does the darkness feel?
  - Are you more aware of how the floor feels under your feet?
  - How about the room temperature? Is it warm or cool?
  - How are the noise levels around you—quiet or noisy?
  - Use your flashlight to guide yourself and turn to come back.

Shine the Light Farther Ahead
- ⊚ Participants walk back with the flashlight beaming 8 to 10 feet (2.5-3 meters) in front.
- ⊚ They can move the light until it's 10 to 12 feet (3-3.5 meters) ahead, if they are willing.

- Maintain core stability—abs in, ribs lifted, and shoulder blades back and down.
- Look ahead and follow the light. Keep the light out 12 feet (3.5 meters) ahead, or at least farther than before.
- How did it go?

◉ Change groups and do the same with them, or go on to Shine the Light on the Wall.

Shine the Light on the Wall

◉ Line participants up about 20 feet (6 meters) away from a wall with a tandem line (optional) in front of them that leads toward the wall.

◉ Invite participants to hold their flashlight next to one ear with the light shining directly on the wall in front of them.

- The light on the wall is your visual target. Walk toward the light on the wall.
- Keep knees soft, abs in, ribs lifted, shoulder blades back and down, chin lifted, and head retracted.
- Let your visual target guide you.
- Do you feel like you're walking on the tandem line? (Yes, likely.)
- How is this working for you?
- Do you feel you can make it to the end without looking down? (Sure)

Give It More Balance))

Try tight tandem walking (heel of one foot nudges toe of previous foot) with flashlights beamed on the wall. This is much more difficult, but it's easier than it seems because it uses a visual target. Let participants choose their own level of challenge here. Remind participants to let the target guide them. It helps!

Keep It Safe))

Whenever you turn down the lights, watch for dizziness, anxiety, or any other signs that the darkness makes participants feel unsafe or uncomfortable. When the lights are first dimmed is an especially good time to have appropriate balance support nearby in case anyone gets dizzy. Once the lights are low, ask if they are still comfortable. Give participants the option of opting out or just watching. Lazer lights can be used instead; they can be seen in well-lit rooms.

Live It))

If participants use visual targets where they are headed, getting there will be much easier. Looking ahead can improve posture, balance, and gait.

TURN DOWN THE LIGHTS

Dimming the light reduces visual input, causing you to direct more attention to input from the other sensory systems. But there are more ways than one to reduce visual input. This activity will give you a few new ideas for manipulating vision for better balance.

Benefits))

- Facilitates somatic and vestibular awareness.
- Applies to other activities.

Set It Up))

Make sure the exercise space is safe and clutter free and that balance supports are available where appropriate.

How to Do It))

You'll need to plan ways to safely reduce the amount of light in your facility. Dimming the lights, pulling the shades, or having participants wear sunglasses are all effective ways to reduce lighting and vision and engage the vestibular and the somatic system.

- Stretching
- Seated exercises
- Some standing or moving activities, such as Belly Button Training or Side Stepping (intermediate to advanced difficulty)
    - Walking on a treadmill (Intermediate)
    - Standing on a balance pad (Advanced)
    - Traffic School (Intermediate)
    - Words on the Wall in the Hall (Advanced)
    - WalkAbouts (Intermediate)

Give It More Balance))

Balance training using reduced vision directs attention to the other two sensory systems (somatosensory and vestibular). Here are some cues to use that can help participants notice increased somatic awareness.

- Anytime that you're standing: Notice the ground beneath you (e.g., carpet, hardwood, inclined, smooth, bumpy, slippery, sticky, grass).
- When doing walking activities: Notice the sequence of your foot patterns moving you over the ground. Do you notice how your heel strike rolls to midfoot and off your toe?
- During stretches: Can you feel the stretch in your muscle? Where? How much?
- When doing strength exercises: Where do you feel the effort? Where do you feel the resistance?
- When standing still: Notice where you feel your body weight over your feet.
- What other changes come to mind?

BALANCE

Keep It Safe))

Let them choose the activities they feel comfortable doing. Dim lights may cause dizziness, especially in participants with vestibular dysfunction. Always begin with seated activities—standing and moving are intermediate and advanced activities. Looking up or over their shoulders can be a fall risk, so always be careful when reducing vision.

Live It))

More kinesthetic and vestibular training can be added to almost any activity with just the flip of the light switch!

BALANCE

MAKING WAVES

This simple activity offers two ways to reduce vision.

Benefits))

- ⊙ Facilitates somatic and vestibular awareness.
- ⊙ Identifies participants with possible vestibular dysfunction.
- ⊙ Links to other activities.

How to Do It))

- ⊙ Participants sit with tall posture in chairs with arms.
- ⊙ They cup their hands over their eyes. They can see out, but not well and only between their fingers.
    - Turn the head left, center, right, and center. Dip the chin, lift the chin up, center, dip, turn, and lift etc.
    - Do slow head turns while nodding. These are the waves.
    - If dizzy, slow way down, that may work. If dizziness persists or they are uncomfortable or wobbly, stop. If not dizzy, try going a little faster.
    - Do trunk circles. These are small circles done with the trunk. The body is held erect and moves in small- to medium-sized circles from the hip. Go both directions.
    - Sway the trunk in figure-eight patterns. Change directions.

Give It More Balance))

Have participants close the spaces between their fingers a bit more. With eyes closed and sitting tall, do the following:

- ⊙ Make waves. Making waves is doing slow head turns while nodding the chin up and down.
- ⊙ Do trunk circles.

Keep It Safe))

Not all vestibular difficulties can be helped with activity. These suggestions may help them adapt, but will not fix a permanent problem. Use chairs with arms; If participants get dizzy, they may temporarily lose their balance and fall to the side.

Live It))

Practicing these differences in vision will help the vestibular system work better during everyday situations such as in darkened rooms, head turning, and changes in position.

BALANCE

BALANCE PADS OR MATS

In general, the firmer and flatter the surface, the easier it is to balance on. Add softness or an incline and there is a balance challenge. For your participants, standing on balance pads is probably similar to us trying to stand on a water bed. The compliant surface gives way under their feet, taking away many of their proprioceptive tools and requiring constant balance adjustments. Balance pads or mats force them to use much more visual and vestibular input to stay balanced. An example of a visual tool you might use to help them reestablish balance is a stationary visual target at horizon level. Engaging and integrating the sensory systems is good balance training.

Benefits))

- ◉ Facilitates and integrates vestibular and visual inputs for balance.
- ◉ Provides challenging activities for balance integration.
- ◉ Uses variety of pads to suit individual ability.

Set It Up))

Provide adequate balance supports as discussed under the safety section of this activity. Corners of a room, with a walker in front, or near a handrail are good places for balance pads. If possible, provide balance pads in a variety of densities, shapes, and sizes.

How to Do It))

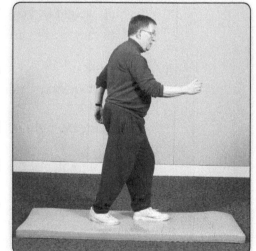

- ◉ Participants step up onto the pad, using the provided balance supports.
- ◉ They take time to get situated and steady.
- ◉ Get their permission to continue. (It may take a while for them to be ready.)
- ◉ Cue them for proper posture:
    - Abs are braced and shoulder blades back and down.
    - Ribs are lifted to lengthen the spine, the head is retracted, and the chin is level.
    - Shoulders are over the hips, hips are over the ankles.
    - Knees are soft.
- ◉ Cue participants to find a stationary visual target at horizon level and try to keep their balance.

When participants are ready, try the following movements. Within each category, movements progress from easy to more difficult. Get one move down comfortably before progressing to the next

Arm Movements

- ◉ Participants should have soft knees. Their eyes face ahead.
- ◉ They stand quietly, hands on their chest.
- ◉ Use the following cues:
    - Lift one arm out to the side; when ready, lift it overhead.
    - Put it back down.

- Do the other arm. Lift it to the side, up, and back down. Take your time.
- Put both arms out to the sides, then tilt them right and then left (like an airplane about to make a turn). Then lift both arms overhead, like sliding down a chute.
- Lift the arms in opposite directions: one forward, one back, then one up, one down.
- Add more trunk movement: Both arms make moves like an airplane. Big turns right, then left, dip, swirl, and rise.
- Do a few small arm swings, and then bigger arm swings.

Sways With Arms on Hips

⊙ These sways are kind of like standing weight shifts. Participants will probably begin by trying to shift weight using their hips. That's not what you want. Cue them instead, to sway from their ankles, not their hips. You'll probably need to help them keep their body straight from ankle to shoulder by lightly touching their hip and shoulder to keep it aligned. It takes some learning for them to be able to sway from the ankles.

⊙ Use the following cues:
- Shift weight toward the toes.
- Shift weight left, then right.
- Shift weight toward the heels (this is tough; watch them closely).
- Shift weight in a circular pattern.
- Can they do a figure-eight pattern?

Leg Movements

⊙ Do one or two sways, side to side, to get used to shifting your weight from one leg to the other.
⊙ Sway left, lift the right heel. Sway right, lift the right heel. Get comfortable with that.
⊙ Take little steps in place. Start with two steps, then progress to four without losing your balance.
⊙ Do little knee bends.
⊙ March in place (Intermediate).
⊙ Lift knee with abs pulled in (Advanced).
⊙ Lift one foot off the pad and move it about a bit (Very difficult).
⊙ Do the Hokey Pokey—add a shake to the previous foot movement (this is the most difficult).

Slow Head Turns

If participants become dizzy from this activity, help them step off the mat or pad. This may be an inappropriate activity for them.

⊙ Look left, then right.
⊙ Look down, then up.
⊙ Do the same wearing sunglasses or in dim lighting (Difficult).

Same Moves on Land

After performing a few of the previous activities, help participants carefully step off the balance pad and then do the same motions on the ground. They should immediately notice and appreciate the firm, solid ground and feel much more stable now. It's amazing how easy the firm ground feels after a balance pad. I say it's like getting your sea legs back!

Give It More Balance))

- Provide distractions.
  - Read while standing on the pad.
  - Juggle a ball or tap a balloon in the air (difficult).
- Change to a softer balance pad.
- Use a different pad under each foot.
- Wear sunglasses.
- Close one eye.
- Use a balance mat (this is a giant balance pad, about four feet by six feet).
  - Walk across it.
  - Walk with big steps.
  - Walk with arm swings.
- Use a foam balance beam.
- Use hedgehogs (bumpy half-domes, available from fitness catalogs and Web sites) placed beside a handrail or with a walker, at least to start.
  - Walk across six to eight of them, stepping-stone style.
  - Stand on two that are parallel or offset and try to get your balance for a moment or so.

Keep It Safe))

Balance pads, mats, and hedgehogs are for individuals or small groups where they can be used as a take-turns activity. Also, people with diabetes or peripheral neuropathies should not use balance pads. (Inadequate feedback from their feet already limits their perception of the ground, much as a balance pad does.)

If you do choose to use them, start with the firmest, largest pads. Look for pads with nonskid backing. For frail populations, large, very firm pads are the safest choice. The pad should be big enough for them to stand on with both feet. Always provide plenty of balance supports, including support on all three sides and you or a walker in front. For participants with walkers, place the pads inside the walker with a sturdy chair, a wall, or a corner behind the person. For participants without walkers, use corners, too, with a sturdy chair in front, or place the pad next to a handrail, and with yourself nearby.

Finally, prepare them for the activity. Before you begin, discuss what they'll be doing and let them feel the pads so they will know what to expect. Let them make their own choices.

Live It))

Activities on balance pads may make participants feel as if they're walking on eggshells, but the practice can engage and improve the vestibular and visual systems. Walking on eggshells is good balance practice.

HEAVY HANDS

Arm swings are important to gait. They add rhythm, flow, lift, and momentum. Unfortunately, arm swings often diminish or disappear as people age. Reasons for this include loss of strength, loss of balance confidence, and the use of walkers or canes. If hands are heavy, they're easier to swing. This activity uses rolled-up magazines to make hands heavy and facilitate arm swings. Old magazines are in almost anyone's budget, which makes this activity doable for any group.

Benefits))

- Facilitates arm swings.
- Uses proprioceptive tools.
- Uses inexpensive props that are easy to find.

Set It Up))

You'll need two magazines per person, one for each hand. They should be heavy enough that participants can feel the effect while doing arm swings (National Geographic or other glossy print magazines work best because they are heavier). Roll the magazines lengthwise. There's really no need to tape them into a roll. Half-pound or one-pound (0.2 or 0.5 kilograms) weights can also be used.

How to Do It))

The Start

Give each participant two rolled-up magazines or the light hand weights. Participants should hold one in each hand.

The Moves

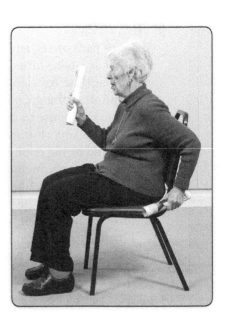

Seated Arm Swings

- Participants sit tall and brace their torso: Abs in, ribs lifted, shoulder blades back and down.
- Use the following cues:
    - Bend your elbows to about 90 degrees.
    - Begin to swing your arms.
    - Try to lift your elbows to shoulder height with each swing.
    - Can you feel the lift it gives or the pull across the trunk as each arm rises while the other is back?
    - Can you feel how the added weight assists the motion?
    - Keep going!
    - Is everyone keeping their abs braced? Good.
    - Explain that arm swings are minor perturbations (little balance disturbances), so participants should brace their core muscles. It will help them to keep stable while their arms swing.

BALANCE

Standing With Arm Swings

◉ Now those that can stand without their walkers, should try arm swings standing and walking.

◉ Brace the core muscles to prepare for the big arm swings. (See When Push Comes to Shove on page 107).

◉ Begin arm swings while simply standing with a braced core.

◉ The motion is the same as above, arms are bent and moving forward and back alternately (reciprocally).

◉ Exaggerate the arm swings so a lift is felt across their midsection.

Walking With Arm Swings

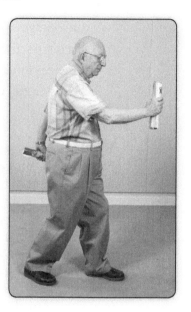

◉ When participants feel ready, they start walking. Here are some cues to use.

- Walk tall with core muscles braced.

- Chose your own stride and just let your arms swing naturally.

- Soon you should feel the lift from the swinging arms. Do you?

- Take bigger steps.

- Can you notice that the arm swings help increase stride length?

- Keep walking until you have a sense of how this should feel more naturally.

- Put away the magazines and walk tall with arm swings.

- Try longer strides with arm swings.

Keep It Safe 》

Cue stable torsos and shoulders over hips frequently; it helps. Let participants determine how much their arms swing and how big of steps to take. The standing and walking variations of this activity are not appropriate for participants with walkers. However, they can still join in with their walkers by walking tall with their ribs lifted and abs braced.

Live It 》

Arm swings provide lift and momentum to walking. They can help participants lengthen their strides.

WALKING STICKS

One important aspect of walking tall is keeping the shoulders over the hips and not leaning forward. Arm swings are useful to walking tall and gait, too; they provide extra forward momentum. Walking sticks are props that you can use to cue participants to walk with more lifted, upright torsos. You will find that both the weight and length of walking sticks are useful for facilitating arm swings and upright posture. Walking sticks also help participants feel the proprioceptive and balance differences that occur when they use upright posture and arm swings.

Benefits))

- Encourages upright posture with abs braced and ribs lifted.
- Facilitates arm swings and forward momentum.
- Engages inner senses of balance.
- Helps participants look ahead rather than down.

Set It Up))

You'll need a few pairs of walking sticks; participants can take turns. One brand is called Exerstriders. I have also used the inexpensive bamboo sticks that you can buy at the beach. They aren't perfect, but they'll work to make your point.

How to Do It))

Teach participants how to use the walking sticks properly. The technique to use is a simple alternating motion. With each arm swing they reach out with the pole and tap it lightly on the ground as they move toward it and past it. Meanwhile they'll bring the other stick forward to tap the ground with it. It's a reciprocal motion between arms and legs, similar to planting ski poles: Reach, tap, and go by. Reach, tap, and go by. Practice yourself before class if you are unfamiliar.

Hands Low

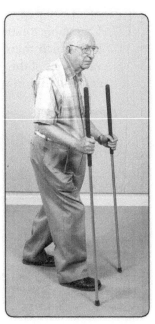

- Ask participants to place their hands on walking sticks at waist height. This low-hands position is common among seniors, especially when walking with canes or walkers.
- Invite them to walk across the room 8 to 10 feet (2.5-3 meters). As they walk across the room, talk with them about how this feels.
    - Can they feel a slight forward bend in their posture? (Yes, when their hands are low and in front.)
    - Can they sense that the stick takes some of their forward weight? (Provides some support.)
    - Ask them to remember how this hand position felt throughout their body.

Hands High

- Participants place their hands on the walking sticks at shoulder height.
- Repeat the walk across the room.
    - Try to walk a little taller, keeping your shoulders over your hips, abs braced, ribs lifted, eyes forward, and head retracted.
    - With your hands higher, can you feel how holding the poles higher helps support your effort to walk tall?
    - Is walking upright a little easier?
    - Is this position easier on your back?
    - Can you feel that the walking sticks help lift your torso into a taller position?
    - Walk across the room again, this time using your tall, ribs-lifted posture and keeping your eyes on the horizon.
    - How does that feel? Do you notice a difference walking with ribs lifted?
    - Were the walking sticks helpful?

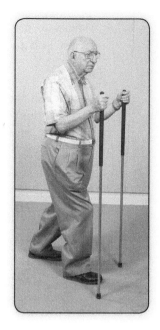

Walk With Arm Swings

- Take the walking sticks away.
- Discuss what arm swings can add to gait (i.e., momentum for forward motion, help in bringing the next leg forward).
- Ask them to walk tall again across the room. Tell them that as they walk this time, you want them to use big, exaggerated arm swings and see if they feel any differences.
    - Walk tall and create big arm swings.
    - Keep elbows bent at 90 degrees.
    - With each arm swing, lift your hands to about shoulder height—the same height where you held the stick in Hands High.
    - Do big arm swings. Be careful, but do your best!
    - Can you feel the *talling* effect of arm swings?
    - What else do you notice?
    - Rhythm and flow?
    - Lift?
    - Speed?
    - Forward momentum?
    - Grace? We can hope!

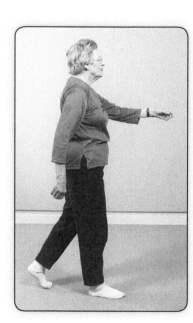

Keep It Safe))

Participants should never lean on the poles for balance support. Inexpensive walking sticks do not have a solid rubber stop on their ends, which means they could slide if leaned on and so are not particularly safe.

Live It))

Participants can give their stride a little lift with walking sticks. Walking tall and using arm swings feels good and helps lift their gaze. It improves their posture, is better for the back, and keeps them moving forward.

KEEPING YOU ON YOUR TOES

Walking on the balls of the feet takes extra balance skill. This activity will keep participants on their toes!

Benefits))

- Improves proprioceptive awareness.
- Teaches participants to maintain balance over a reduced base of support.
- Strengthens lower legs.

How to Do It))

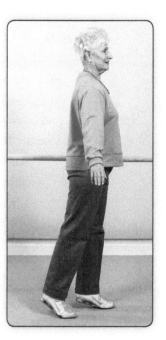

- Participants shift their weight to their toes, but do not lift their heels yet.
- Use the following cues.
  - Adjust your balance to this position for a few seconds (they should notice their weight is mostly on the toes, which dig in a bit). Do this a few times until it is comfortable.
  - Lift your heels and find your balance over the balls of your feet. Hover a moment there.
- Repeat several times so that balance on the toes seems stable for them.
- When they're ready, invite participants to walk on their toes beside a handrail or other balance support. They can hold onto the support as much as they want.
- Use these kinds of cues:
  - Shift your weight to your toes; regain your balance there a moment.
  - Lift your heels and hover a moment.
  - Are your knees soft? Abs in?
  - Ready to walk? Do you have a plan? (What do they know that will keep them balanced?)
  - Start walking. Try to take 10 steps.
  - Stop. Lower your heels and shift your weight back onto the whole foot.
- Rest and repeat.

Give It More Balance))

- Can participants walk with only a light touch on the handrail? What about not touching the support?
- Tip-Toe Hopscotch: Place agility dots or masking-tape *Xs* on the floor in an easy or modified hopscotch pattern. Participants can tip-toe through these.

Keep It Safe))

Provide plenty of hand holding and balance support. Let participants choose what they are willing to try. Be ready to help, especially the first few times.

Live It))

Tip-toe walking is good balance practice because it requires walking on a small base of support. Posture, strength, and attention to balance all come into out to play.

BALANCE

Heel walking compliments toe walking, and heel–toe motion is desirable for gait training. Heel walking tends to pitch the body backward, which can be a scary feeling and may in fact cause a fall. So be careful with any backward movements.

Benefits))

- ⊙ Improves postural control of backward momentum.
- ⊙ Strengthens lower legs.

How to Do It))

- ⊙ Participants stand with one foot a little in front of the other, shoulder-width apart.
- ⊙ Stand beside or behind the participant while the participant holds onto appropriate balance support.
- ⊙ Use the following cues.
    - Knees should be soft and core braced.
    - Shift weight to your heels (hold the chair).
    - Lift your forefeet (one at a time if it's easier, front one first).
    - Balance on your heels.
    - Get used to how that feels. Hold onto the support until you have good balance.
    - Start walking. (It will feel awkward at first.)
    - Try to take 6 to 10 steps and then stop.
    - Rest, relax, and do it again.

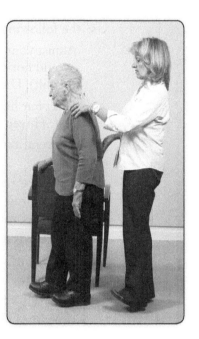

Keep It Safe))

Provide plenty of balance support and one-on-one attention. Overlap forearms with participants for greater balance safety with heel walking. They should only do what they are comfortable doing.

Live It))

Heel walking is more difficult than toe walking, but both are good practice for balance and require postural control. Controlling backward momentum is a difficult but practical balance challenge.

HEEL-TOUCH AND ROLL-UP

In walking, each step should begin with a heel strike. Then weight rolls across the foot, and off the ball of the foot. This heel–toe flowing motion is the focus of this activity.

Benefits))

- Practices aspects of normal gait mechanics.
- Improves functional range of motion at the hip, knee, and ankle.
- Practices one-legged standing.

Set It Up))

Provide appropriate balance support for each participant, such as a sturdy chair or a handrail.

How to Do It))

Participants stand beside their chair with one hand on the chair back for balance support. Feet are shoulder-width apart and offset (one foot forward, one back; the foot closest to the chair should be the back one). Their knees should be soft and their torso stable. Teach this activity in two parts.

Part I: Roll Forward and Up on Toes

- Use the following cues.
  - Rock forward and back a few times (between front and back feet).
  - Notice that when you rock forward you rock up onto your toes. (Onto balls of feet with the heels lifted.)
  - Notice that when you rock back; toes come up a bit.
  - And your weight is mostly on the back foot. Can you feel that?
- Repeat a few more times, but in a more exaggerated manner. Can they feel the rolling heel–toe motion? Then, cue the following:
  - Rock forward. Roll up onto your toes and lift heels. Hold a moment.
  - Rock back; toes lift.
  - Notice how it feels to roll across the heel and up onto the toes.
  - Rock back, and lift the toes in the back position. Good.

BALANCE

Part II: Add a Knee Lift

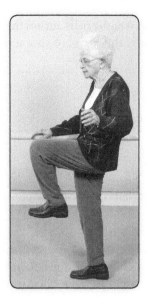 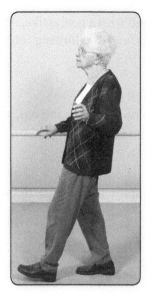 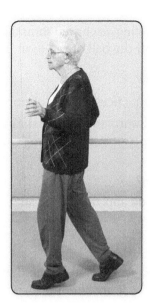

◉ Use the following cues.
- With one hand on the handrail, rock forward, rock back, and then lift the front knee as part of the rocking-back motion.
- Balance for just a moment on the back leg, with your knee lifted.
- Touch the front heel down, and roll forward onto it, heel–toe style.
- Rock and roll all the way across the foot and up onto your toes.
- Rock back and lift the knee again. Hold a moment and balance.
- Repeat it all together: Rock back, knee lift, and hold; roll forward, heels up.
- Rock back, lift the knee, and hold; roll forward, heels up.
◉ Have participants walk to the other side of the handrail and repeat with the other leg.

Give It More Balance))

◉ Hold the knee lift a few seconds.
◉ Hold onto the balance support less tightly.
◉ Intermediate: Lift the outside arm up and directly overhead during the roll-up.
◉ Advanced: Place hands on hips, so there is no touching the chair.

Keep It Safe))

Take it slow and easy. Keep participants close to their chairs, and watch them for their confidence and comfort level. Again, it is the rocking and rolling that makes this one-legged standing so easy and natural.

Live It))

Rocking and rolling provides good movement cues and a certain rhythm; it's very much like gait, too. If the weight shifts are complete and rhythmical, participants can likely balance themselves on one leg, if even for a moment longer than previously thought.

ROCK FORWARD, KNEE LIFT

This gait activity, Rock Forward, Knee Lift is the most similar to walking. Bringing the rear leg forward to take a step, and rolling the body weight across the foot from heel to toe is the foot motion you want participants to practice.

Benefits))

- Works on gait, including swinging the rear leg forward.
- Improves internal sense of balance via attention to weight shifts (somatic learning).
- Practices one-legged standing.
- Improves functional range of motion at the hip, knee, and ankle.

Set It Up))

Provide balance support for each participant—a sturdy chair, handrail, or walker.

How to Do It))

- Use the following cues.
    - Stand at the side of your chair, holding onto the chair with one hand. The feet are offset; the foot closest to the chair should be forward.
    - Rock forward and back a few times.
    - When you're ready, rock forward and lift the rear knee up and forward.
    - Hold for just a moment.
    - Put the lifted foot back down to where it started behind you, toe to heel, then rock back, again.
    - When you stop, most of your weight should be on the back leg again.
- Repeat the sequence several times.
- Do the other leg from the other side of the chair.

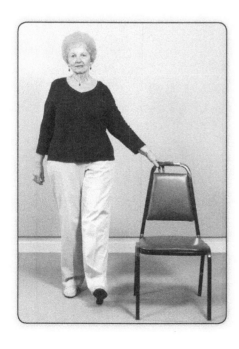 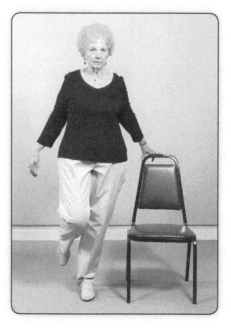

Give It More Balance))

⊙ Do more repetitions.
⊙ Give it some rhythm. Count a rhythm with them, call the cues with a clear cadence, or use music.
⊙ Hold onto the chair only loosely.
⊙ Intermediate: Add Rock Back, Knee Lift to the sequence: Rock forward knee lift; rock back, knee lift.
⊙ Intermediate: Increase hold times at the end of movements.
⊙ Intermediate: Try Rock and Walk from the Rhythm and Moves section (see page 322).
⊙ Intermediate: Lift the outside arm as the knee comes up and forward.
⊙ Advanced: Do the easier versions without touching the chair.

Keep It Safe))

Take it slow and keep participants close to their balance supports.

Live It))

Rock and roll for the 80- and 90-year-olds—who would have thought it? These activities mimic important footfall patterns and weight-transfer elements of gait. The rhythm and rocking make gait flow better and make one-legged standing much more doable.

COUNTRY-WESTERN HEEL AND TOE

Everyone knows what country-western leg swings are about: heel touches forward, toe touches back, and whooping "Yee-haw!" And so it is with this activity for gait training and balance. The leg swing and foot motion of this activity can help with the leg swing and foot motion of walking, and the brief time spent on one foot is balance practice.

Benefits))

- Practices sequential movements that may have some carryover to gait.
- Improves core stability.
- Practices one-legged standing.
- Uses music.

Set It Up))

Provide balance support for each participant (sturdy chair, handrail, or walker). Find a slow to moderate country-western song that has a nice heel–toe beat.

How to Do It))

First, teach just the heel-touch.

Heel-Touch

- Have participants stand beside their chair with their feet parallel, shoulder-width apart. They can touch their chair with one hand and put their other hand on their hip. Knees are soft, cores are braced.
- Have them place one heel out in front. Say, "Heel" (use leg farthest from the chair).
- They draw it back and place it beside the other again. Say, "Together."
- Repeat a few times, using one word for each motion (heel, together, heel, together).
- Keep the pace slow and deliberate.
- Participants move to the other side of the chair and change legs.
- Repeat the sequence.

Toe-Touch Back

- Those who feel they can, may add a toe-touch back.
- Participants stand beside their chair with feet parallel and shoulder-width apart, knees soft.
- Have them touch one heel out in front (cue "Heel").
- Have them swing the leg back and touch the toes on the ground behind them (cue "Toe"). (See Step and Stop on page 237.)
- Repeat several times at half-speed. (Heel, pause, toe, pause; it's a stop-and-start rhythm.)
- Participants switch legs.

Add Music

- Play music.
- Do the heel-touch, feet together version first.

- ⊙ Those who want to can progress to heel–toe leg swings.
- ⊙ Call the movements at half-speed.
- ⊙ Participants can stop and start wherever they want. Be their model, but let them find the rhythm.

Give It More Balance))

- ⊙ Hold onto the chair loosely.
- ⊙ Change legs every few times (stay on same side of the chair).
- ⊙ Put hands on hips. (Intermediate to advanced)
- ⊙ Advanced: Add reciprocal arm swings (the left arm swings forward when the right foot is out).

Keep It Safe))

Let participants choose what they want to do and find their own pace.

Live It))

This activity is helpful for gait and balance and is fun to do with music.

BALANCE

AGILITY LADDERS

Former British Prime Minister David Lloyd-George once said, "You can't cross a chasm in two small jumps." I think what he meant is that big steps can be scary but are sometimes necessary to get where you want. Big steps often take you from where you safely stand to a spot that's way over there. In this activity, participants discover how step height can help lengthen their stride. They will also recall elements of Belly Button Training and the knee lifts practiced previously. Prior learning will definitely help them take this next big step.

Benefits))

- ◉ Improves stride length, strength, and balance.
- ◉ Practices transitions (moving from one position to another).
- ◉ Generates and controls momentum.
- ◉ Builds on previous activities.

Set It Up))

You will need masking tape or chalk to create an agility ladder with about 12 rungs spaced progressively farther apart, 12 to 30 inches (51-76 centimeters) at the widest. Put the ladders next to a handrail for balance support. If a handrail is not available, plan on holding one or both hands (or forearms and elbows) as participants step through the ladder.

How to Do It))

The easiest way to increase step length is to increase step height. That means a bigger knee lift before taking a big step. Also remind participants about Belly Steps (see page 242) and how their trunk (belly button) needs to follow their foot in order to take a successful big step.

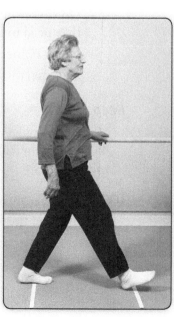

BALANCE

- ◉ Participants will need to take turns on the ladder. Have them start at the end with the rungs closest together.
- ◉ Instruct participants to begin each step on the ladder with a big knee lift and to follow the step with their torso, as they did in Belly Button Training.
- ◉ Cue them also to set visual targets and look a few steps ahead on the agility ladder; two or three rungs ahead is a good start. Looking down at each step will not be helpful.
- ◉ Use the following cues.
  - Look a few steps ahead.
  - Knee lift and step forward to the first line. Land heel–toe.
  - Move forward to the next line, using the same knee lift and step motion. Keep going.
  - How's it going? What worked?

- Did the knee lifts help you get farther?
- Did it help to focus on your torso moving toward the stepping foot?
- How about looking ahead—did the visual targets help?
- Do a few steps where your foot moves out but you don't move the torso forward. Can you feel a difference? (It's a big difference!)
- Do it again, moving the torso forward. Does that work better?
- Try it with no knee lift.
- Try it with a knee lift.
- Big difference? (For sure!)

Agility Ladder—Sidestepping

- This is an intermediate to difficult activity where participants step through the ladder moving sideways.
- Use the same techniques—big knee lift, belly moves with stepping leg.
- Participants sidestep through the agility ladder between the rungs.
  - Abs are braced, ribs are lifted, shoulder blades are back and down, and knees are soft.
  - Step together, step.
  - Step together, step.
  - Knee lift, step with trunk following, and transfer.
  - Knee lift, step, and transfer.

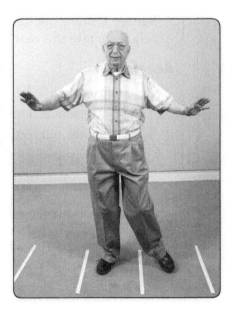

Give It More Balance))

- Use less support (hold both hands lightly, hold just one of their hands, or hold one hand lightly).
- Intermediate: Take four steps and stop (they have to control momentum).
- Go slower on some passes and faster for others; slow will be more difficult and they need to control the change of pace.
- Reach to the side with each step: Step, reach; step, reach.
- Side step through with hands on hips or out to the side.

Keep It Safe))

Make sure you can supervise participants closely. Hold their hands and forearms. Do the activity individually for the first several times, and with a handrail until they are willing to try it on their own.

Live It))

Crossing over the physical chasms in life is easier with big knee lifts and eyes on the goal.

AGILITY GRIDS

Agility grids are preplanned stepping patterns. Repeating the preset patterns make certain components of gait more symmetrical.

Benefits))

- Practices agility skills.
- Improves gait symmetry.
- Requires postural control.

Set It Up))

Make a grid or grids using masking tape or chalk. Decide on stepping patterns for each. Think of it like hopscotch for your grandpa. Hopscotch can be a pattern, but we don't want them jumping between squares. The squares should be wide enough for a foot to land in and long enough that the forward pattern is similar to a step length. I usually make a grid about 4 to 6 spaces (foot spaces) across and 10 to 12 spaces long. It depends on how much space, time, and tape you have. Then put markers (dots, numbers, or *Xs*) to mark the pattern you want them to use.

The easiest pattern would be right down the middle— a right-left, right-left walking pattern. Intermediate might be wide-wide, narrow-narrow stepping patterns, or a mix. Advanced skills might call for cross-over steps. Over time you can add dual tasks, by having them keep a rhythm to their steps, recite an old jump rope song, or toss a ball from hand to hand.

How to Do It))

Easy Grids

These patterns are similar to a normal walking gait.

Moderate Grids

These grids require bigger steps and more complicated stepping patterns.

Hard Grids

This grid requires cross-over stepping patterns.

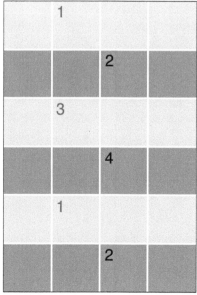

Easy grids

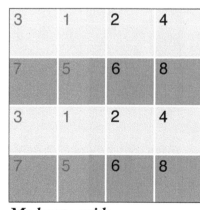

Moderate grids

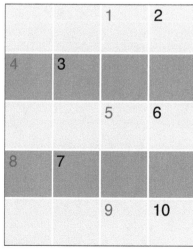

Difficult grids

BALANCE

Give It More Balance))

- Have them go through the course at a cadence.
- Challenge them to do it a little faster.
- Have participants recite a nursery rhyme or count backward by 4 from 101.
- Have them walk through the grid kayaking with a stick.

Keep It Safe))

For groups, make two grids, one easier than the other. Everyone should be able to try at least one grid. Be available to hold hands or put them along a railing. Participants should only do what they are comfortable doing.

Live It))

Agility grids are not unlike maneuvering through the aisles of grocery stores, places of worship, or theaters. These grids will increase balance confidence in real-life situations and help with everyday transitions.

PUDDLE JUMPING

Kids jump into puddles and teenagers prefer to drive through them; both do it with wild abandonment. Grown-ups jump over them. It's such fun! The art of staying dry makes a good ABLE Bodies balance practice activity.

Puddle Jumping requires a plan. It also requires greater step height and length. Participants must commit to the forward move. They need to initiate the movement with a big knee lift and follow through (as in Belly Button Training). They will land best if they use a heel–toe motion. Coming to a stop after a big step means they'll need to explore how to stop forward momentum of their center of gravity. Have fun with this activity; it may become a productive favorite.

Benefits ⟩⟩

- Increases step length and height.
- Practices momentum control.
- Requires a cognitive plan.
- Develops transferable skill for everyday life in a fun, easily adaptable activity.

Set It Up ⟩⟩

You will need some targets to be imaginary pieces of dry ground; masking tape or agility dots work best. Agility dots, available from fitness equipment stores and Web sites, are preferable because you can easily move them to suit participants. Some dots also have nonskid features on one side. They would be safest to use. Do not use paper dots or other materials that may slip out from under participants' feet. Practice with the materials yourself so you can be sure the targets do not skid.

Near a handrail, put out some agility dots in a stepping pattern. Place them at distances apart that you know they can do. After a few passes, you can increase the distance between them. Here are four basic patterns:

- Offset, in a left–right walking pattern, similar to stepping stones
- Straight line
- Curve or figure eight
- Random (straight, offset, changing distances and shapes)

How to Do It ⟩⟩

Practice the Stepping Motion

- Participants practice beside their chairs, first.
- Provide them the opportunity to check out the difference that knee height makes to step length.
  - Knee lift and start step.
  - Move to forward position, land heel–toe.
  - Bring up the back leg beside the other. Safe landing!
  - Repeat a few times (use various knee heights).
- Once they move away from the chairs, your close supervision or taking turns is necessary.

Puddle Jumps

- Start with the puddles set up by a handrail.
- Taking turns, participants take big steps across the dot pattern, one dot at a time.
- Stay nearby so you can help as needed.
- Use the following cues.
  - Stand with both feet on one dot.
  - Target the dot on which you plan to land.
  - Make a plan that will get you there. (They should be thinking of what techniques they can use.)
  - Knee lift—get good height for the greatest distance!
  - Step out to the targeted dot.
  - Follow the foot forward with your torso (as in Belly Button Training).
  - Land heel–toe.
  - Bring the other foot beside the forward foot.
  - Stop and settle (abs in and ribs lifted helps; as does When Push Comes to Shove).
  - Look for the next dot and make a plan.

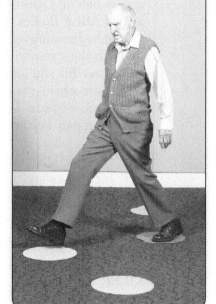

Give It More Balance))

- Hold their hands instead of having them use handrail.
- Can they jump puddles on their own? (Set dots away from handrails. Still have them take turns. You stay close for safety.).
- Use more difficult patterns or distances.
- Dim the lights.
- Combine with another task, like singing a nursery rhyme.
- Use this concept in other activities; for example, add puddle-jumping dots to the River Fun games.

Keep It Safe))

Use nonskid materials as stepping targets. Test them ahead of time on your floors. Stay nearby. Encourage participants to plan ahead for their challenge.

Live It))

Balance training should be imaginative, fun, and as engaging as possible. This activity carries over to real-life situations. Big knee lifts and following the traveling foot will help carry participants over the great divides of life.

LIFE'S LITTLE HURDLES

Hurdles are an advanced challenge. They make a good next step after Agility Ladders. To clear a hurdle, participants must lift their knees high. High knee lifts increase step length but are a greater balance challenge. The fall risk and length of time spent on one leg is greater with higher knee lifts. Two stepping patterns are used here: sidestepping and heel–toe stepping over the hurdles.

Benefits))

- Improves mobility and agility.
- Improves leg strength and range of motion.
- Increases stride length and step height.
- Facilitates heel–toe motion.
- Facilitates preplanning.
- Practices momentum control.

Set It Up))

You will need four to eight hurdles. Look for brightly colored, lightweight hurdles that are no more than 4 to 6 inches (10-15 centimeters) tall. Most hurdles can be set flat or high. Ease participants into hurdles by starting with the flat side down until they are familiar with the tasks.

How to Do It))

Sidestep Over One Hurdle

Participants will sidestep over a hurdle, one foot at a time, and then step back. Tell them to leave enough room for both feet on each side of the hurdle.

- Remind participants they will be using the tactics of Plan Ahead, Belly Button Training, and Knee Lift, Abs In as they step over the hurdles.
    - Plan Ahead means think of useful tactics and step wide enough so there is room for both feet when side stepping.
    - Belly Button means their belly follows the moving foot.
    - Knee Lift, Abs In will help them keep stability when lifting knees.
- Here are some cues to use for sidestepping over the hurdles.
    - Master one hurdle first.
    - Knee lift and step over with one foot (plan to step far enough to make room for the other foot).
    - Transfer your weight (and belly button) to that side and foot.
    - Move the other foot over and get stable (stand tall with abs braced and ribs lifted).
    - Don't make the next move until you're ready.
    - Knee lift, step over, transfer weight, feet together, and stabilize.
    - Repeat until you find a rhythm for stepping over and back.
    - See how much the knee lift helps?
    - Did thinking about Belly Button Training help?

Sidestep Over Several Hurdles (Flat-Side Down)

Place four to six hurdles in a row, about 18 inches (46 centimeters) apart, flat side down. The goal is to sidestep over the flat-side down hurdles, one at a time to start. (Think Step and Stop, see page 237.)

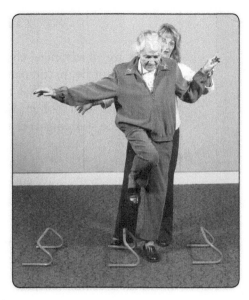

- Let participants figure out their footwork on their own.
- Encourage them to find a pattern and use a rhythm.
- Use the following cues.
   - Step one foot over, feel the weight transfer, and bring over the other foot.
   - Step, together, step, stop. (One hurdle cleared.)
   - Step, together, step, stop. (Next hurdle cleared.)
   - Posture check—are you standing tall and stable?
- If you need to act as a spotter, stand behind the participant and hold their wrists.

Sidestep Over Tall Hurdles

Turn the hurdles tall-side up.

- Participants sidestep over the hurdles, one at a time, just like the previous activity (step, together, step, stop).
- Cue higher knee lifts and weight-transfer awareness (Belly Button transfers).
- Connect more steps.
- Cue good posture.
- Cue pattern and rhythm.
- Add more balance by connecting more steps and using shorter stops.

Heel–Toe Walking Over Hurdles

Instead of sidestepping across hurdles, participants will step perpendicularly over the hurdles in a heel–toe manner. Their goal is to clear each hurdle using a rolling heel–toe foot motion. Your job is to help them discover how best to do that. Practicing previously learned skills in a new environment is a way of linking new learning to older learning. Here are a few suggestions worth reviewing to help facilitate success at hurdles: Knee lifts, foot flexion, and Belly Button Training.

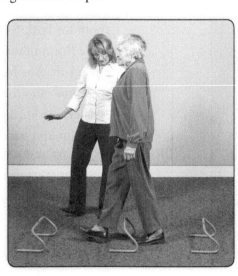

- Knee lift: Training for knee lifts helps with both step height and step length. The knee lifting activities practiced previously might be helpful (Knee Lift, Abs In; Marching in Place; and Rock Forward, Knee Lift). Practice some good knee lifts before starting these hurdles.

- Foot flexion: As they lift the forward-stepping leg, cue them to flex that foot. This readies the foot to clear the hurdle (not snag it) and to land, prepared to roll from heel to toe. Practice knee lift with foot flexion.
- Belly Button Training: These techniques also may help participants clear hurdles. Once they put their foot down, they need to move over it. The momentum of moving forward will help generate the next step, and the next, and so on. Practice knee lift, foot flexion, and Belly Steps.

Head for the hurdles and do a row of them, maybe flat side down at first, then tall side up.

- One participant crosses at a time, near a handrail or with you holding their hands.
- Slow but with cadence works best: knee lift, belly step, knee lift, belly step.
- Can you get them to look ahead?

Give It More Balance))

- Move the hurdles a little farther apart.
- Add a few more hurdles.
- Play some music.

Keep It Safe))

Participants should take turns. You should stay close, hold their hands, and talk them through the activity.

Live It))

Life's Little Hurdles can be fun *and* they improve agility and gait. Practice variations in gait and agility challenges using various patterns and rhythms.

BALANCE

HEDGEHOGS

Hedgehogs are also known as *agility domes*. They are brightly colored half-domes with a bumpy top. The dome is air-filled and compliant, making them difficult to balance on. The bumps stimulate sensors on the bottoms of the feet, providing more information about what's going on beneath the feet. The goal of this activity is for participants to walk across the backs of the hedgehogs.

Benefits))

- Increases kinesthetic awareness.
- Provides a difficult transitional challenge.
- Takes courage and builds confidence.
- Uses colorful, fun toys.

Set It Up))

You'll need a clear, safe area, near a handrail. I also recommend having an extra walker for participants to share. Hedgehogs or agility domes normally come in 6- and 10-inch (15- and 25-centimeter) sizes. You will need enough to place them 12 inches (30 centimeters) apart in a walking pattern (as if they were footprints) alongside a handrail.

How to Do It))

One at a time with you by their side, guide your participants across the hedgehog path. Get them to keep putting one foot in front of the other. Use the following cues:

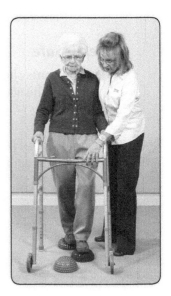

- Take your time.
- Knees should be soft and posture upright.
- Place your foot on one hedgehog and just keep traveling right over to the next hedgehog.
- Your weight just moves towards and then over each hedgehog, from one to the next.
- Can you look ahead two or three hedgehogs? It will help keep you moving forward smoothly.

Give It More Balance))

- Place hedgehogs farther apart.
- Place hedgehogs in a straighter line.
- Put a few hedgehogs into River Fun activities (page 334) or obstacle courses (only if you can be nearby).

Keep It Safe))

Understandably, Hedgehogs are an advanced activity. But with a walker and you by their side, many participants of intermediate skill can cross over hedgehogs. It's a real "Wow! I did it!" confidence builder. I think all participants should try it with a walker first, and it should always be closely supervised by you.

Live It))

This tough activity takes balance control and integrates several systems of balance. These toys can really boost balance confidence.

TRAFFIC SCHOOL

Every day participants must navigate the world in very physical ways. They go through doorways; they make turns. They hurry to catch up with friends; they slow down so as not to spill their coffee. They step over mud puddles and curbs. They change directions and pace. All of these situations challenge their balance. Staying active means maintaining the ability to navigate in normal situations. The challenges of ABLE Bodies' Traffic School include Change of Pace; Red Light, Green Light; and all kinds of fun ways to practice changes in pace and direction. You can do the activities separately or mix them up as participants improve. Lengthen the time spent walking to build cardiorespiratory endurance. Traffic school can make a great WalkAbout, too (see chapter 8).

Benefits))

- Practices everyday challenges in walking.
- Integrates many components of balance.
- Builds endurance in a fun and social way.

Set It Up))

- You need only a large room, clear of tripping hazards. Allow room for participants to spread out, change directions, or form a London Bridge.
- Props are optional. However, you can create some props, such as direction arrows, cones, a stop sign, a green light, a red light, and a yellow light.
- Plan ahead for the challenges you'll use. The activity will go better if you have a list.
- Plan the flow of traffic and the order of challenges.
- Anticipate traffic flow and walkers.
- Pull out your drill sergeant's voice.

How to Do It))

Have participants line up on one side of the room. For greater challenge, split the group and put half at each end of your room—they will be walking past each other to further complicate the challenge. Stand where you can face the group and they can see your hand signals as well as hear your voice.

Change of Pace

Explain to participants you will be asking them to walk across the room at varying speeds. Their mission is to follow your commands (smile when you say that) to slow down or speed up. They should change pace, accelerating or decelerating as quickly as they safely can. Use the following cues:

- Get ready, get set, go!
- Walk fast.
- Walk slow.
- Walk very slow, even slower than that.
- Speed up, walk fast, faster.
- Slow down, down, down, and stop.

BALANCE

Red Light, Green Light

Explain that when you announce or signal a green light, their mission is to cross from one side of the room to the other as quickly as they can. When you announce or signal a red light, they should stop as quickly as they safely can. You may also use a yellow caution for slowing down. The object of the game, of course, is to see who gets across the room first. Speak loudly and clearly, facing the group.

- Ready, set, go!
- Go carefully!
- Red light! (Hold up your arms or the red signal.)
- Green light! (Bring your arms down or hold up the green signal.)
- Violators will be prosecuted! (Or whatever—make it fun.)
- Caution (yellow light). Slowly lower your hands, palms down, like saying "whoa, slow down!"
- Blinking red light (stop, go, stop, go).

Continue until they cross the room. Make times between lights unpredictable. Have some fun!

Changes in Direction

Explain to participants that they will be following commands to make turns left or right. There may be a traffic circle to go around (this could be a small group of chairs you have set up for them to circle). Only do left and right turns at first, and do not ask them to turn while walking fast. They should comply as quickly as they safely can with the traffic challenges. Speak loudly and clearly, facing the group.

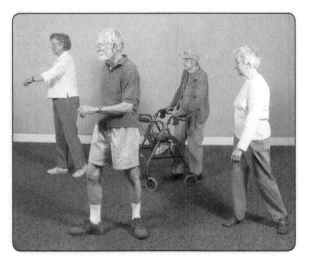

- Start walking.
- Walk faster.
- Slower.
- Turn right and keep walking.
- Speed up.
- Slow down, turn left, and stop.
- Go around a traffic circle at the end of the room.
- Keep going.

Window Shopping

This activity is simply walking with head turns. As participants walk across the room, they window shop—every four to six steps, have them look left or right. Watch them for signs of getting dizzy. Let them know it could happen and if it does, they should stop and get your help. Use the following cues.

- Start walking.
- Look over there—is that a donut shop with the lights on?
- Look to the left—there are some nice dresses and suits at that store.

- Look at your neighbor.
- Look down "Did someone walk their dog this morning, yuck!, step over that!"
- There's a shoe store on the right – is that your size?
- It's a bird, it's a plane, it's Superman! (It's a cue to look up)
- Keep walking and Window Shopping.

Pivot Turns and Corners

This advanced variation involves pivots and walking into and out of corners or other tight spots. This activity may be especially helpful, though difficult, for participants with Parkinson's disease (PD). Sometimes PD participants freeze and cannot take a step when they walk into corners or through doorways. Use the following cues.

- Walk ahead.
- Walk faster.
- Turn left and keep walking.
- Do a pivot and keep walking.
- Keep walking. Pivot and stop.
- Walk to a corner of the room.
- Walk right into the corner and pivot out of the corner.
- Walk away fast.
- Walk slow, slower, very slowly.
- Can you stop with just one foot on the ground?

London Bridge

This intermediate activity gives participants something to duck underneath. It's a balance challenge to lower their frame over their feet to pass under a bridge-like obstacle.

The bridge can be made of participants holding their arms up as people go under. Ask several participants to form a bridge by holding their arms over a pathway. These bridge tenders can then have some fun lowering or raising the bridge as they see fit for their buddies walking underneath. The bridge could also be a cloth or a bar you set up ahead of time. If you have an actual overhanging stairway or other piece of architecture, they can duck under that, too. Variety is the spice of good balance training.

Prepare the people who will be going under the bridge. Before they duck, cue them to brace their core, bend their knees, and drop their hips back. Demonstrate this for them and then have them practice these mechanics before they begin. Use the following cues.

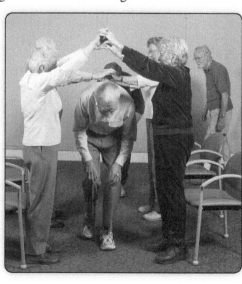

- Group A: Form a bridge!
- Be a sturdy bridge. Your friends are going under.
    - Feet are set, knees soft, abs braced, and ribs lifted.
    - Join hands at the top.
- Group B: Under the bridge we go!
    - Feet are wide set, knees bent, and abs braced.
    - Lower yourself and start walking under the bridge.
    - Good job! Keep moving until the whole troop passes through.

- Group B, be the bridge; group A, get ready!
- A participant who doesn't want to go under could be a toll collector at the bridge entrance. Each traveler must high five him before going under.

Traffic Circles

Traffic Circles are just another way to be creative while lightly jostling your participants a bit. They can be just a few sets of circles of chairs that they circle around; or the activity can turn into Opposing Circles and High Fives (see page 255). You might also create traffic jams. In traffic jams, people walk close, starting, stopping, accelerating, slowing, moving right, moving left, and maybe even waving, yelling, or talking on their cell phones. Be careful and keep it safe for your group's ability.

Keep It Safe))

Be sure to speak clearly, facing the group. Use hand and voice commands together so that your instructions are clear. Many of your participants are hard of hearing. It's perfectly okay for anyone to opt out at any time. Find ways to make opting out easy and not embarrassing. Give alternatives, or have someone less able help you in some way. For instance, they could stand by their walker and be a toll collector, whose hand each person must tap. Explain that slow traffic happens and others must deal with that too. Pass on the right.

Live It))

Life is full of surprises, just like traffic. There will always be a need to make changes in pace and direction and time for window shopping. Practice helps participants be ready, willing, and ABLE.

BALANCE

SHAKE A LEG

Reminiscent of the Hokey Pokey, keeping your balance on one leg while the other is moving is difficult. Try it yourself! Limb movements disturb balance. Practicing such a feat, though, helps participants better control their balance.

Benefits))

- Facilitates kinesthetic sense for balance.
- Practices balance recovery and postural control.
- Uses visual targets.
- Incorporates one-legged stance.

How to Do It))

Have participants stand beside their sturdy chair with one hand touching the back of the chair. Participants with walkers should use their walker for their balance support in front and a chair should be placed behind them.

Belly Button Weight Transfers

Use the following cues.

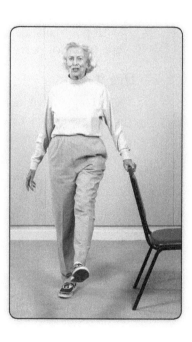

- Transfer weight (belly-button style) onto one leg and then back to the other.
- Repeat a few times, until it feels comfortable.
- Transfer weight to one leg, hold, and steady yourself.
- When you're ready, lift the other leg and pull that knee up in front of the down leg.
- Do you notice that bringing the knee up to the front and center of the supporting foot better balances your weight more directly over the supporting foot?
- Hold steady a moment on one leg.
    - Keep your gaze steady, ahead at the horizon.
    - Find a visual target to concentrate on there.
- Touch the foot back down and shift the weight back onto both legs
- Repeat.

Shake a Leg

Participants come into a one-legged stance and get steady. When they're ready, practice these variations. They can set their foot down every once in awhile to rest and regroup. Use the following cues.

- Point the toe and flex the foot of the up leg.
- Do ankle circles.
- Good job! Try it again.
- Next, bend and extend the knee. Do it again.
- Be careful—go slow.

- Rest time! Put your foot down. Rest, recover. Balance on one leg again.
- Lift the leg out to the side and bring it back.
- Cross your body with it.
- Push it back behind you.
- Put your foot down. Rest, recover. Balance on one leg again.
- Switch legs to train both.

Give It More Balance))

- Vary the motions randomly instead of doing the same motion two or three times.
- Decrease length of rest time.
- Dim the lights or wear sunglasses or Heads-up glasses.
- Advanced: Do the activity standing on a balance pad.

Keep It Safe))

Make sure participants carefully find their balance over each leg before they move the other. Remind them to keep their gaze steady and on the horizon. Switch legs frequently to provide more rest. Provide lots of balance support—sturdy chairs, maybe on both sides; walkers; corners of rooms; and so on. Place a chair behind participants with poor balance or those who use a walker. Let them decide what they are willing to try. Monitor participants closely.

Live It))

One-legged balance is tricky business, but participants use it many times a day undertaking everyday tasks such as climbing stairs or stepping over obstacles. Shake a Leg is good balance practice for postural control.

WALK IN THE PARK

A walk in the park is about distractions. When you take a walk, you're enjoying time to yourself. You may be looking at wildflowers, wildlife, or kids playing in the park. You may be talking with a friend or distracted by your dog's behavior. The point here is, you're not concentrating on your walking or balance. You're environmentally distracted and balance is automatic. Using distractions or dual tasks is a balance training tool for many ABLE Bodies activities, including this one.

Benefits))

- ⊙ Engages and integrates systems for balance.
- ⊙ Practices gait under varied conditions.
- ⊙ Negotiates obstacles.
- ⊙ Encourages everyday mobility.

Set It Up))

You'll need a clear, safe room to walk across; a route plan, including various obstacles, lighting conditions, and paths; and various distractions:

- ⊙ Something easily read while walking, such as large-print magazines, newsletters, a funny story or joke you've printed in a large font, or a list for treasure hunting.
- ⊙ Medium-size ball to juggle or toss.
- ⊙ Sunglasses or Heads-up glasses.
- ⊙ Planned obstacles.
- ⊙ Masking tape (for marking curbs and circles).
- ⊙ A short step (more like a real curb).
- ⊙ Items and a list for a treasure hunt.
- ⊙ Dog leash (a rope used to simulate the pull of a pet after a squirrel).

How to Do It))

Talk with participants about why this activity is helpful for balance and gait. Give them their mission and then get started.

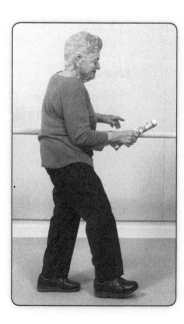

- ⊙ Give them each a large-print magazine or a page that is easy to read as shown here.
- ⊙ Set up a treasure hunt (so they must walk with head turns to spot items). Make it as complicated or easy as you have time to do. Hunt for pictures of birds, animals, people (celebrities, presidents, police officers), and places (fountains, places of worship, homes). Clip the pictures from magazines and then spread them around the room at various heights. You can give them a list of items (read and walk), announce the items as they walk, or ask them to remember the list (cognitive task). Only use a few items, especially the first time, such as three animals, so you learn what works and how they like it.
- ⊙ Walk and juggle. Give participants one ball to toss from hand to hand, or if they have pockets, have them move their keys from one pocket to the other.

- Jump (actually, take a big step) over a puddle or two (agility discs or taped circles).
- Trudge through knee-deep snow (use their imagination; it's slow, big knee lifts with arm swings that help them while trudging forward).
- Manage an escaping pet (as they walk by you, grab the leash, and tug it).
- Walk around a public fountain (tape on the floor).
- Walk along a curb (tandem line by a handrail).
- Step up onto a curb (small step you've put out; have them use Belly Step Up, from Belly Button Training).
- Walk with head turns to spot real or imagined sights.
- Walk under a bridge (go through a doorway).
- Vary the path pattern, directions, and pace.

Give It More Balance))

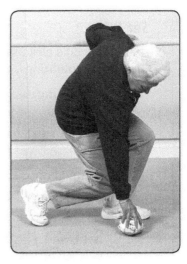

- Walk up a few stairs or step over a few obstacles.
- Pick up leaves or pinecones (or wadded-up paper balls as shown here).
- Look up to spot a bird in a tree.
- Look backward over the shoulder. (Walk along a handrail, one hand holding on. Look back over the outside shoulder.)
- Walk at dusk (dim the lights).
- Walk at high noon (wear sunglasses).
- Walk sideways.
- Advanced: Take off a sweater or put one on.

Keep It Safe))

Keep it simple. Use just a few options for the treasure hunt; too many can cause problems. You can present a variety over time. Cue participants to make plans and ask them what might help. Provide handrails and other touch supports (walls, counters) liberally.

Live It))

Hopefully, these tasks will help them get out there and enjoy their world and community. Practicing outside walking indoors can make that task a little easier.

IT'S A REACH

Reaching is an everyday skill, but it can pose a balance risk. Tipping points change with foot and body positions. This activity educates participants to reach smarter and safer. By redistributing their body weight they will be less likely to loose their balance when reaching for what they want.

Benefits))

- ◉ Teaches participants about their tipping point and how to control it.
- ◉ Creates safer reaching techniques.
- ◉ Links with Venus de Milo Arms and Anchors A-Sway (see Posture Affects Function and Balance, page 101) .

Set It Up))

You will need the following for this activity:

- ◉ Large, sturdy table (the top provides the reaching distance).
- ◉ Objects for them to reach. Some examples are car keys, remote controls, or prizes such as candy kisses, small toys, or movie coupons
- ◉ Masking tape

Strategically place the objects on the table, some close, others farther away. Put the more desirable items almost out of ordinary reach. Use masking tape to place a line on the floor. They must stand behind the line in order to reach for the objects of desire.

How to Do It))

Warm up and stretch the shoulders with shoulder rolls, reaching stretches, and neck stretches.

Reach With Knees Straight and Feet Parallel

Use the following cues.

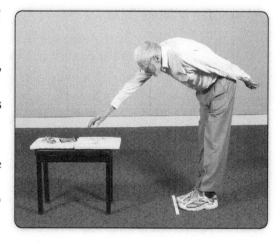

- ◉ Stand with feet parallel, toes behind the line, and knees straight.
- ◉ Reach for an object, keeping your knees straight. (Hinge forward from hip.)
    - Reach a little farther.
    - Do you feel your weight shift toward the table when your knees are straight?
    - Can you begin to feel a tipping point? (They will)

Reach With Hips Back and Feet Offset

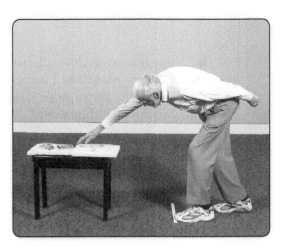

The assignment for participants is to notice how this position works and how it affects their personal tipping point. Use the following cues.

- Stand with feet offset and shoulder-width apart (one foot forward, one back). The front foot is on the line.
- Bend your hips and knees. (Hips move backward so that they are over or beyond the back foot.)
- Now reach for the object you'd like.
    - Do you notice any differences with your feet offset?
    - Has your tipping point changed? Where is it now? (It's farther back.)
    - Why do you think it changed? (More of their weight is behind the line.)
    - Can you tell your weight is redistributed?
    - Reach again. Does this feel better? Safer?
    - Use your Venus de Milo arms to reach even farther (use length from ribs and shoulder extending toward the object).
- Compare the choices.
    - Repeat with straight knees and parallel feet, as you did earlier.
    - Repeat again with offset foot position and hips back.
    - Do you feel the difference? Did one feel like you could reach farther more safely?
    - Good, grab some goodies!

Give It More Balance))

- While participants are reaching in the correct position (offset feet, hips back), have them reach the other arm backward.
- Ask them if that helps. (It's an even better redistribution of weight.)

Keep It Safe))

Use a sturdy prize table; it may be needed to help arrest lost balance. The pictured table is too short and unstable to provide adequate balance support. A dining room table works great. Participants should only reach as far as they feel is comfortable and safe.

Live It))

Tipping points change with foot and body positions. Participants can safely reach farther with their best foot forward and their hips back.

HAT TRICK

Reaching overhead, such as into a closet for a hat, may be a fall risk for many frail elders. Again, foot positioning makes a difference. So does which way they pull the item off the shelf. This challenge helps participants with overhead reaches.

Benefits))

- Provides progression for horizontal reaching (It's a Reach).
- Enhances balance and posture awareness.
- Experiments with techniques and posture.

Set It Up))

You'll need a hat box or reasonable facsimile, something lightweight and easy to grab; a high shelf (real or imagined; imagined ones are safer); and balance support for your participants.

How to Do It))

Warm up and stretch the shoulders with shoulder rolls, reaching stretches, and neck stretches.

Tug an Overhead Arm Backward

Use the following cues.

- Stand Lucy Goosey style
    - Unbraced abs
    - Straight, locked knees
- Keeping one hand (or one leg) touching a balance support.
    - Reach one arm up and overhead.
    - Tug the arm backward. (The tug should be strong enough to cause their weight to shift backward a bit, but not strong enough to cause an imbalance.)
    - Did you feel that? Did it tug your whole body backward? (It should)
    - Explain why: When core muscles are not braced and knees are locked straight, overhead arm motion can cause exaggerated weight-shift changes and affect your balance.

Braced Torso

Participants will do the raised arm tug again, but this time they'll brace their abs for the tug.

- Pull your abs in and up, shoulder blades back and down.
- Keep your knees soft.
- Lift one arm and pull it back.
    - Feel a difference this time? (Yes)
    - Did you rock backward a little less? (Yes)
    - Did a stabilized torso help you keep your balance? (Yes)

Offset Feet

Participants do the raised-arm tug again, but this time they add offset feet.

- ◉ One foot is forward, one back. Feet are shoulder-width apart.
- ◉ Keep your knees soft.
- ◉ Pull your abs in and up, shoulder blades back and down.
- ◉ Lift the arm again.
    - Reach up and forward with it.
    - Then and tug it firmly back.
    - Feel any differences when the feet are offset?
- ◉ An explanation: Offset feet gives us more room in which to rock or move forward and back safely. This is because our center of gravity (our belly button) is staying between a wider base of support (offset feet). When our feet were side by side our safe rocking space was only the length of our feet. We effectively lengthened our base of support in the direction of our reach with offset feet.

Hat Box to Chest

Now they are ready to reach for those hat boxes with braced abs and offset feet. Tell them that this time there will be one more change. Once they reach their hat box, instead of pulling it back overhead they should lower it to their chest. This way there is less momentum to pull them backward and more that directs the pull toward their center of gravity.

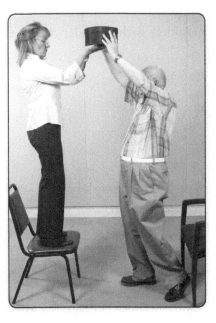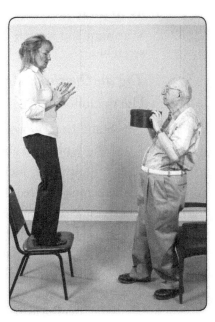

- ◉ With braced torso, soft knees, and offset feet, reach up for the hat box.
- ◉ Can you feel yourself rock forward onto the forward foot?
- ◉ Grab the box using your Venus de Milo Arms, if necessary. (Does Go Go Gadget come to mind?).
- ◉ Keeping your abs braced, pull the box down toward your chest (not overhead).
- ◉ Did you feel yourself rock to the back foot as you came down? Perfect!
- ◉ Can you notice the extra distance you can safely rock forward and backward when your feet are offset?

Give It More Balance))

- For comparison's sake, have participants rock with the feet side by side (there's more balance risk here, so be careful).
- Rock again with offset feet.
- Ask participants if they feel the difference in the range of motion (offset feet create a wider base of support).

Keep It Safe))

- Place walkers or chairs in front of participants for extra backup.
- Let them decide how far they want to reach upwards. This is where having imaginary shelves is handy.

Live It))

Torso stability, foot position, and arm movements all affect balance stability during everyday tasks such as reaching.

BALANCE

PUT YOUR BEST FOOT UP AND GET OFF EASY

Going up and down stairs or curbs are some of the scariest situations for frail adults. These limitations can seriously limit mobility, opportunities, and independence. Oftentimes, too, one leg functions better than the other. These two activities, Put Your Best Foot Up and Get Off Easy, provide easy rules for negotiating stairs or curbs when legs do not function equally.

Benefits))

- ◉ Teaches an easy way to remember which foot to use when.
- ◉ Practices an everyday mobility skill.

Set It Up))

Place a single step beside balance support. Four inches (10 centimeters) is a good first step height. You can add risers later.

How to Do It))

Discuss the safest way to go up and down stairs—up with the good foot and down with the bad foot. Ask participants to volunteer whether they have one leg that works better than the other. It's common, so you'll likely get lots of responses. This activity is for them.

Put Your Best Foot Up

Use the following cues.

- ◉ Place your best foot on the step.
- ◉ Shift your weight (think Belly Button Training) toward and over the foot on the step. (Belly Step style.)
- ◉ Push down on that foot and lift yourself onto the step.
- ◉ Bring the other foot onboard. Stop and get your balance. Step back down carefully.
- ◉ Practice several times. Change feet if the other leg is capable.
- ◉ Stay on top of the step for the next activity.

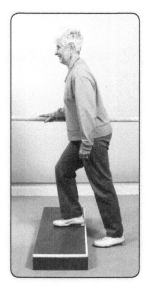

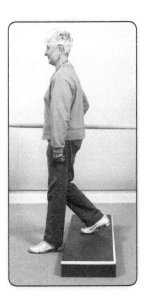

Get Off Easy

Now they'll practice stepping off with the weaker leg. Explain to participants that the stronger leg should stay on the step to control the lowering of their weight. This technique makes it easier to get off the step. Use the following cues.

- ◉ Start on top of the step.
- ◉ Lower your weaker leg to the floor. Toe down first is usually easiest.
- ◉ Keep your weight on the strong leg until the other foot touches down.
- ◉ Transfer your weight down to the floor.
- ◉ Are you aware you can control the descent with the stronger leg? That is why you leave the stronger leg on the stair. Step down with the weaker leg because the other one maintains control.
- ◉ Lift the leg back up and try it again.

BALANCE

Keep It Safe))

Supervise participants closely for wobbliness. Provide plenty of balance support. Watch for signs of pain in their faces when they step up or down. If they look uncomfortable or wince, then remind them that they should modify or stop the activity if it hurts.

Live It))

Participants should put their best foot up first when stepping up onto a curb or stair. Getting off easy means stepping down from a stair or curb with the less capable leg.

PICKUP LINES

Picking up an object from the floor without losing balance is a difficult challenge for most frail adults, but it's a common everyday task. This activity will help them with this task.

Benefits))

- ◉ Practices an everyday task.
- ◉ Links to other skills (Anchors A-Sway, Belly Button Training, It's a Reach).

Set It Up))

Use masking tape to create a line parallel to a sturdy balance support such as a handrail. You will also need an object for participants to pick up, such as their keys or a plush toy.

How to Do It))

The Start

- ◉ Explain that this activity is similar to retrieving a golf ball on the fairway.
- ◉ Demonstrate the golf ball pick-up technique.
    - Place an object in front of the chosen support leg.
    - Reach down for the object with the opposite hand.
    - At the same time, lift the other leg up and behind you. Bend the supporting leg to make the reach.
- ◉ Let them know that the first version you have for them is easier than that. Demonstrate what you want them to do.
    - Place an object on a low chair (instead of on the floor), a few feet out in front of the participant.
    - Participant will stand beside railing, feet shoulder width and widely offset.
    - Front leg should be the one closest to handrail. Front foot should be aligned on the parallel line.
    - The support-side hand stays on the handrail.
    - They will be reaching with the other hand.
    - Participant will keep both feet on the ground while retrieving object.
- ◉ Remind participants to keep their torso braced.

The Moves

- Practice the form of it first. Pick up an imaginary object. Then go for a real object or toy.
- Place the object in front of them (or on a low chair) on the line.
- They should reach down and retrieve the object.
- Then stand back up, tall and upright.
- Can they reach an object that is lower, maybe on the ground?
- Can they do the same reach and lift the outside leg up to hip height as their arm drops?
- After each reach and retrieve they need to stand back up, tall and upright.
- Have them keep one hand on the handrail.

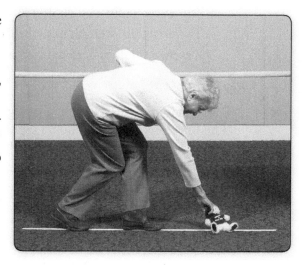

Give It More Balance))

- Ask them if they notice where their belly button is in relation to their supporting foot (it should be right above it). Do they understand why that's important? (Better balance when center of gravity is over a support.)
- Pickup Line From a Beam: With you beside them, those who are willing can try the activity standing on a poly beam or a large balance mat. This is advanced but doable; they will be surprised at their capability.

Keep It Safe))

Make sure they hang onto the handrail and practice parts of the activity before doing the whole thing. You can make the activity much more doable by putting the object on a box or chair to start.

Live It))

Safely picking up objects from the ground, such as dropped keys or remote controls, involves creating counterweight. Foot and leg positioning help with that. With Pick Up Lines they should have an easier time reaching for objects on the ground.

BALANCE

MULTIDIRECTIONAL LUNGES

This activity expands Clock Stepping, which was shown in chapter 6 (page 192).

Benefits))

- ⊙ Enhances agility and coordination.
- ⊙ Develops leg strength in multiple planes of movement.
- ⊙ Practices multidirectional stepping for safer everyday mobility.

Set It Up))

Create an imaginary clock by placing lines of tape on the floor in a starburst pattern. The lines represent most hours on a clock. Each line should be about a yard (meter) long to allow for various lunge lengths. Participants stand in the center of this clock.

How to Do It))

- ⊙ Rock around the clock.
    - Participants step out to do a lunge on each line.
    - Between each lunge, they return to the center.
- ⊙ Progress to doing three different lunges before returning to the center. (Move from one point on the clock to the next—don't go back to the center between lunges.)
- ⊙ Progress to where you can call out all directions randomly.
- ⊙ Small lunges at first, then deeper lunges when they are ready.
- ⊙ Do frequent posture checks (no forward leaning, trunk stays upright, front knee is over front ankle when lunging).

Give It More Balance))

- ⊙ Challenge participants to step farther out on the radiating lines.
- ⊙ Make lunges happen a little quicker.
- ⊙ Challenge them to reach opposite hands out past their lunging knees.
- ⊙ Cue with a cadence that creates a pace they must follow.
- ⊙ Consider using music. The rhythm will help them anticipate the next move.

Keep It Safe))

This is an advanced activity. Start with the easiest marks first. Numbers to the side and front, then back, and then those that require crossing over. Perfect one movement before moving on to another. Hold their hands or forearms as needed.

Live It))

Multidirectional lunges are difficult, but they will help participants handle unexpected balance challenges.

FIGURE EIGHTS, RECIPROCAL MOVEMENT, AND KAYAKING

Figure-eight patterns involve reciprocal movement about a central point. With reciprocity, where there is a push, there is an offsetting pull. Many activities incorporate sequential, reciprocal motions. For instance, when you walk with arm swings, one arm swings forward while the opposite leg swings back. There is a push and a pull to the rhythm around the core or trunk. Reciprocal movements help transfer momentum during gait.

For ABLE Bodies training, some figure-eight patterns are practiced by walking in a figure-eight path. Others, such as seated kayaking, are practiced from a chair. Controlling large reciprocal forces is a part of the balance challenge. This series of activities provides good balance training for everyday living. Kayaking is an excellent choice for individuals with Parkinson's Disease. The flowing, body-twisting motions are helpful for easing rigidity.

Benefits ⟩⟩

- ◉ Uses and improves figure-eight movements.
- ◉ Enhances balance control for opposing motions.
- ◉ Practices sequential everyday movements.

Set It Up ⟩⟩

Expect that you might use poles or sticks for kayaking, sunglasses or heads-up glasses to reduce vision, and agility poles or chairs to set a kayaking course.

How to Do It ⟩⟩

This series of activities can be progressed from seated to standing to seated on an agility disc or a ball to moving, depending on which level is an appropriate challenge for your participants.

Kayaking Arms

To teach this arm pattern, give participants a lightweight pole to use as their kayak pole. The goal is to teach them to kayak with their arms and shoulders using a dip-turn-lift motion. Ideally, the upper body will turn in the opposite direction of the knees and head. Try using these cues:

- ◉ Sit Tall on your chair with your torso stabilized and your feet flat on the floor. Knees face forward. Hold your pole in both hands, palms facing down.
- ◉ Lift the pole to shoulder height.
- ◉ Dip the pole low to one side and pull the stroke down and back.
- ◉ Lift again to center.
- ◉ Kayak to the other side and return to center.
- ◉ Begin to link strokes and develop a rhythm.
- ◉ Keep going until you've completed sets of 8 to 12 strokes.

Kayaking Knees

When participants kayak with their arms on their right side, have them point their knees left.

- Paddle on right, knees point left
- Paddle on left, knees point right

Kayaking Head

When the arms dip and row to the right, have participants turn knees AND head opposite. Try these cues:

- Dip the pole left.
- Head and knees push right. Finish kayak stroke on left.
- Dip right.
- Head and knees push left. Finish kayak stroke on right.
- Link the moves.
- Develop a rhythm.
- Say the Pledge of Allegiance while kayaking (Or another dual task).
- Sit with feet tandem and heels lifted.

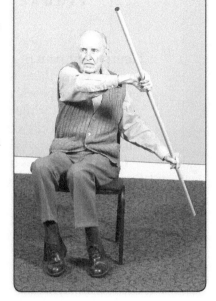

Kayaking While Walking

This is a difficult activity for most. Be cautious and stay close by when doing this moving activity. Participants should pretend they are kayaking down the river.

- Start with Kayaking Arms while standing (for balance support, one leg should touch the back of their chair).
- Participants should maintain good core stability.
- When they are ready and you are close by, have them begin walking and kayaking.
- Walk in a straight line first.
- Then have them walk through your Kayak course, using a figure 8 pattern.

Give It More Balance))

- Add sunglasses or heads-up glasses, or dim the lights.
- Sit on a balance disc.
- Kayak through the course with Heads-up glasses on.
- Kayaking is a natural addition to River Fun.

Keep It Safe))

These movements can be tiring. Let participants choose their challenge. If anyone's back hurts, that person should stop and make some adjustments, such as doing smaller motions. For standing and walking variations, be near the participants.

Live It))

Offsetting motions can cause little perturbations that participants can learn to control with rhythmic motions and counter rotations. Practicing will help improve gait, balance confidence, and other everyday skills.

FIGURE-EIGHT OBSTACLE COURSE

Figure-eight walking patterns require changes in direction and momentum. You can easily add difficulties with small changes in pace, patterns, obstacles, lighting, and so on. It's easy to be creative with this activity.

Benefits))

- Integrates many balance systems and skills.
- Uses visual targets.
- Enhances postural control.

Set It Up))

Set up an easy, widely spaced figure-eight or slalom course. It can be two to eight agility poles, cones, or even chairs set in a row; for large classes use two groups of chairs set in a circle. The design should accommodate participants with walkers. If your course will have other challenges, prepare for those.

How to Do It))

Participants will weave their way through the course. There are endless variations you can try.

EZ Eights

EZ Eights are easy courses. Obstacles are wide apart so there is plenty of room to pass between them, and they're easy to negotiate (no doorways to go through, no steps to walk up and over). Lighting should also be comfortable and bright, not dimmed. EZ Eights involve normal walking (no sidestepping or big arm swings).

Use the following cues.

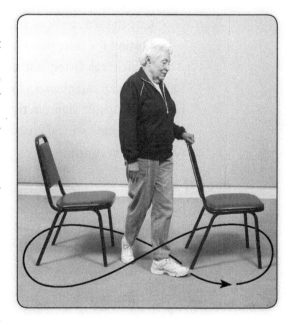

- Observe the upcoming course and any obstacles.
- Make a plan.
- Start weaving through the course.
- Look ahead to the next turn.
- Look ahead two turns.

To give this exercise more balance challenge, you can try the following:

- Vary chair position—offset some chairs and set others closer.
- Walk faster.
- Recite a poem or sing "Happy Birthday" while walking.
- Add arm swings.

BALANCE

Tighter Eights

Tighter Eights can be an intermediate or difficult activity. You will need to supervise closely, and participants should probably take turns. Tighter Eights and variations are created by making the basic figure eight tighter or otherwise more difficult.

- Use fewer poles. (The 180-degree turn at the ends happens sooner and more frequently.)
- Make pathways smaller and tighter.
- Provide tight spaces in which to maneuver.
- Make part of the pathways go through a doorway (place chairs on both sides of the doorway; they'll go around one chair, through the door, then around the other chair).
- Set it up so that one end of the figure eight requires them to turn in and out of a corner or walk close to a wall.
- Set a chair in a corner where a pivot is needed to come back out (advanced).
- Vary stepping patterns (big steps, long steps, marching, on toes, side steps).
- Dim the lights or provide sunglasses or ski goggles (it's a slalom course).
- Add a cognitive task, such as counting backward by 5 from 100 or recalling old addresses or cars.

To give this exercise more balance challenge, you can try the following:

- Make it a timed event; encourage them to go faster each pass.
  - Cue them to walk as fast as they safely can.
  - During the next pass cue them to take big steps.
  - Which was faster, fast steps or big steps? (Probably big steps were.)
- Randomly call out changes in direction or pace.
- Have participants sidestep through.
- Have them walk with their back to the chairs, hands touching the chairs.
- Ask them questions as they walk or sidestep through.

Keep It Safe))

The more difficult the course, the more supervision is needed. Tighter figure eights may cause some people to become dizzy. Keep the course fairly simple and progress slowly, providing plenty of supervision.

Live It))

Figure-eight practice helps participants integrate many aspects of balance. It covers many everyday walking challenges.

ALLEMANDE LEFT

This intermediate activity uses a fun weaving motion borrowed from square dancing. The hands become a visual target as participants weave from one person to the next. Allemande Left also engages the vestibular system because the peripheral vision is disturbed by passing objects. You could combine this activity with other musical themes for a dance day, such as a class with Country-Western Heel and Toe, Box Steps, Step-Together-Steps, and Step-Together-Step-Turns.

Benefits))

- Integrates many systems and aspects of balance and movement.
- Introduces visual targets.
- Challenges the vestibular system.

How to Do It))

Explain that this is a square-dance activity. Partner up participants, one pair for each side of a square. Here are some calls and cues you can use:

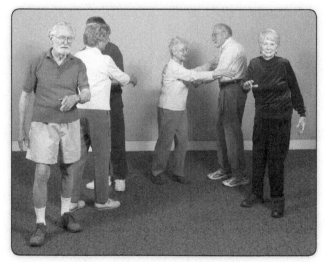

- Bow to your partner. (Partners bow.)
- Bow to your corner. (Corners bow.)
- Allemande left. (Participants turn away from each other and weave around the square, clasping hands with each person.)
  - Watch for the next hand—it's your visual target until you grasp it.
  - Clasp one hand, and then look on to the next hand.
  - Keep weaving your way around the square and back to home.
- All promenade. (Partners link arms and walk in a circle until back to home.)
- Allemande right.
  - The next hand is your visual target.
  - Watch for the hand—see the hand and target it until you grasp it.
  - Keep moving around the square, spotting the next hand.
- All promenade! (Partners link arms and walk in a circle until back to home.)

Give It More Balance))

Advanced: Add a do-si-do, a pass-and-return square-dance movement. Participants pass shoulders around their corner or opposite person. This movement is advanced because it involves backward walking on the way home.

Keep It Safe))

This activity can get a little confusing really fast. People may hurry to keep up. Keep the pace slow enough that participants are comfortable.

Live It))

Allemandes are a series of handshakes with friends that make balance training, and handshakes, more fun.

WALK THE LINE

Walk the Line is a series of activities that involve lines on the floor in patterns that particularly improve lateral balance. Some of the activities will work easily in groups with just a single piece of tape behind each person's chair. For other activities, participants need to be up and away from their chairs. For those activities, participants should take turns.

Benefits))

- ◉ Improves lateral (side-to-side) balance.
- ◉ Increases abductor and adductor strength.
- ◉ Uses narrow base of support.
- ◉ Teaches visual targeting.

Set It Up))

You will need several rolls of masking tape, in wide and narrow sizes and in various colors, if available. In lieu of creating lines, sometimes you can find lines in the design of the carpet or flooring in your classroom. If you can have class outside, consider using sidewalk chalk. It is bright and fun. Whatever you use, have the lines ready for participants ahead of time.

How to Do It))

Over and Back

Place a line about 18 inches (46 centimeters) long behind each chair, perpendicular to the chair back. When you put the tape down, put a tab on each piece of tape (roll over a small piece at the end). This makes it much easier to take it back up.

This is a lateral stepping activity that can be used to practice everyday stepping skills as well as to strengthen hip abductors. Participants stand on one side of the line, facing the chair. They should lightly hold on to the back of their chair with both hands to start. Use these cues.

- ◉ Stabilize your torso—shoulder blades back and down, abs in, knees soft.
- ◉ Step over the line with both feet.
- ◉ Step back.
- ◉ Keep going.
- ◉ Is your torso still stabilized? Are your knees still soft?
- ◉ Imagine the tape is 4 inches (10 centimeters) high.
    - Lift your knees a little higher.
    - Step over, stop. Step back, stop. (The stop lets them find their balance between steps.)
    - Repeat a few times.

You can increase the balance challenge by doing the following:

- ◉ Take wider steps.
- ◉ Follow a rhythm. (Count in sets of 4 or 8 and participants try to keep time with your count.)
- ◉ Hold the chair less tightly.
- ◉ Hold the chair with just one hand.
- ◉ Put hands on hips (advanced).

BALANCE

Big Steps

This activity increases stride length, practices everyday transitions, and requires planning. Participants must estimate how big of a step they think they can take. Turning around to take the next big step is an everyday mobility skill, too. This activity done behind chairs uses same piece of tape as Over and Back, above.

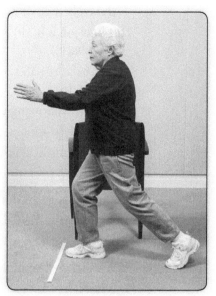

- Participants stand facing the line behind their chair, one hand on the chair back.
- Invite participants to step back from the tape as far as they estimate they can take one big step. Use these cues:
  - Stabilize your torso—shoulder blades back and down, abs in.
  - Keep one hand on your chair.
  - Take the step! Land it and bring the other foot beside it.
- Have participants turn around carefully and set up to take their big step again.
- Once they've done a few big steps successfully, cue them to use bigger knee lifts and a heel–toe motion or add an arm swing.
  - Lift your knee as you get ready to step.
  - Use that knee height to help get your heel out across the line.
  - Can you land heel–toe?
  - Do it again.
  - Knee lift, heel–toe.
  - Follow the foot out there (think Belly Steps, page 242) and move your torso toward that line, too.

Step-Ball-Change

This intermediate activity practices a crossover stepping pattern. It lets participants practice balancing over a narrow base of support, strengthens hip abductors and adductors, and requires weight shifts. This activity done behind chairs uses same piece of tape as Over and Back, above.

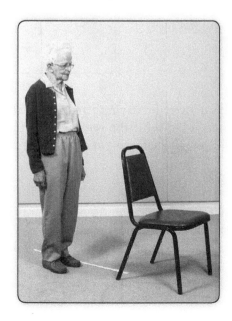
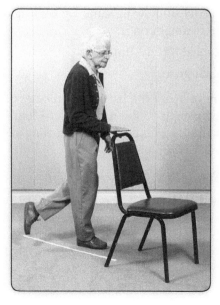

- Participants stand an arm's length from the back of their chairs, with both feet on the right side of their taped line. Torso is stable and knees are soft.
- Their job is to do a step-ball-change across the line. (It's a crossover step forward, then back.)
- For balance safety, when one foot crosses the line the same-side hand can touch the chair.
- Use the following cues:
  - Right foot steps across the line.
  - Transfer your weight to it.
  - Step back to the starting position. That's one step-ball-change.

  Do six to eight repetitions with one leg, and then change sides.

You can increase the balance challenge of this activity by adding the following:

- A complete weight shift, such that the unweighted foot lifts slightly.
- A cadence or count
- Music

Watch for signs of wobbliness with this activity. Participants who use a walker should use it for this one. Participants who have had recent hip surgery should not do this activity. Take it slow and easy, especially at first.

Pendulum Legs on a Tandem Line

This intermediate activity is essentially a leg lift from back to front that ends up looking like the movement of a pendulum. It lets participants practice static balance over a narrow base of support, strengthens hip abductors, and uses weight shifts. To set this one up, the taped line should run parallel to the back of the chair, about a yard (meter) long.

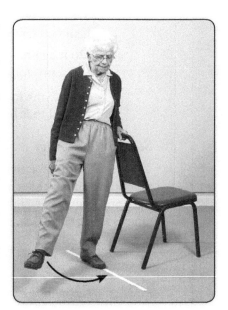

- Participants stand on the line behind their chair, one hand on their balance support and knees soft.
- Cue them for proper posture: tall standing, abs in, ribs lifted.
- Participants swing the outside leg forward and transfer most of their weight to it.
- Participants swing same leg back again and put most of their weight on it.
- Repeat 8 to 12 times.
- Change legs.

You can increase the balance challenge of this activity by having participants transfer all their weight to the new forward leg. When it lands lift the rear heel off the line. When the leg swings back again, they should put all their weight on that leg and lift the now forward knee.

The Straight and Narrow

This is the first Walk the Line Activity away from chairs; plan on participants taking turns. Participants will practice walking (dynamic balance) over a narrow base of support to strengthen their hip abductors and to practice visual targeting skills. They can pick either the straight or the narrow challenge.

- You'll use three 12-foot (4 meter) lengths of masking tape to create this three-line walking path. Two lines should be laid down 10 to 12 inches (25-30 centimeters) apart to form the outside dimensions of the path. The third line will run down the middle. To make the lines distinctive, use a wider width and a different color for the middle line. Place the path an arm's-length from a handrail or be available yourself for balance support.

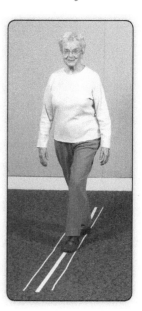

- On the first pass, give participants a choice. They can walk this path either by staying between the two narrow lines or walking on the wide center line. They can try it a couple of times if they like.

- On the second pass, they should walk it with the abs braced and shoulder blades back and down.

- Ask them if walking tall and more upright helps.

- On the third pass, have them keep their knees soft and put their arms out to the side.

- Ask if those changes made a difference.

- On the fourth and fifth passes, have them experiment with slow and fast walking speeds and see which is easier.

- By now, they know this path pretty well. This time ask them to walk their chosen path with these skills together: good posture, soft knees, arms out to the side, and reasonably quickly, plus one more.

- Stand at the end of the path and provide a horizon-level, visual target (it can be a picture, a spot on the wall, or your hand). You want them to walk the line without looking down.

- Remind them that their brain knows what their feet are doing, even without seeing the feet. Ask participants to look directly at the target, not down and at the line. If this is too difficult, get them at least to look toward the end of the line. Brace their abs, soften their knees, hands to the side, Go! You can use the following cues as they are needed.
    - Only look ahead at horizon level.
    - Torso braced, shoulder blades back and down, ribs lifted.
    - Knees soft, arms out to the side.
    - Gaze ahead at the horizon.
    - Walk quickly along the Narrow path.
    - What changed when you used the visual target for guidance? (Makes it easier to stay on the path.)

You can give this activity more balance challenge by doing the following:

- Challenge them to try walking the center line, the Straight path.
- Encourage them to use less support from the handrail.
- Try it with music. "New York, New York" is a great one.
- They can carry a glass of water with both hands. No spilling!

Walk and Waddle

The task of this activity is to walk along two widely set lines. Left line, right line, left line, right line—each step is a transition from side to side. The resultant big sways create a lumbering gait, a kind of walk and waddle.

- Put down two tape lines that are 8 to12 feet (3 to 4 meters) long and 12 to 24 inches (30-61 centimeters) apart, depending on participants' ability. Place the lines near a handrail or row of chairs for balance safety.

- Have participants practice Walk and Waddle beside their chairs.
    - First practice wide lateral swaying from one foot to the other.
    - Then practice waddling steps (big, wide stepping motions) from side to side, near their chairs. You want them to get a feel for the side-to-side swaying, before they get out on the floor.
- Head to the lines, stay near them, and take turns. You can use the following cues.
- First pass.
    - Step on the right line.
    - Transfer your weight to that leg and then push off from there so you can land on the left line.
    - Move along, allowing yourself to lumber from side to side.
    - Feel your legs push you back to center.
    - Lean right. Push left.
    - Lean left. Push right.
- Add arms, on the second pass, if you think they are ready.
    - As you lean right, reach your right arm left. Then vice versa (lean left, reach right).
    - The arms help correct the sideways movement.
    - Arm swings give momentum that helps bring you back to center. Can you feel that?
- Add music.
    - Try to walk and waddle to music.
    - See if the music can help you make your movements bigger, more like diagonal lunges.
    - Can you step to the right and reach an arm over to the left and vice versa?

Holiday Lines

Curved or complex lines add a change in direction to straight-line activities. They are just a little more difficult but probably won't seem so because they are more engaging and fun. This activity lets participants practice dynamic balance over a narrow and ever-changing base of support. The activity lets them practice changes in direction, strengthen hip adductors and abductors, and use visual targeting skills.

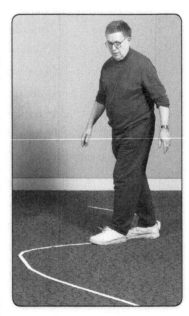

- Pick a theme and make a masking tape image on the floor for them to follow. Examples might be a heart, shamrock, Easter egg, bunny, chick, flower, flag, fireworks, ship, airplane, rocket, Christmas tree, Star of David, cloud, autumn leaf, basketball, football, baseball bat, race car, covered wagon, stop sign . . . or just a simple wavy line.
- Participants walk along the outline of the image.
- Cue them like other Walk the Line activities to keep the abs in, ribs lifted, and shoulder blades back and down. Knees soft and arms out to the side. Gaze ahead at next turn.
- For more challenge dim the room, give a dual task, or try sunglasses or heads-up glasses.

H-Lines

Maintaining standing balance with offset feet or tandem feet is difficult. Bracing the core muscles, imagining yourself glued to the floor, and establishing a visual target are all techniques that will help with this task. This activity lets participants practice static balance over a narrow base of support, improves kinesis, and refreshes earlier concepts (When Push Comes to Shove and visual targeting).

- Before class, make an H-line out of masking tape for each person. Simply tape down a big letter *H*. Make the parallel lines 8 to 10 inches (20-25 centimeters) apart. Be sure to tab each piece of tape so it pulls off quickly when you are done.

- Appropriate balance support may include using walkers with a chair behind or placing chairs on three sides of the participant.

- H-line Challenge 1 is standing with parallel feet. Participants stand with feet side by side on the parallel sides of their H-line, toes behind the crossbar. Use the following cues.
  - Place your feet on the parallel lines and look directly ahead. Take a deep breath.
  - Exhale, blow out all your air, and draw your shoulder blades back and down. Brace your core muscles.
  - Push down with the palms of your hands and mentally glue yourself to the ground.
  - Don't just place your feet there; plant your whole self there (as learned in When Push Comes to Shove).
  - Keep shoulder blades back and down, knees soft.
  - Hold the position 10 to 20 seconds, breathing normally.

- H-line Challenge 2 is standing with offset feet. Participants stand on parallel lines with feet offset, the preferred foot in front of the crossbar. Give them a few tries to figure out which foot they prefer to have forward (kinesthetic learning). Their task is to practice the When Push Comes to Shove stance in an offset position. Use these cues.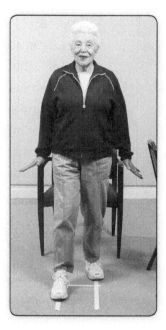
  - Inhale, exhale, look directly ahead, and bend your knees slightly.
  - Push your shoulders down and glue yourself to the floor.
  - Keep most of your weight over the back foot.
  - Hold steady for 5 to 10 seconds, if possible.
  - Step off your lines and take a break.
  - Try it with the other foot forward.

- H-line Challenge 3 is standing with tandem feet. After a brief rest, invite those who are willing to step on the H-line, tandem style. Not everyone will be willing or able to do this one. Those that aren't up to this challenge can do Challenges 1 or 2 again. Monitor participants closely and provide extra balance support.
- Once your participants are on their marks, use the following cues.
    - Bend your knees a little.
    - Transfer most of your weight to the back foot.
    - Look straight ahead; find a visual target at horizon level.
    - Inhale, exhale, brace your core muscles, and glue yourself down.

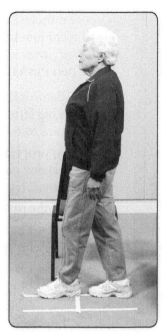

You can give any of these three foot positions more balance challenge with the following:
- Lift an arm up.
- Lift arms out to side.
- Close one eye.
- Do arm swings, while holding the position.
- Recite or read a poem.
- Tell a joke.
- Get them to laugh at one of your jokes.

Live It))

There are all kinds of line challenges. Most are about maintaining balance over a narrow base of support. The narrowed base means more balance is required, particularly lateral balance. Lateral balance helps prevent falls. These activities especially strengthen the inner and outer thighs, which are critical to preventing falls to the side. Visual targeting is also an important aspect of walking the straight and narrow situations in life.

RHYTHM AND MOVES

Music is part of every culture and it's wonderful right-brain stuff. Music evokes thought and imagery, memories and emotion. Rhythm and melodies elicit almost automatic body movements such as toe tapping, head nods, and sways. I think that it is these qualities that make musical activities both fun and effective. Rhythm has a way of prepping people for movement, helping them anticipate when, where, and how to move. Musically inspired movements tend to involve the whole body, too, which is one more great reason for using music to help with balance and whole-body coordination. This section remains my favorite.

Benefits))

- Coordinates whole-body, sequential movements.
- Helps transitions feel easier, almost automatic.
- Uses previously learned dance skills.
- Enriches the mind–body connection.
- Benefits participants of all levels.

Set It Up))

Gather music from the participants' generation for these activities. It's difficult to get quality songs from the 30s and 40s; but by the 50s, there seems to be more available through Web site distributors. Select songs that match the activities you choose. "Theme From *A Summer Place*" by Percy Faith is an excellent waltz that works great for sidestepping. *My Girl* by The Rolling Stones is great for Rock and Walk; try *Blueberry Hill* by Fats Domino or *Don't Fence Me In* by Bing Crosby for box stepping and Patti Page's *Tennessee Waltz* for Tai Chi and lots of other slow activities. You'll discover that certain songs work better for certain moves.

How to Do It))

Do any set of movements one at a time at first. Combine them as participants improve.

Toe Taps and Head Nods

- Begin seated. Select some toe-tapping music (I've liked *Do You Believe in Magic* by the Loving Spoonfuls and *I Walk the Line* by Johnny Cash). Try these seated moves.
  - Toe taps
  - Head nods
  - Arm swings (with stabilized torso)
  - Seated marching (with stabilized torso, march in place)
  - Heel–toe foot tapping
  - Marching and arm swings combined
  - Heel–toe stepping with arm swings combined

Increase the balance challenge of this activity with the following:

- While seated, participants close their eyes.
  - Arm swings and head turns to music
  - Heel–toe foot tapping

Some Simple Standing Moves

When doing any standing musical activities, be safe. Participants should be within an arm's length of their chair, near a handrail or their backs should be to a wall. For frailer adults, use a chair on either side of them or use a walker. Abler classes can stand beside a chair or handrail, maybe with one hand on their hip. If they can free stand, have them stand in front of their chair with one leg touching it. Ideally, they'll follow your moves as you lead them, but allow them to find their own rhythm and make their own choices for what they feel safe doing.

- ◉ Stand with good posture and appropriate balance support. If you're ready for another song, pick a slower one than above (*Begin the Beguine* by the Limelighters, or *The Birds and Bees* by Jewel Akens) and do these moves.
  - Sways
  - Small steps in place
  - Marching in place
- ◉ Do advanced standing activities.
  - Marching with higher knees
  - Marching with wider steps
  - Arm swings and marching
  - Look left, look right, while marching

Box Step

This multidirectional stepping pattern practices weight shifts and agility. It is a set of simple steps that form a square. You can give it more balance challenge by pairing up participants, to box step like two dancers would.

- ◉ Select some good box-step music from their era. I like *Blueberry Hill* by Fats Domino and *Don't Fence Me In* by Bing Crosby.
- ◉ Participants practice steps that form a square. The outside foot takes the step. Practice first without music, then with music. Use these cues:
  - Sidestep right, together
  - Forward step right, together
  - Sidestep left, together
  - Back step left, together

Waltzing Matildas

Sidestepping is a foot pattern in waltzing; hence the name *Waltzing Matildas*. When you add music to sidestepping, that's when participants are most involved with their whole body. Soon they want to twirl and arabesque; sidestepping becomes a whole-body waltz.

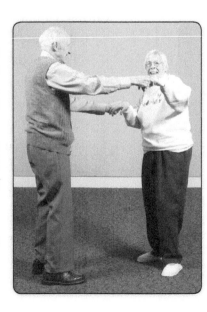

- ◉ Music is a must for this activity, of course. I like "Theme From *A Summer Place*" by Percy Faith. It is so lilting and smooth. But you could also use the original "Waltzing Matilda" song, too.
- ◉ Pair up participants into dance partners.
- ◉ Prepare for crowd control—space everyone out so couples can sidestep several steps before changing directions.

- Practice sidestepping with no music.
    - Step together, step. Step together, step.
    - Change directions and repeat.
    - Use bigger steps.
    - Step together, step, etc.
- Turn on the waltz music.
    - Step together, step. Step together, step.
- Cue pairs to add arm swings to the music.
- Cue them for bigger, deeper steps (add a knee bend to each side step).
    - Step, knee bends and then straightens as they finish the sidestep.
    - Step, knee bends and then straighten. Step, etc.

Watch as these basic step-together movements become fluid, whole-body moves. Instead of moving just the legs, the entire body gets involved: Arms, torso, head, and emotions. It is remarkable and fun to see the transformation. Use these cues.

- Step together, step.
- Feel the flow. Step together, step.
- Notice how your whole body creates the movement.
- Feel the sway and enjoy!
- Sing or count along.

You can give this activity more balance challenge by doing the following:

- Dim the lights. (Romantic, as it should be.)
- Add turns, progress to the next activity.

Step Together, Step Turns
- Begin with just sidestepping, then add turns.
    - Step together, step. Step together, step.
    - Step together, step turn.
    - One partner turns underneath one hand and arm of the other partner. The guiding partner can use his/her other hand as balance support for the turning partner.

Rock and Walk
Rock and Walk is similar to the movement of normal gait. Heel–toe motion and weight transitions rule this activity.

- Pick out suitable music with a rocking melody. I like *My Girl* by the Rolling Stones; it helps that most participants know the words and like it too. I also recommend the great rhythm of *Hackensack* by Fountains of Wayne.
- If you plan to do the tandem line option, put down 2 or 4, 12-foot (4-meter) lines of tape on the floor, about 4 feet (1.5 m) apart. You'll want to have one person on each line and the people holding outstretched hands. Plan that you will be one of the people on the line, holding hands with participants who will take turns doing the Rock and Walk with you.
- As a warm-up, do some heel–toe rocking a few times with feet shoulder-width apart. Three great practice activities could be Heel-Touch and Roll-Up; Rock Back, Knee Lift; and Rock Forward, Knee Lift.

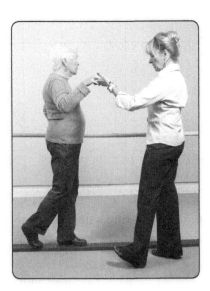 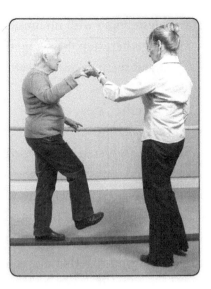

◉ Then pick one volunteer to join you on the tandem lines. You're ready to cue up the music.

◉ You and your participant get on one line each. One foot forward and one foot back.

◉ Hold hands at about shoulder height and wait for the music.

◉ Start the music! Here are some cues to use:

- Rock forward, rock back, in time with the music.

- Keep rocking until it feels comfortable.

- Keep your eyes on the horizon.

- Use full heel–toe motion.

- Ask if your partner can feel the heel–toe weight shifts. (Weight crosses from the heel through the foot to the toe.)

- Rock forward, rock back. Rock forward, rock back.

- Listen, and when you sense the music says "now," take a step. Land on the line.

- Rock forward and back again two or three times.

- Rock until the music leads you to the next step. Take the next step with the music.

- Then rock back and forth again, until you're ready for the next step.

- That's Rock and Walk!

- Feel the rhythm of your rocking.

- Feel how the music can guide your movements, and tell you when to step.

- Notice how the front foot lifts naturally when you rock back and how the rear leg is ready to lift toward the next step when it's time to step.

- Rock three times, step; rock three times, step.

- It's Rock and Walk!

- Ask how they liked it? Was it fun, did they get it?

- Next Partner? I've done it with a partner on each side. I've also had good luck letting them be each other's partner instead of me being the only partner. Use your own sense for what will work with your group. Any way you do it, this one is amazing and fun.

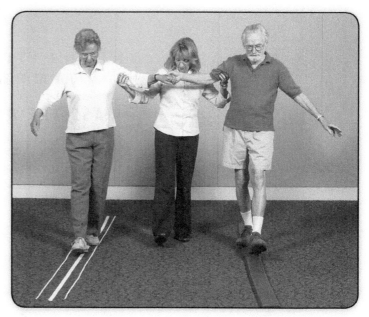

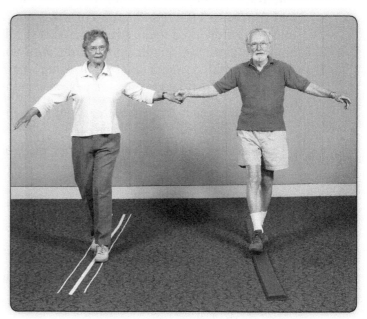

Give It More Balance ⟩⟩

- ⊚ Relax and feel the flow.
- ⊚ Turn down the lights or wear sunglasses.
- ⊚ Do it on a poly balance beam.

Keep It Safe ⟩⟩

Music should have the appropriate volume and cadence. If it's too loud, participants will feel distracted by it. If it's too soft, it's hard to feel the rhythm. The pace should be moderate; the melody inviting and, easy to follow. Balance support should be ample. Hold their hand or provide a handrail.

Live It ⟩⟩

Music and rhythm enhance anticipatory skills and improve sequential movements, including gait. Music evokes pleasant memories and can make balance training fun and relaxing.

PASS THE DUCK

Pass the Duck is a little like a cross between Musical Chairs and Hot Potato. Music is played and participants pass a heavy object from person to person until the music stops. Their balance training goal is to keep their core stable while passing the heavy object.

Benefits))

- Develops core strength and stability.
- Uses music and is fun.

Set It Up))

I'm from Oregon, where the university mascots are the Ducks (University of Oregon) and the Beavers (Oregon State). For this game, I purchased ducks and beavers from university stores and then sewed 3 pounds (1.5 kilograms) of beans into each stuffed animal mascot. You might do the same with your local mascots. You can also use a medicine ball, 2 to 4 pounds (1-2 kilograms) max. If your budget allows, these mascots make wonderful prizes for the last person standing (seated, actually).

- Arrange chairs in a circle. Start out with enough for everyone. If you have a big class, do two circles of chairs.
- Select suitable music you think they will enjoy.

How to Do It))

Explain to participants that the purpose of this game is to develop their awareness of posture and core stability. They will try to pass the duck using their arms only, keeping their torso stable and tall, while only their arms move. They should keep their elbows close to their sides.

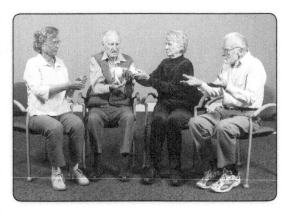

- Use the following cues.
  - Sit tall on the edge of the chair.
  - Elbows are bent and held close to your sides.
  - Abs are braced, ribs are lifted, and shoulder blades are back and down.
  - Practice how you will pass the duck. Keep your back still, no twisting. Only the forearms should move much at all.
  - Good job! That's how you want to do all the passes. Ready?
- Start the music and start passing the duck.
- Stop the music. Whoever is caught holding the duck is out of the game. Remove one chair and keep going.
- Eventually eliminate all but the winner.

Give It More Balance))

- Call out changes in the passing pace (e.g., slower, faster).
- Have participants sit closer to the edge of the chair with feet tandem and heels raised.
- Have participants gently toss the duck to each other (instead of pass).

Keep It Safe))

Nothing should hurt. Trunks stay still; only the arms move.

Live It))

Passing the duck will help participants keep their torso stable for long periods of time while they are busy having fun.

BALANCE

SEATED BALLOON OR BEACH-BALL VOLLEYBALL

This activity can be done by just one person, or it can become a fun group activity.

Benefits))

- Improves eye–hand coordination.
- Develops reaching skills.
- Strengthens back extensors.

Set It Up))

You will need balloons or beach balls. Set out groups of four or five chairs in small circles.

How to Do It))

- Give the groups a goal. First group to 10 volleys without their balloon hitting the floor is a good first goal.
- Use the following cues.
    - Which group can do it first? Ready, set, go!
    - Keep the abs in whenever you reach.
    - Use your Venus de Milo arms!
    - Tap the balloon to your neighbor on the right.
    - Tap the balloon to your neighbor on the left.
    - Keep your eye on the ball when you are waiting for it.
    - Tap it to where you want it to go.
    - Make the push with your whole arm.

Give It More Balance))

- One Big Happy Audience: The group should be sitting fairly close together. Send out one or several balloons over the group. Their mission is to keep all the balloons in the air as long as possible.
- Divide the room in half. The contest is between the right side and the left side.
- Play while singing. Try the song *Row, Row, Row Your Boat*. Each group starts at a different verse. They must sing and keep the balloons up. It's chaotic and fun.
- Use glow-in-the-dark balloons. This is an intermediate activity because the lights need to be turned down low, which may make some people dizzy. Warn them of this possibility.
- Put up a net using see-through fabric or even a rope. Two to four people on each side will keep it lively.

Keep It Safe))

Know your group. Start easy, and stay easy enough for everyone to play.

Live It))

Physical activity should be fun. Eye–hand coordination is good skill practice and the beach ball makes it fun and social. It's a chance to laugh and work as a team.

BOP THE HEDGEHOGS

This tossing activity is easy enough that anyone can have fun playing it. Tossing involves balance. Whenever you toss an object, your center of gravity is slightly disturbed and you must control the forward momentum to keep your balance. Bop the Hedgehogs is a tossing game that helps participants learn to maintain balance and control momentum when letting go of an object. The use of visual targets helps improve eye–hand coordination, and core stability makes a difference, too.

Benefits))

- ◉ Focuses on balance, postural control, and core stability.
- ◉ Develops eye–hand coordination.
- ◉ Allows almost anyone to participate in a fun and easy activity.

Set It Up))

You will need tape to create a line for participants to stand behind, and you will need objects to toss and targets to hit. Soft objects and rings are good for tossing because they won't hurt someone if they bounce. Plan on having each participant toss at least three objects. Hedgehogs are the target, but you can also use other items for targets, such as agility dots, boxes, barrels, bull's-eye targets, and so on. Make it your own and enjoy!

How to Do It))

Put down a line for participants to stand behind. Put the targets out front. Assign point values to the targets, if you like. For example, red hedgehogs are 10 points, yellow are 5, and so on.

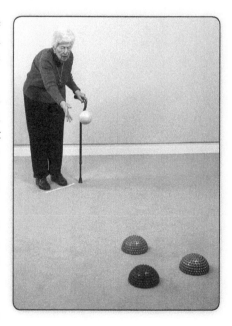

- ◉ Have participants practice a few throws. Underhanded is the safest and easiest for most, but let them decide. Coach them to keep their balance using core stability (an offset foot position will increase balance). Also practice how to extend their arms over the start line (offset feet and drop the hips back to act as an anchor). They will probably have fun being creative with their throws.

- ◉ Give each participant three objects to toss. Participants try to hit the targets with as much accuracy as they can. If it is too easy, make it more difficult. Here are some cues to use:
  - Stand stable.
  - Make a plan—what can you do to hit the target? What balance lessons will you apply?
  - Wind up your arm for the toss (pull it back).
  - Keep your eye on the target all the way through to the release.
  - How did your first plan work? Try again. What will you change?

Give It More Balance))

- Throw from a balance mat.
- Throw while standing on toes. (Advanced)
- Play the game on grass.
- Toss from one leg. (Advanced)

Keep It Safe))

Let participants determine the challenge level. Stand near the throwing line at first. Allow those with walkers to bring them to the start line.

Live It))

Hedgehogs are cute and make fun targets for tossing games that improve postural control.

BALANCE

CHAIN GANG

This is a passing game. Balloons are passed overhead, around the sides, and even through the legs. All of these motions are balance disturbing. Working on the Chain Gang is about keeping good balance while being challenged by all kinds of limb movements. It can be easily adapted for different abilities.

Benefits))

- ◉ Uses core stability to control balance and changes in momentum.
- ◉ Practices changing posture with balance control.
- ◉ Allows socializing while balance training.

Set It Up))

Choose several rocks (various objects) for each group to pass. I like balloons, balls, and fuzzy dice. None should be heavy and all should be large enough to pass easily. You will also need two rock boxes for each team's rocks. Place a rock box at the front and back of each line. Each line of participants fills a box of rocks.

How to Do It))

Divide the class into teams of four to eight. Each team forms a straight line. Some teams can sit in chairs and other teams can stand, if that works for your class. Each team is a designated chain gang. They must empty their box of rocks at the front of their line by passing the rocks to the box at the back of their line. To do so they will pass the rocks chain-gang style as you instruct them. Some passes will be overhead, some to the left, some to the right, and so on. Use cues such as these to prep them for the activity:

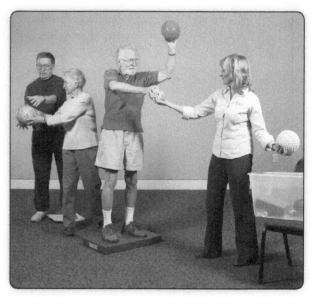

- ◉ What can core stability do for you while passing objects?
- ◉ Keep knees how? (soft)
- ◉ How are the feet? (offset or wide)
- ◉ Torsos are . . . ? (braced: abs in and up, shoulder blades back and down)
- ◉ When you reach for an object, how will you do that?
    - Keep your eyes on what? (the prize, the object they want to grab)
    - Keep your abs how? (braced, with arms doing as much of the work as possible)
    - How can you make your arms longer? (Venus de Milo arms)

Hand the first objects to each line. They will start at your signal. Each team must pass all the objects from front to back. Your instructions will tell them how. After all the rocks make it to one end, pass them back to the other end. Here are some ideas to cue passes:

- ◉ Pass on the right (everyone passes along the right side of their line).
- ◉ Pass on the left (pass the next rock along the left side of the line).
- ◉ Pass left, then right (alternate passing left and right from person to person).

- ◉ Pass right, then left.
- ◉ Pass overhead (carefully, with trunk braced).
- ◉ Pass through the legs, only if you think they are able, or overhead.
- ◉ Pass under, over, under, over.

Give It More Balance))

- ◉ Have the team sing *Row, Row, Row Your Boat* or the *Chain Gang*, if they know it.
- ◉ Play on a lawn, which is a naturally uneven surface.
- ◉ Those who are willing can stand on a balance pad.
- ◉ Use lightweight medicine balls.

Keep It Safe))

Until you are sure how this activity will go, keep it simple. Difference in heights can make it difficult to do overhead passes; the tall person nearly falls over trying to reach the short person. Teams will want to race each other. That's always fun, but do some practice rounds first.

Live It))

Core stability gives balance stability. Trying to keep the core still while moving the limbs helps participants stay balanced and is fun, too.

YOU SHOOT, YOU SCORE!

This advanced activity uses bouncing, dribbling, passing, and lifting skills. It's probably been awhile since your participants have bounced, dribbled, or passed a ball. This activity involves some distraction; they are walking and playing with a ball. It also integrates many aspects of balance, including gait, visual targets, core stability, agility, and coordination.

Benefits))

- ⊙ Practices mobile agility and coordination.
- ⊙ Uses visual targets in a challenging, fun activity.

Set It Up))

You will need stability balls or lightweight, soft playground balls in medium to large sizes, enough for one per person.

How to Do It))

Have participants stand with their back to a wall or in a corner, which gives them something to fall back on. Cue them to keep the knees soft and torso braced.

Bounce the Ball

Use the following cues.

- ⊙ Bounce the ball once and catch it.
- ⊙ Keep the knees soft and torso braced. Do it again.
- ⊙ If all goes well, bounce it several times in a row.
- ⊙ Change hands and bounce the ball with the other hand.
- ⊙ Can you change hands with each bounce?

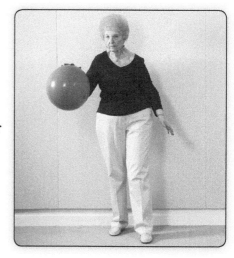

Toss and Catch

- ⊙ Play toss-and-catch games.
  - First toss and catch the ball while seated.
  - Keep the torso stable but moveable.
- ⊙ Stand for the toss and catch.
  - Wall is behind you.
  - Feet are offset toward your partner.
  - Torso is stable and knees are soft.
  - When you catch the ball, pull it toward you, not overhead.
  - Rock back a little as you catch it. (Helps absorb the momentum.)

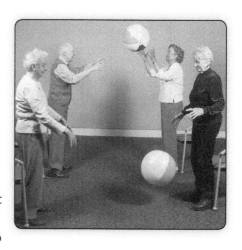

Dribble, Pass, and Shoot

Dribbling involves bouncing a ball and walking at the same time. It is difficult for many participants, but they may show improvement quickly. Participants bounce the ball in place with both hands. Then they walk and dribble. Provide a box for them to shoot baskets in.

Keep It Safe))

It's not professional basketball—keep it simple. Participants should only try the parts of this activity that they want to. Different participants will want to do different skills, but they all score!

Live It))

Not only are participants keeping balanced while their limbs move, they are keeping balanced while being perturbed by external objects, like balls.

BALANCE

SOCCER DRILL

Eye–hand and eye–foot coordination are both good skills for everyday mobility. This soccer drill will instill confidence in those who are successful. They will make comments such as "I did it!" and "It's been a long time since I kicked a ball."

Benefits))

- Improves eye–foot coordination.
- Uses dual tasks.
- Builds confidence.

Set It Up))

Create a soccer ball by wadding up a few pieces of newspaper and taping them into a ball. Tape it up pretty good so that it keeps its shape. These kinds of balls roll better and slower than real balls or balloons. Place an 18- to 20-foot (5.5- to 6-meter) tape line on the floor along a wall or handrail to provide a visual guide for the kicker to follow. At the end of the room, set up a net of some kind. It can be two chairs with a net at the back or just a line to kick the ball across—that's their goal.

How to Do It))

The task is to dribble a ball (using the inside of the foot, soccer style) along the tape line and across the goal line. Use the following cues.

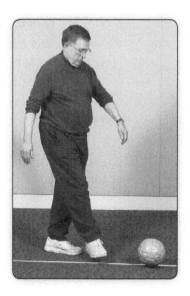

- Use gentle kicks.
- Keep core stable.
- Kick with a sweeping motion from the inside of your foot.
- Follow the line toward the goal.
- Keep your eye on the goal as you approach it.
- Use a sweeping movement to sweep the ball in the desired direction.

Give It More Balance))

- Partners pass the ball back and forth between two or three participants. They're a team. They work the ball up the field and score together!
- Change kicking legs more frequently.
- Make it more like a real soccer game and have two small teams of two to three people each (advanced).

Keep It Safe))

This is a more difficult activity in terms of fall risk. Take turns with the soccer drills.

Live It))

Soccer drills build self-confidence. Your participants can still play soccer!

RIVER FUN

River Fun is the grand finale. It combines lots of learning into a few goal-oriented activities. The river of balance is your stage for some drama and excitement.

Benefits))

- Adapts easily for various participants.
- Offers social, imaginative, fun activities for game days.
- Integrates many skills involved in balance.

Set It Up))

You will need many of the following items for these activities:

- Tape
- Agility dots
- Poly beams
- River treasures, such as stuffed toy frogs or prizes they can easily pick up
- Boxes on which to set river treasures
- Foam beams
- Variety of balance pads
- River stones or hedgehogs (both are available from catalogs and Web sites)
- Sunglasses
- Heads-up glasses

How to Do It))

Create a river challenge to match participant ability. Use masking tape for the river banks. (Make sure the tape is flat on the floor so there aren't any tripping hazards.) The banks should be close together at one end and get progressively farther apart so that the shape resembles the letter *A*. At least one of the shorelines can be wavy. There should be at least two bridges (one of tape and the other a balance beam) crossing the river. Place the appropriate items and other balance challenges inside the river.

Lazy River

Lazy River is the easiest River Fun challenge. Here are some suggestions:

- Walk along a straight shoreline (sidestep or tandem-walk the shore).
- Follow a wavy shoreline.
- Cross the river at its narrowest end with a single step.
- Cross the river at a wider point. The wider the crossing point, the more the step will begin to resemble a lunge step (belly steps).
- Cross the river on stepping stones (agility dots) or narrow bridges (tape line).
- Try not to get wet feet! Walk up and down the river only stepping on agility dots, taped *X*s (river rocks), and other dry features.

Category 3 River

This river has intermediate challenges that are a bit more difficult than the Lazy River.

- Poly beam: Place a poly beam across the river. Participants walk across, pretending it is a narrow bridge over the river.

- Easy-to-reach river treasures: Place some of the treasures on boxes or on chairs. (Having the objects higher off the floor will make them less precarious for participants to reach.) As participants explore the river and its banks, they can reach for treasures. They can stand on the banks or on river rocks (agility dots or taped *Xs*) and try to pick up their treasures.

- Take lunge steps across the river: Participants go where they think they can cross without getting their feet wet.

- Work their way up the river: Participants start from the lower banks and then work their way up the river, using lunge or belly steps to cross. Cue big steps and belly button training.

Category 5 River

Advanced River Fun activities add more challenges. They also require more supervision. Be available to spot participants. You might create two rivers at this point so one is easier and the other is harder. That way everyone can make their own choice and everyone can play.

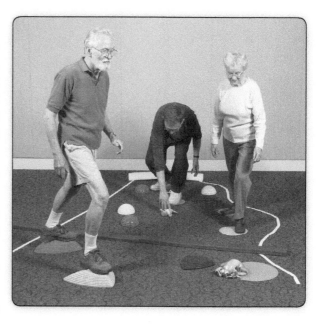

- Poly beams: Cross the river on poly beams (firm beams).

- Foam beams: Cross the river using foam beams (soft, compliant beams, such as balance pads).

- Balance pads: Place a few in the river (use a variety of densities).

- Hedgehogs: Cross by stepping on the hedgehogs.

- River treasures: Reach for river treasures placed on the floor or banks. (You could also include a high place, such as a waterfall or cliff, where they can reach up and find a treasure.)

- Kayak up the river, avoiding all the obstacles and staying in the water.

Give It More Balance))

- Space discs, stones, or hedgehogs farther apart.
- Leave more space between the beam bridges and shore.
- Sing, count, do multiplication tables, or carry something while navigating the river.
- Create an alligator pit. In the Alligator Pit, the theme and hazards change. Hedgehogs make great hidden alligators—they add the elements of time and anxiety (participants need to hurry to safety!) to make it more difficult. Depending on your group, use various kinds of bridges, dots, and river stones for participants to use as they navigate the pit.

BALANCE

Keep It Safe))

Participants should take turns so you can be available for balance safety and for giving cues. Everyone should have an escort in the perilous waters of balance. Always create more than one way to cross the river so people of all levels can play. Encourage, laugh, help plan, and help play. Participants know they should only do what they are comfortable doing.

Live It))

River Fun helps participants put together many of the skills they are beginning to master in balance class. It's a safe, fun place to try out those skills.

Cardiorespiratory Endurance

Cardiorespiratory training develops both power and stamina. The breath in your lungs becomes the spring in your step as oxygen delivery drives this energy system. Increasing cardiorespiratory endurance, or stamina, in your participants will have a positive effect on their everyday lives. Increased energy levels may reduce fatigue-related injuries (Nelson et al., 2007). And staying active will be easier with energy reserves that can keep up with aspirations, goals, and to-do lists. Active adults tend to be more independent, have more lifestyle options, and have a better quality of life (Mazzeo et al., 1998).

ACSM protocols for older adults and aerobic activity are discussed in more detail in chapters 1 through 3 and should be reviewed to proceed (Mazzeo et al., 1998; Nelson et al., 2007). To develop stamina, a person needs to accumulate 20 to 30 minutes of moderate, continuous work almost every day. Any moderate, continuous activities that target large muscle groups can be used for cardiorespiratory training. Intensity should be between light and somewhat hard, relative to an individual's aerobic fitness. On a 10-point scale, where sitting is 0 and an all-out effort is 10, moderate would be a rating of 5 or 6 and produce a noticeable increase in heart rate and breathing. The order of progression recom-

mended is to first increase frequency, then duration, and finally intensity. A 5-10 minute, light warm-up and a similar cool-down with stretching that suits the chosen activity should be a part of any regular cardiorespiratory program (Mazzeo et al., 1998; Nelson et al., 2007).

The protocol is slightly different for frail adults; it is necessary for them to first have adequate strength and balance before beginning cardiorespiratory training (Mazzeo et al., 1998). Most ABLE Bodies participants fall into this category; it is reasonable for the first several months to focus on flexibility, posture, core stability, strength, and balance. You should embark on a cardiorespiratory training program for these participants only when it is apparent they are willing and their exercise tolerance and balance confidence is improved. It may take months before some participants are ready for aerobic activity. Strength and balance take time to develop. You and they must be ready, willing, and able to progress. Review chapters 1 through 3 for more guidelines for beginning, selecting, and progressing aerobic activities.

Cardiorespiratory fitness can be taught as a separate class, or more gradually by making existing classes gradually more aerobically productive. This would be done by linking exercises, providing shorter rest periods, using more difficult exercise selections, and more. There are many more ideas to consider in chapter 2 under the sections Selecting Cardiorespiratory Activities (page 28) and Progressing Endurance Activities (page 38). Most of the activities in chapter 8 can be part of either scenario. Select activities you feel will help craft the best classes for your participants. I'm sure you will do great!

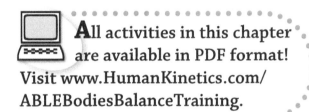 **A**ll activities in this chapter are available in PDF format! Visit www.HumanKinetics.com/ ABLEBodiesBalanceTraining.

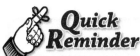 **Quick Reminder**

As always, progress only as well tolerated by your participants. Nothing should hurt; participants should be willing and able to continue; and show no signs of dizziness, nausea, or excessive fatigue. Provide adequate balance support, especially when frailer adults are on their feet. Overall, look for a clear sense of both exercise tolerance and balance confidence in your participants as they perform. Watch for signs of tiring; getting too hot, heavy breathing, needing to sit down, pain in their faces, new clumsiness, and complaints or comments like "oh my aching back!" These are good indicators to slow things way down, do some easy seated stretches, rest, or stop. You can review chapter 3 for more information on exercise tolerance.

CARDIO

AFRICAN SAFARI

The goal of this activity is for participants to stay active for up to 10 minutes. Use this trip or design your own trips, such as trips to various countries, childhood tales, or stories common to your participants' culture.

Benefits))

- Provides a fun and imaginative way to be active.
- Keeps participants active for 5 to 10 minutes.
- Introduces heart rate awareness.

How to Do It))

Begin this activity after warming up and stretching. As you go through the scenarios, get participants as active as you can by exaggerating the chosen movements. Use fingers, arms, shoulders, legs, and feet however you can. Be imaginative and have fun! Nearly all of this activity can be done while seated.

Get Ready to Go

You will be taking your participant on a trek to Africa to hunt a lion! But first, they must take their heart rate (thumb side of wrist, 10-second count). Ask them to remember that number. Now they are medically cleared for takeoff.

Start the trip from their home. Begin with seated marching as they walk around their home packing. What will they need? Ask for ideas. Use the following cues.

- Will you need a passport? Pretend you're going upstairs and getting a passport out of a drawer. Lift the lid of your imaginary, very large suitcase and put the passport in.
- How about a safari hat? Pretend you're walking to another room. Reach up high into a closet. Oops, you can't quite reach it with the left arm, so reach with the right arm (stretch it out with Venus de Milo ribs and arms). Snag the hat and walk it over to your suitcase.
- Pack a few more items, such as underwear that's still in the dryer downstairs, a toothbrush, and maybe a wallet that fell behind the nightstand. Find or retrieve the items and put them in the suitcase, one at a time.
- Close the suitcase, drag it off the bed, and haul it with great effort down the stairs.
- With great aplomb, open your front door, and lug that heavy suitcase out to your car. Pop open the trunk and load your suitcase.
- Open the car door and hop in, get settled. You're off on your great safari!

Drive to the Boat Dock

- Put your keys into the ignition, push in the heavy clutch, and start the car. It takes two tries. That's two clutch pumps!
- Begin to drive the car. Use lots of arm motions to steer. Bounce and sway.
- Lean over and turn on the radio.
- Check out the neighborhood, Smell the Coffee at your local coffee shop.
- Drop your cell phone on the floor and retrieve it. Chatter awhile and drive.
- Whoa! Stomp on the breaks—you almost missed a stop sign. Put the phone down.
- Reach over and pick up the stuff that slid off the seat.

CARDIO

- Look over your shoulder. Did anyone see that?
- Make some turns and have some other adventures on the way to the port.
- Arrive at the boat dock and park.
- Get your backpack from the trunk and put it on using great, big arm motions.
- Haul out that heavy suitcase and hand it off to a valet.
- Keep marching (while seated).

Get on Board

- Keep marching.
- Walk up a rickety plank to get on board. Use big, wide steps and let your trunk sway wide, too.
- Your arms walk/climb along the handrail keeping you steady.
- Now it's finally time to say goodbye. Hug all your family and friends.
    - Some family members are small. Bend down to hug them.
    - Some friends are tall. Reach high to hug them.
    - Wave good-bye! Big arm waves!

On Board the Ship

- Play shuffleboard with imaginary big, long sticks.
- Now you're getting seasick. Oh no! Rock back and forth in a wretched way until you've lost your lunch over the rail. (Be careful they don't hit their head on a table.)
- Ah, now you feel better. Go swimming—use the breaststroke, sidestroke, and fancy diving, too.
- Ballroom dance the night away. Some grand ballroom waltzing and a little jiggy.
- Wake up early and stretch.

Arrive in Africa

- De-board the ship using the same rickety plank. Big wide steps (while seated), body sways, and arms climb along the railing.
- Meet your guide with a big handshake.
- Climb in the jeep.
- Put your backpack and camera behind you in the private jeep, with the backpack on one side and the camera gear on the other.

Start Driving

- You're the driver because you like to be in control. Bounce along in the jeep over rough terrain.
- The steering wheel is oversized. Use big arms and make some big turns.
- Stop once or twice and survey the terrain. You're looking for big game.

Spot Something

- You think you spot something. Get out of the jeep. Reach back in for your camera bag.
- Start tromping through tall grass. Push the grass out of your face.

- Trudge through a swamp (while seated), use big knee lifts with feet that keep getting stuck in the mud.
- (Instructor roars loudly.) It's a lion! And it's coming straight for you!
- Drop your camera and run.
- Come to a tree and climb up it (stand up, if able).

Take Heart Rate

- Your heart rate should be elevated well over that resting rate you took earlier. Is it? Are you breathing harder?
- All that and you barely moved from your chair! Now back to that nasty lion.

Throw Coconuts

- Turns out you're up a coconut tree. (It's the only one in Africa.)
- Pick a coconut from your tree. (Reach up and unscrew a coconut.)
- Throw one at the lion. It misses.
- Use the other arm to get another coconut. Throw it!
- Climb a little higher.
- Dig through your pack for your extra camera and take a picture.

Resolve the Situation

The lion leaves or the guide arrives, whichever scenario you choose. Then they can climb back down and walk back to the jeep. Later that night, they can dance around the fire or help local citizens clear fields or build a school. It's your story now. When you're done, debrief them:

- Did you have fun?
- Were you amazed by the change in your heart rate?
- We stayed mostly seated, right?
- And it wasn't that tough? Fun, doable, and amazing aerobic results. Perfect!

TRIP TO THE OLYMPICS

Take the class with you to the Olympics. Many aspects of this activity can be done seated.

Benefits 》

- Uses fun and imagination to create new ideas in movement.
- Keeps participants active for 5 to 10 minutes.

How to Do It 》

In this activity, participants are novice athletes with Olympic fantasies—they want to try out all the Olympic sports they can. Perhaps you can ask them for their favorite events or events they'd like to try. Your goal is to involve as many major joints and muscle groups as possible in the chosen activities. Ideas are presented here for both upper- and lower-body exercises. If you like, all of these activities can be done while seated.

Opening Ceremonies

- Imagine the grandeur and excitement. Lift your head up and look around; breathe in all the sights, sounds, and excitement. Turn your head right and left to see; get jostled by the crowd; get out of somebody's way who is in a big hurry. Wow, this is amazing!
- March in the stadium. Big knees marching. You're an athlete! Big, puffed-up chest.
- Carry the flag as the athletes march in.
- Wave to the crowds, turn your whole body to wave all around.
- Grab your camera from a back pocket and snap pictures.
- Turn and twist, looking all around to take in the sights.
- Light the torch. Stand or sit tall with a torch held high in one hand. Then in the other hand.

Swimming

- Get ready, get set, (whistle!) dive in the water at the bell.
- Swim multiple events or work on just one. The crawl (freestyle), breaststroke, backstroke, or any stroke that can be done fluidly. (Make the race close—competition gets people to push themselves.) Swim vertically (upwards) to strengthen back extensors.
- Work on the breathing in the crawl stroke. Change arms and breathe out the other side. Inhale, exhale, and take big breaths.

Diving

- Climb the big ladder. Arms and knees climb a ladder.
- Jump (imaginatively, not literally). You can do any dive you want!
- Use your arms to create a dive—swan, half-twist, or whatever you can do from your chair.

Volleyball

- Warm up your hands and fingers for the match (rub them together, wriggle and crunch the fingers, flex and extend them, do wrist circles).
- Serve the ball.
- Reach up and spike the ball to win the point.

CARDIO

- Change arms and spike again with that arm.
- Dig out a save from the right side of the chair (two straight arms get under a low ball and pop it up).
- Dig out a save from the left side of the chair.
- Set up a ball so your neighbor can spike it.
- Jump to block a ball that's flying over the net.

Basketball

- Play some Olympic basketball from the chairs using an imaginary ball.
- Dribble with one hand and then with the other.
- Pass the ball behind your back and dribble some more.
- Pass the ball to your neighbor on the right, then the left.
- Use your back to block another player trying to get by you.
- Catch a pass.
- Quickly move among the other players to get to the basket.
- Shoot a basket. You shoot, you score!
- Reach up for a rebound. Get it and then use your elbows to create some space for you and the ball.

Kayaking

Sometimes it's best to separate upper- and lower-body activities. Kayaking is an excellent upper-body activity using long, double-paddled oars. Participants dip one oar in the water, drag it back, lift it out of the water, and then dig it in on the other side. Pull it back and up again. Dig right, pull back, up and center. Dig left, pull back, up and center. (This activity gives participants a chance to use reciprocal arm motions and to develop core stability.) Be sure to cue them to keep the back tall and straight, with their abdominals braced. Can they feel their strength?

- Carry the kayak overhead to the water and put it in the water. Climb in and get comfortable. (To add more torso difficulty and balance challenge, ask participants to cross their ankles and hold their legs off the ground as they paddle.)
- Put on your helmet and life jacket.
- Practice the arm movements in the practice pool.
- When ready, paddle to the starting line.
- Backstroke to keep the kayak from moving forward until the gun fires.
- Bang! You're off! Head down your course!
- Look for and conquer obstacles. Turn to look at your fans in the crowd.
- At the end, hold your paddles overhead in triumph. You did it!

Curling

Curling is a fun upper-body activity that builds both core stability and balance. The quick, sweeping motion with a broom while the torso is held still is an awesome strength challenge for the torso. The quick motions are disturbing to balance, making the activity a great balance challenge, too. Get used to curling while seated, and over time progress to trying the activity standing.

Hand participants an imaginary broom or a real stick if you have one.

- Sit at the edge of the chair, knees wide apart.
- The first stone is thrown and you're ready with your broom—sweep, sweep, sweep, sweep, sweep. (Cue them to use core stability with those strong, fast strokes!)
- Get out of the way and check the results. Looks good! Wait for the next stone.
- Here it comes—sweep, sweep, sweep.
- Continue until your stone hits your imaginary goal. Great job!

Other Upper-Body Events

Use your imagination. Gymnastics, badminton, javelin throw, synchronized swimming, archery, shooting, judo—you can include just about any activity that's fun and physically engaging. If you can imagine the possibilities, you can come up with a story.

Skating

Skating is an excellent lower-body and core-stability activity. Speed skating provides a good opportunity to practice side-to-side weight shifts. If participants are sitting, have them sit on the edge of their chair. If they're standing, have them stand behind their chair with one or both hands on the chair. The following cues are for speed skating, but try some figure skating, too—it takes upper- and lower-body grace.

- Everyone's at the starting line. Stretch, move side to side, practice the arm swings, and put on your game face.
- Assume the ready position.
- The gun goes off! Start the race.
- Right, left, right, left, with nice, even strokes (instructor calls the pace).
- Come to the first corner: right, right, right, right, right, and straighten it out.
- After a bit of straight, round the next corner: left, left, left, and so on.
- Sprint for the finish!

Track and Field

You can create both upper- and lower-body activities from track and field events. Pick a couple of activities. Long-jump arms and throwing the javelin or discus are good events for the upper body, whereas the 100-meter dash will engage the lower body. The hurdles, done from a chair (big, reciprocal arms and legs), involve both the upper and lower body.

Skiing and Snowboarding

Imaginary skiing engages both the upper and lower body. Imagine a slalom race—that means lots of turns. If participants can stand, they place their feet shoulder-width apart. Have them imagine skis on their feet and ski poles in their hands. For safety, they can stand in front of their chairs or to the side with one hand on their chair.

- Starting gate: Crouch low and then explode out of the gate (keep one hand on the chair).
  - Head down the ramp and to the jump.
  - Imagine you fly 400 feet (122 meters) standing tall over your skis. Then land with a bit of a knee bend and start your turns. On to the slalom course!

- Slalom ski turns: Practice a turn or two first. As the knees bend and point right, the left arm reaches out (pole plants) and pulls back as you complete the turn.
- Cross-country: Stand with one foot forward, one foot back in front of a chair. Big arm swings are offset by slight knee bends for each stroke. Pace it easy and just feel the motion. Easy does it—it's a long race up hills and around turns. Save a few sprints for the finish.
- Snowboarding: Get on a snowboard, with one foot forward, one back. Picture the motions in your mind and then board down a hill.
    - Let the hips and torso oscillate over the board.
    - When you're ready, crouch and go for a jump.
    - Pretend to do a tip touch and come back down.
    - Bow as you collect your medal.

Fencing

Fencing benefits both the upper and lower body. Participants stand beside the chair with one foot forward, one back. They hold their saber in one hand and keep the other hand on the chair as needed for balance support.

- Put your face shield down. It's show time.
- Raise your saber and circle it overhead.
- Circle it in front toward your clever opponent.
- Lunge (knees both bend) and push the saber toward your opponent.
- Pull back the front foot so you're standing with your feet side by side.
- Lunge again (step forward with one foot) and push the saber out again.
- If you're confident of your balance, do the next lunge with one hand on the hip instead of the chair.
- Be Zorro for a moment—lunge forward and make a Z with your saber.
- Pretend to fight many bad guys, some coming at you from the right, some from in front.
- Watch out! You turn in time to see another opponent coming at you from behind.
- Surprise—you're ambidextrous! Move to the other side of the chair and fence with the other hand.
- Conquer all and take a Gentlemen's Bow. Give the crowd a big wave.

WALKABOUTS

WalkAbouts are as basic as their title. The term refers to a type of wandering journey by Australian aborigines, but it is also used by Queen Elizabeth II to describe her public greet-and-meet walks outside Windsor Castle. ABLE Bodies WalkAbouts are similar; they allow participants to walk around the room and talk with each other as they warm up for class. WalkAbouts gradually turn into miniature obstacle courses as you begin adding a few simple everyday balance challenges. Be creative, but keep it simple. You just want them walking and practicing a few everyday skills, such as stopping and starting, changing direction and speed, turning, overcoming obstacles, and so on. Even short amounts of time spent walking can offer cardiorespiratory benefits, especially for frail participants. Encourage the more fit participants to do several laps for better results.

Many groups, especially frailer groups, would rather begin with stretching. It may be tough to get a committed group of preclass walkers; most participants may be intent on getting settled in their particular chair before class. Consider making name tags for the chairs so participants can save their spot. The majority of ABLE Bodies endurance training comes by way of WalkAbouts and by gradually increasing connected minutes of exercise.

Benefits))

- ⊚ Adds an aerobic component to classes.
- ⊚ Practices everyday living skills.
- ⊚ Includes balance challenges to keep it interesting and engaging.
- ⊚ Practices recently learned skills.
- ⊚ Enhances listening and reaction skills.

How to Do It))

Plan WalkAbouts ahead of time. You can use the classroom space, but going to new areas, such as a hallway or outside on nice days, is always fun, too. The more you've done ahead of time, the more available you'll be to help participants. Your WalkAbout plan should include a floor plan with appropriate safe floor space and balance supports for safety (e.g., handrails, chairs). You should also plan for resting chairs and benches—it's always necessary to have some backup balance supports.

Anticipate traffic jams, which happen easily and create fall risks. Changes in direction are good for balance training but require planning and caution. Participants' abilities will vary widely, and many will use walkers and canes. If participants generally use walkers, encourage them to use their walkers here, too, and you need to plan for the extra congestion they will cause.

Some participants will have problems hearing commands. Be aware of noise levels in the room, especially when everyone is walking, talking, and having fun. Plan ahead so that all participants will be able to hear you. Do you need a microphone, or is there a specific place where you can stand and be heard best? Music may help with pacing, rhythm, and motivation; it has a way of keeping the group moving. However, it can also cause annoyance and confusion. In some situations adding music can be too much. Ideally, if you do choose to add music, do so softly and gradually; you'll learn from the participants what they prefer. Check with them about the volume and music choices. Have your selections cued ahead of time so you won't be distracted by changing music.

Keep WalkAbouts simple—resist the temptation to do too much at once or too soon. Chaos, defined as an out-of-control situation, can happen all too easily when too many people are doing too many things. Plus, this activity is for cardiorespiratory improvement. Adding several balance toys or challenges will slow that progression down and change the dynamics. Two kinds of balance challenges per course are probably about right.

The first goal is to just get participants up and moving before class. Slower people can walk inside the circle and faster ones can pass on the outside, which is a longer path. The first several weeks you offer a WalkAbout, do plain walking for 3 to 5 minutes. Let people go as slow as they need. Involve yourself—get in and walk and talk with them. Thank them for coming, and use their names. See how it goes the first few times and learn how you can make it go more smoothly.

After a few weeks, encourage a moderate pace. Moderate means they can walk and talk easily at the same time. Look for signs that they can do this with ease and confidence. Cue them to walk and talk with friends. They should appear comfortable and engaged. Socialize with them yourself—it's a simple way to monitor their intensity.

Over more time, add a bit of an obstacle course. Try ideas in Traffic School (chapter 7) for starters. Changes in pace and direction, commands to follow, and head turns add dual tasking and other balance aspects to WalkAbouts. If you plan to use any tape, chalk, cones, dots, or hurdles, give participants a few laps to observe the course first. Then when they're ready, they can play. It's always their choice.

Here are some cues you can use for WalkAbouts.

Start Walking

- Start slow, and stay slow if you'd like. Just keep walking at a pace that suits you.
- Stop and sit awhile if you like.
- There's no race; no hare and no tortoise. Walk at your own pace.
- Walk and talk. Share some news. Talk with your friends, have some fun, and keep going at your own pace.

Now you've got participants up and going. From here you can add changes to how they walk.

Focus on Posture

- Walk tall, everyone! Pretend there's a string from the crown of your head to the ceiling.
- If you have a walker, move closer to its front bar. It will be easier to walk tall that way.
- Walk with your stomach pulled in a little.
- Does that feel better for your back? (It definitely should.)
- Where are your shoulders?
    - Over your hips?
    - Or over your toes?
    - Which feels better?
- Did everyone notice how those changes in posture felt?
    - Slump walk
    - Bent Over Posture (chapter 5)
    - Tall walk
- Share the differences you feel. Just call out your answers! We'll all listen.

CHANGE OF PACE

This activity is described in Traffic School (chapter 7). Here it is used for cardiorespiratory workouts. Changing pace is more difficult than maintaining pace; it includes controlling momentum. Call out various speeds. Be careful about using the fast or fast-stopping commands at first. Here are some examples:

- Walk slow. Walk slower. Walk very, very slowly.
- Step by step, inch by inch, slowly we turn.
- Pick up the pace. It's time to get going!
- Walk fast. Walk faster. Walk as fast as you safely can.

You can increase the balance challenge of this activity by doing the following:

- Stop: Use stops only during slow paces at first. Then stop during a more moderate pace. For advanced participants, do fast stops.
- Change directions: Call out changes in direction several times. If the room is big enough and you have good crowd control (participants are spaced out), use left and right turns as direction changes, too.
- Stop and go: Intersperse these two commands here and there. When you say *stop*, they should stop as quickly as they safely can. For *go*, they should get going as quickly as they can.

For more able groups, consider the following ideas for WalkAbouts. These increased balance challenges require closer supervision. Have participants take turns so you can be available to hold hands, or have plenty of balance support nearby, such as handrails or a set of chairs.

- March (beside a handrail).
    - Big steps with abs in
    - Little steps
    - Big again
- Add music.
- Walk in opposing directions (see Opposing Circles, page 255).
- Walk with head turns (beside a handrail). This one is tricky; they may get dizzy or clumsy. Often participants turn their whole body or lose their footing when they turn their head. See chapter 7 for more on introducing this movement.)
- Use arm swings.
    - Use big arms swings.
    - Bend the elbows (it's easier).
    - Can they feel the momentum arm swings add to their walking motion?
- Take big, long steps (similar to lunge steps).
    - Cross an imaginary chasm.
    - How much distance can one step cover? Are both legs equally good at covering distance?
- Add bridges, tunnels, and corners. Look around, find something that you can walk under, such as an overhanging wall or a stairway. Participants can also form a bridge that lowers or raises as participants duck under to pass through.

- Use corners in the room. As part of the balance challenge course, walk into and out of a corner. See if they can use a pivot step out of the corner.

- Combine arm swings with marching, then with big steps, and then with big, long steps. For advanced groups, add a head turn to big, long steps.

- Do figure eights. Put out cones or place chairs for participants to go around in a figure-eight pattern. Some days use patterns that are tight; for example, they'll need to pass between a wall and a chair. Or, advanced participants can go through the pattern while sidestepping.

- Dim the lights. Turn them down just enough to dim the room and get their attention. There should be no other obstacles in a dim room. A good progression in a dim room could be to give them flashlights and have them point the lights farther and farther ahead in their path until they are looking more forward than down as they walk. You could place objects for them to find with their flashlights—birds on the walls or ceilings, squirrels on the low walls, the telephone, the light switch, the bucket you've stocked with candy!

- Side Steps Walking.

- Walk tandem lines: Use masking tape in a straight line that participants try to walk along.

- Walk squiggling tandem lines: Use masking tape to create long, wavy lines.

- Step only on agility dots: Set out agility dots or masking tape *X*s in a pattern that calls for big, long steps or a wide stepping pattern.

- Add a step to walk up and over. Participants will step up onto the step and then off. Cue them to make it a part of their stride if they can.

- Add a balance pad to step up and over.

- Step over hurdles. Set out a few small hurdles, 6 inches (15 centimeters) or lower, to step over. If you have no hurdles, put down a brightly colored object such as a book or shoe box.

Keep It Safe))

Most variations need a handrail, row of chairs, or other balance support. Watch participants for signs of being overly tired, dizzy, or otherwise not tolerating the activity well. Let them know they should be able to walk and talk, and remind them to pay attention to how they feel. Share responsibility with them; they are capable of monitoring how they feel.

Be prepared to manage traffic problems. Canes, walkers, and many differences in walking speed, seeing, and hearing abilities means you need to plan for traffic. Keep people spread out. You might have a slow lane (inside lane) and a faster lane (outside lane); you can tell participants to be courteous and careful passers. Keep the area clear of obstacles and equipment.

CARDIO

GAMES

Playing games keeps participants on their feet and keeps up their heart rate, adding a cardiorespiratory component to classes. Teamwork will make the classes more social, providing connections among participants and additional inspiration—no one wants to let the team down.

Benefits 》

- Engages participants in a fun, social activity.
- Adds motivation and effort through competitive aspects.
- Builds teamwork.

How to Do It 》

Make sure you are prepared with a plan for which you've done a trial run with staff or friends. Whatever the game is, make sure the props are ready to go. Know the rules, and try to troubleshoot what could go wrong. Consider the various ability levels and what each person can do safely in a class setting. It's easy to have a good idea of how a game works, but it helps to do a dry run. Kinks happen, and the more you work them out ahead of time, the better the games will flow. For cardiorespiratory effects, pick games that take time and keep people involved. If you're using teams, for example, smaller teams will be more aerobic because there will be shorter rests between turns.

Four Corners

Participants walk to the four corners of a room depending on how they answer questions. You should see waves of movement with each answer. In addition to moving around, participants will get to know new things about each other. Participants go to a specific corner depending on how they respond to questions about these kinds of topics:

- Participants who had only male children, female children, no children, or five or more children.
- Participants who were housewives, teachers, leaders, or in the medical field
- Participants who like green, red, blue, or yellow
- Participants who played tennis, played golf, swam, were spectators, ballroom danced, square danced
- Participants who had a family member who fought in a war, went to the Olympics, homesteaded
- Favorite seasons
- Favorite food groups

Relays

Relays are another team activity that can add a cardiorespiratory component to your normal exercise class. For greater aerobic conditioning, make the relay routes longer and teams smaller. You can also do relays back to back to keep participants going. Rearrange teams and start again.

Try to keep the teams as evenly skilled as possible. If one team wins all the time, move some members out or give them a tougher route or task the next time.

CARDIO

ABLE Bodies Balance Training

Get Up and Go Relay

The format of this relay race is similar to the Rikli and Jones Get Up and Go test (Rikli and Jones, 2001), but this version is a lot more fun! Most participants move much faster in a game than they will for a test.

- Form relay teams of four people per team. Each team member sits on a chair.
- Place an agility cone (or a piece of furniture) about 8 to 12 feet (2.5 to 4 meters) in front of each team.
- To win each team must send all four players, one at a time, down and around the agility cone and back. Each player must wait for the player in front of them to sit down before he or she rises to go. The team that can do this the fastest wins.
- The winning teams can challenge another team and so on. You can handicap the winning team with a balance beam, tandem line, or make them all use walkers.

Traditional Games

Traditional games are a great way to add a cardiorespiratory component to your class or for participants to do on their own. The main idea is to get out and have a little fun while putting balance and mobility training to the test. Try miniature golf, bocce ball, shuffleboard, and table tennis. As with the relays, try to keep the teams as evenly skilled as possible. If one team wins all the time, move some members out or give them more challenges the next time. Have fun with it!

Other Games

You can use games from other chapters, such as Pass the Duck and Bop the Hedgehogs, and you will also find yourself making up new games. Once you get going, you'll have many ideas to contribute to participants' fun and continued success.

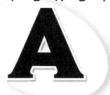

Sample Balance Training Sessions

ow! What a journey we've had together through all these chapters, tools, and activities. It is my hope you've enjoyed the journey and your head is swirling with new ideas you can't wait to try. You've probably learned lots. Your classes will have new infusions of your fresh ideas. They will be fun, interesting, and exciting. You can challenge participants to learn with their mind and body. Their positive results will bolster their self-confidence and their well-being.

So, maybe you're wondering just where and how to start. This appendix provides 16 progressive session plans to help instructors, trainers, and others get started using ABLE Bodies techniques and activities.

The materials do not span any certain timeline. They can be spread out over months, or weeks. You can start at Session 1 and work through all the sessions and it should take however long it takes. One session is not necessarily one class, though it could be. One session could be spread out for several class periods. In our initial study, every regular session was supplemented with short practice sessions led by university interns, who focused on main points and strength training so we could meet minimum ACSM protocols for strength training (Mazzeo et al., 1998) twice each week. It worked out well for us and over the 16 weeks we were able to demonstrate significant improvements in strength and balance (Scott and Rosenberg, 2005)

The sample sessions begin from day one, where you first meet a new class and the activities are easy. From there, each sample session weaves in something to represent all five ABLE Bodies components. The sessions use a variety of activities that gradually progress in difficulty. The plans are complete, including suggestions for participant homework (activities they can do on their own) and for practice sessions described earlier (little classes between classes).

All of the sessions have been used successfully in assisted living and retirement communities and they were designed specifically for frail elders. The recommended group size for these sessions is 8 to 12 participants. Each plan takes approximately 45 to 60 minutes.

SESSION ORGANIZATION

Each session is presented as a recipe, so to speak. The list of ingredients is the supplies and activities. Some preparation is needed ahead of time. Each class starts with a warm-up to get their bodies ready, not unlike preheating an oven. Then the action plan will give step-by-step instructions for how to put the components together. There are optional dashes of this or that, and ideas for serving the activity with a bit of flair. You'll want to add your special touches, too!

Each session plan is built on a template with the following parts:

▶ Supplies—What you need to bring along for that session. Each session will prompt you to bring the following:

- Written session plan.

- Equipment list: everything that is needed for each activity.

- Activity printouts: the descriptions of each activity can be found on the online resource at www.HumanKinetics.com/ABLEBodiesBalanceTraining.

- Participant homework: these are available on the online resource at www.HumanKinetics.com/ABLEBodiesBalanceTraining

- Roster: a way to take attendance. Rosters will help you learn names and track attendance. They show participants you care they attend, and creates an expectation for them to come. Attendance will influence your results; people who exercise consistently typically show greater changes in strength, function, and balance. Finally, rosters are an easy way for awarding motivational rewards: Certificates of completion (see appendix C), stars, stickers, or gift certificates for coffee, movies, merchandise, tee shirts, maybe their own Slo Mo ball or flashlight?

▶ Advance Preparation—What needs to be done ahead of time for today.

▶ Opening—Openings are important; make a good first impression every class. Start on time with a welcome.

- With new groups your opening may also include an icebreaker and a discussion establishing ground rules for safety.

- You'll be reminded to take roll.

- You'll be reminded to make announcements.

- You'll prepare your participants for learning with brief reviews of what they learned previously and previews for what they can expect to learn today. This review/preview time helps participants link to past experiences, prepare to explore new information, and reinforce the topic of the session.

▶ ABLE Bodies Activities—Most every session will include something from each of the five components of ABLE Bodies:

- Flexibility

- Posture and core stability

- Strength for a purpose

- Balance and mobility

- Cardiorespiratory endurance

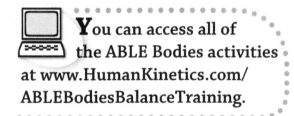 **You can access all of the ABLE Bodies activities at www.HumanKinetics.com/ABLEBodiesBalanceTraining.**

▶ The order in which you present activities from each component may change from class to class. For example, your cardiorespiratory component may be first if that component is used as an active warm up. And you may present strength activities before balance activities, early on, when the strength activities are more difficult than the balance activities. Many activities overlap components, so expect to see activities from chapter 5 under balance on occasion. For example, Posture Affects Function and Balance can be used as a balance or a posture activity. Tall Sits, a core stability exercise, can be used as Strength for a Purpose in early sessions. The point is that at day's end, you've presented a little from each component.

- Closing— Start strong, finish strong. Your Action Plan will prompt these features to ensure a strong finish to your ABLE Bodies session.
  - Finish on time and with a thank you for coming.
  - Give them a Take-Home Message— Leave your participants with one or two things to think about this week. Sometimes it's the theme you used that day, or a brief summary bringing together what you hope they've learned.
  - Throw out a hook—Something that will bring them back next time. A good hook creates curiosity and builds excitement and anticipation for what they will learn next. Hooks will get their minds processing thoughts and preparing a place for your new information before you even arrive next session!
  - Give them some homework—ABLE Bodies Homework is not lots to do. It will consist of flexibility and strength activities, a suggestion to take some walks, and perhaps a concept to ponder. Homework is one more way to bolster compliance with ACSM protocols for strength, flexibility, and cardiorespiratory training. And . . . it keeps participants actively engaged and self processing what they are learning. Be forewarned, getting participants to do their homework is tough; most prefer to rely on class settings for exercise, instead. But some participants will do the homework, and accordingly, their actions will begin to make a difference in their results. Their self motivation will empower them from within. It's good stuff!
  - Leave them laughing with a funny joke or inspired with a favorite quote.

You can access the homework handouts at www.HumanKinetics.com/ ABLEBodiesBalanceTraining.

These sessions will get busy; there is always lots to do. And much depends on how things go that day. You may not get all the way through your planned session in one class. That is okay. Plan A can become Plan B. Simply wind down in a reasonable way and finish on time. Then make written notes so leftover activities can be built into your next session.

PRACTICE SESSIONS

Practice sessions are short and sweet—just the basics, done in 15 to 20 minutes. These added short sessions give your group extra work for better balance. They are another way that your group can meet ACSM protocols for building strength and improving flexibility (Nelson et al., 2007). Basically, practice sessions are the homework activities plus a balance element from their previous session. Practice sessions include:

- Whole-body stretch and/or an active warm-up from chapters 4 and 8
- Four to eight basic exercises from chapters 5 and 6
- Something balance or concept oriented, from the previous class.

Practice sessions may also offer additional opportunity to expand this program. If you are in a facility with other activity instructors who are interested in balance training, consider connecting with them. Practice sessions can help train another staff member, or a promising participant, to use ABLE activities in classes of their own. The new ABLE candidate should shadow each of your classes to prepare to lead the practice session. You will need to shadow their practices too, until you are confident they are comfortable on their own. It's a win/win situation. They will learn new things and you get an extra staff member to help hold hands during your session.

SAFETY

Chapter 3 discusses participant safety in great detail. For safety's sake, please review chapter 3 and be careful out there. The more you learn the better you will do.

TAKE HOME MESSAGE

Have fun with your participants; a little exertainment is good training! Fun, engaging, and challenging classes are the ones they will remember. You are bringing new learning into new places and transforming participants' everyday lives. Now, it's time to dig into these 16 recipes. Don't be afraid to experiment a little. The best recipes are made to order. I hope you will enjoy serving them up!

Feel-Good Posture

Supplies

- Written session plan
- Equipment list (supplies for activities)—No equipment is needed for this session.
- Activity printouts—Printouts are available at www.HumanKinetics.com/ABLEBodiesBalanceTraining
  - African Safari
  - Seated Whole-Body Stretch
  - Feel-Good Posture
  - Parts of the Whole
  - Posture Affects Function and Balance
  - Tall Sits
- Cheat sheets
- Participant homework for session 1
- Rosters and name tags—Bring a roster of names or a blank roster to fill in during class.

Advance Preparation

- Set up chairs. Provide a good view for each participant.
- Create list of emotions for Feel-Good Posture.

Opening

Welcome

Give a warm welcome to everyone. It's the beginning, and beginnings are important. They set expectations—expect great things.

Show personableness and respect. As participants come in, take note of their names. Then use their name somehow in your welcome; it will help you remember their names. Other welcoming behavior includes eye contact, a smile, a nod, or a hello. Also begin to observe physical abilities or limitations. Can they talk while they walk? Can they stand and sit easily? Can they turn their heads comfortably? Do they seem to be able to follow directions?

Attendance/Roll Call

After you take attendance ask them, "What's the best exercise?" Tell them, "It's the one you'll do!" Regular exercise is the only effective exercise. I hope you will come each class.

Icebreaker

Begin by introducing yourself. Share a few things about yourself and then thank them again for taking the time to come and work on their balance skills. Now, try to get them to talk about themselves and get to know each other. Here are a few icebreakers you can use this week or over the next few weeks:

- Count up all the grandchildren and great-grandchildren they have among them.
- Who has skied? Golfed? Played tennis? Fished? Played any unusual sports?
- Are there any artists, carpenters, teachers, nurses, or mechanics? Who had the most unusual job?
- Who had the longest marriage? Shortest? Most recent?

Encourage a few people to share something of themselves. Ask for volunteers to respond to these questions:

- What historical events did they witness?
- Complete the sentence: "One thing I am proud of in my life is _____."

Set Expectations

Ground rules or expectations are important for any group. Discuss how often and for how long your classes will meet. If you expect to miss any sessions, let them know. Then set out your rules. Here are some of mine:

- Classes will start on time and finish on time.
- Everyone will be respectful and courteous of others.
- All activities are optional. Participants choose what they like and are comfortable doing. Choosing only to observe is a valuable option. Your choice will be respected and welcome.
- Participants should only attempt what they are 90 percent certain they can do successfully. (It's our 90 percent rule, see chapter 3).
- Your role as their instructor is to be that other 10 percent from the 90 percent rule. You will be prepared and able to teach, encourage, respond to their progress, provide appropriate balance activities, and be committed to their safety and exercise.
- Safety is a shared responsibility. Their role is to make decisions with which they are comfortable and to let you know if they need help or have problems with any activity.
- Participants should listen to their body and do only what they feel comfortable doing. If their doctor has told them to avoid certain movements, they should avoid those movements. For example, participants with recent hip surgeries should not cross their legs and participants with osteoporosis should avoid flexing their spine.
- Nothing should hurt or make them feel uncomfortable, anxious, or ill.

Announcements

Will you have attendance rewards (i.e., a certificate)? How will they earn them?

Review and Preview

- Review
  - Today is the first class, so you could go over test results if you've done pretesting. Give them an idea of how they did as a group, rather than single any one out.
  - Ask them about their goals for starting this class.
  - Share your goals for the class.
- Preview
  - Today they'll learn a basic flexibility routine that they'll be doing at the beginning of each class. We'll do it the same way each week, so it is easier for them to remember and do on their own. And we will play with ideas about posture. We'll look at Parts of the Whole picture. Posture might be more important than they realized.
  - They'll explore posture and the effect that posture has on emotions and attitude.
  - They'll examine and experience how posture affects important everyday functions.
  - They'll take a trip to Africa.

ABLE Bodies Components

Cardiorespiratory Endurance
African Safari

Flexibility
Seated Whole-Body Stretch

Posture and Core Stability
- Feel-Good Posture
- Parts of the Whole

Strength for a Purpose
Tall Sits

Balance and Mobility
Posture Affects Function and Balance

Closing

On time with a thank you.

Take-Home Message

Posture affects people in many ways. As they experienced today, it can affect how they breathe, how they balance, how they feel, and how they move. Good posture habits are formed through constant repetitions done over long amounts of time. Good posture takes persistent practice. Tell participants to think tall and strong this week and to work on posture all they can. Ask them to notice posture in themselves and others over the next few days. Leave them trying to count how many parts can be adjusted: head, back, hips, feet, and attitude.

Hook

You've got a ball game in mind for session 2. Do they want to play? And for the ladies, you'll have some nice lotions.

Homework and Reminders

Pass out their homework. Welcome them back to school. There is homework, remember? Explain the benefits of homework. When done regularly, homework activities will complement the balance work done in class and help them improve their balance more quickly.

Their homework will vary and progresses over the first 10 sessions, so staying current is going to benefit them. After week 10 homework assignments will stay the same, but doing it regularly will continue to make a difference in their progress.

Fun and Inspiration

- Praise a few specific examples of good work on their part.
- End with a song, a mantra, an inspiring quote, or a funny joke and your thanks for coming along on this adventure in better living through exercise.

That's a wrap! If you got all the way through this material, great! If you were unable to do all the activities, pick up wherever you left off next time. The point of progressive training, after all, is to keep moving at a pace appropriate for your group. Make notes of any difficulties you had or activities you did not get to but would like to do later.

Need a printout of an activity? They are all available at www.HumanKinetics.com/ABLEBodiesBalanceTraining.

ABLE Bodies Practice Session 1

Explain what practice sessions are and announce the times when practice sessions will be offered and encourage them to come (entice them with socializing, fun, and treats).

Supplies

No supplies are needed for this session.

Warm-Up

Pick one of these activities from chapter 8:

- African Safari
- Trip to the Olympics

Flexibility

Seated Whole-Body Stretch

- Take plenty of time teaching these positions.
- Move slowly; give participants time to get into the positions.
- Help participants get a feel for how breathing expands their torso and adds to their stretches. They may also notice that it feels good and helps them relax.

Strength for a Purpose

Tall Sits

- Do three to six repetitions.
- Hold each for 3 to 15 seconds, as suits your group.

Balance and Mobility

Parts of the Whole (just work on a few of the options today)

- Feet—Try, compare, and decide which their bodies prefer between
  - duck feet,
  - pigeon toes, and
  - parallel feet feel.
- Knees—Try, compare, and decide which their bodies prefer between
  - pushed back and super straight, and
  - soft knees with a little bit of bounce to them
- Hips—Try, compare, and decide what feels best between
  - Pull abs up and in to bring hips under shoulders, and
  - Push hips backward and sling one hip out to the side.
- Ribs—Try, compare, and decide what feels best
  - ribs and back curved forward and hunched, or
  - ribs lifted with the spine lengthened.

- Shoulder—Try, compare, and decide what works best
  - rolled forward,
  - pulled way back, or
  - level, even, and pointing to the sides.
- Head—Try, compare, and decide what feels best
  - hung forward (can they feel how this overstretches their neck?),
  - off to one side, or
  - square above their flat, even shoulders with a level chin.

Overall Objectives

- Have fun with your participants.
- Get to know each other.
- Work on learning names and faces.

Coming to Your Senses

Supplies

- Written plan
- Equipment list (supplies for activities)
  - Three scented lotions—simple fragrances that are easy to identify
  - 1 unscented lotion
  - Eight to twelve balls (one per person, if possible). Get a variety of balls: tennis balls, footballs, baseballs, soccer balls, and even round fruit if you can find some that are fragrant (e.g., grapefruit, oranges)
  - A few nonrounded objects, such as fuzzy dice
  - One balloon (or Slo Mo ball) per person
- Activity printouts—Printouts are available at www.HumanKinetics.com/ABLEBodiesBalanceTraining
  - Trip to the Olympics
  - Seated Whole-Body Stretch
  - Supple Spine
  - Whooh, Whoohh, Whooohhh!
  - Thumb Rolls
  - The Ball Game
  - Coming to Your Senses
  - Tall Sits
  - Tall Sits With a Balloon Squeeze
- Participant homework for session 2
- Rosters and name tags

Advance Preparation

- Set up chairs. Provide a clear view and a safe exercise space for each participant.
- Be sure you know how to do each activity correctly; use printouts for any extra help you may need. Instructor should practice Supple Spine ahead of time. It takes a while to get all the pieces right.
- Put lotions and balls out of sight.

Opening

Welcome

On time with a welcome! Invite participants to be seated and thank them for coming.

Attendance/Roll Call

Keep learning and using names.

Icebreaker

If needed, do an icebreaker. Share a personal story, or ask them about something related to the day, the news, their facility, or the class.

Announcements

Make any necessary announcements.

Review and Preview

- Review
  - Did they practice Tall Sits?
  - Could they feel the difference in height when they sat tall?
  - Did they play with all the nuances of posture? Did they get their friends to try any of it? Did they notice the posture of others or read emotions by reading posture?
- Preview
  - Today they'll be learning from their body.
  - Without looking they'll use touch and smell to learn about their environment.

ABLE Bodies Components

Cardiorespiratory Endurance

An active warm up: Trip to the Olympics

Flexibility

- Seated Whole-Body Stretch
  - Use full, deep breaths that expand their ribs and help them relax.
  - Ask them to notice where they feel the stretches.
  - Explain that a good stretch is tolerable tightness in the targeted muscles.
- Supple Spine

Posture and Core Stability

- Whooh, Whoohh, Whooohhh! (this activity gives participants a feel for core stability)
- Thumb Rolls

Balance and Mobility

- The Ball Game
- Coming to Your Senses

Strength for a Purpose

- Tall Sits
- Tall Sits With a Balloon Squeeze

Closing

On time with a thank you!

Take-Home Message

Even gentle flexibility activities, such as Supple Spine, can improve function and feel great. Also, through ball games and hand lotions they learned about their environment from their senses, without their eyes. They felt, smelled, squeezed, and manipulated the balls to get sensory information which they automatically compared to their previous knowledge and came up with the ball type. In real life, they move through the environment using and learning from many senses. Their brains always know what their limbs are doing. Today they noticed that sometimes excluding one sense, such as vision, gets them tuned in to the other senses. Coming to all of their senses helps them to work better.

Hook

Next session they'll be dancing with dragons. Meanwhile, during the practice session this week they'll do Supple Spine again. They should bring a friend—it'll be fun!

Homework and Reminders

Yes, there's homework. Their balance will get better sooner if they do a little extra work on their own. Hand out the homework, review the new assignment, and answer questions. Encourage them to use good posture this week.

Announce when the practice session will be held. The practice session will review a few class activities and practice their ABLE Bodies homework exercises, so they can be sure they are doing them correctly.

Fun and Inspiration

- Praise something special that participants did today, such as great attendance, arriving early and ready, being quick learners, volunteering, taking a chance, and so on.
- End with a song, a mantra, an inspiring quote, or a funny joke and your thanks for coming along on this adventure in better living through exercise.

Make notes of any difficulties you had or activities you did not get to but would like to do later.

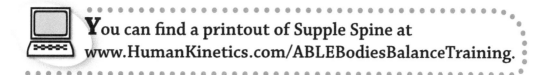

You can find a printout of Supple Spine at www.HumanKinetics.com/ABLEBodiesBalanceTraining.

ABLE Bodies Practice Session 2

Supplies

No supplies are needed for this practice session. However, you should practice Supple Spine ahead of time. It takes a while to learn.

Active Warm-Up

Today, the focus is on stretching and flexibility. So keep the active warm up simple. Use some simple and big shoulder rolls, then add arm rolls to the side. Turn those into arms reaching up, over head, and down towards the floor. Then do a few big, wide yawns that stretch their chests and backs. Do they feel warmed up now?

Flexibility

- Seated Whole-Body Stretch
- Supple Spine

Posture and Core Stability/Strength for a Purpose

- Tall Sits: Emphasize stabilization of the core muscles. Do three to six of these, holding each for 3 to 15 seconds, as suits your group.
- Whooh, Whoohh, Whooohhh!
- Thumb Rolls

Balance and Mobility

None needed today, Supple Spine was plenty.

Overall Objectives

- Appreciating flexibility and how it affects function was our main goal. Ask them if it is a little easier to turn their heads, now? Perfect!
- Continue to get to know your participants' names and personalities. Answer any questions.

Enhancing Balance

Supplies

- Written plan
- Equipment list (supplies for activities)
  - Balloons or Slo Mo balls, 1 per person
  - Masking tape, in two widths (wide and medium)
  - Tennis balls, 1 per person
  - Small, heavy ball, 4 to 5 inches (10-13 centimeters) in diameter, 1 to 2 pounds (.5-1 kilogram)
  - Piece of paper
  - 6-12 agility cones (if cones are not available, you can use furniture or chairs to mark routes)
- Activity printouts—Printouts are available at www.HumanKinetics.com/ABLEBodiesBalanceTraining
  - WalkAbout
  - Smell the Coffee
  - Seated Whole-Body Stretch
  - Rock the Pelvis (from Supple Spine)
  - Torso as a Cylinder
  - The Straight and Narrow
  - Tall Sits With a Balloon Squeeze
  - Forklifts
  - Show Me the Money
  - Seated Toe Raises
  - Seated Heel Raises
  - Ducks and Pigeons
- Participant homework for session 3
- Rosters and name tags

Advance Preparation

- Set up chairs. Provide a clear view and a safe exercise space for each participant.
- Be sure you know how to do each activity correctly. Use printouts for any extra help you may need.
- Make sure all the supplies are ready and available.
- Make sure the WalkAbout area is clear and safe.
- Set up the course for the WalkAbout (see chapter 8).
- Put down masking tape for The Straight and Narrow near a handrail.

Opening

On time with a welcome!

Attendance/Roll Call

See if you can remember all of their names by now.

Icebreaker

Answer any questions.

Announcements

Make any necessary announcement.

Review and Preview

- Review: Last session the emphasis was mostly on their sense of touch—light touch, firm touch, and learning about the shape of objects by how their hands wrapped about it.
- Preview: This week, they'll gain confidence in knowing where they are situated in space. They'll dance with the dragon. But first, let's get their bodies warmed up and ready to move.

ABLE Bodies Components

Cardiorespiratory Endurance

Use an active warm-up such as WalkAbout. Explain that a WalkAbout is just walking and talking around the room, generally before class, and sometimes around some obstacles or simple balance challenges. It is optional. If they don't feel safe or comfortable walking or if they think it will be too exhausting, they may choose NOT to do this walk. Then ask those who are willing to take just one or two laps around the room, along the path you have laid out with agility cones or furniture. There are no obstacles or course changes. The activity should take no more than 5 minutes. Observe them for signs of fall risks or other difficulties.

Flexibility

- Smell the Coffee
- Seated Whole-Body Stretch

Posture and Core Stability

- Torso as a Cylinder
- Rock the Pelvis
- Practice the hip rocking section from Supple Spine to help them find neutral spine. Neutral spine is a comfortable tall sitting position. Hips are level and position is comfortable.

Balance and Mobility

- The Straight and Narrow—Remind participants to walk their chosen path with good core stability and to begin looking ahead a bit farther.

Strength for a Purpose

- Tall Sits With a Balloon Squeeze
- Forklifts
- Seated Toe Raises
- Seated Heel Raises
- Ducks and Pigeons

Closing

On time and with your thanks for coming!

Take-Home Message

Two things should be memorable from today: Kinesthetic and posture. We all have an inner sense of kinesis; our body naturally keeps track of where it is in space. Even without vision, our inner sensory systems know where their limbs are in space and exactly what they are doing. And using good posture with core stability can really make a difference in our stability. They should continue to think about these wonderful attributes over the next week.

Hook

Next week they'll explore flexibility and core stability a little more. They will meet a modern-day Venus de Milo and push each other around a bit. We may even go back in time to a play with a teeter-totter.

Homework and Reminders

Hand out the homework. Review their new assignment and answer questions. Remind them to use good posture this week. Announce when the practice session will be held for their benefit.

Fun and Inspiration

- Praise a few specific examples of good work on their part.
- End with a song, a mantra, an inspiring quote, or a funny joke and your thanks for coming along on this adventure in better living through exercise.

Make notes of any difficulties you had or activities you did not get to but would like to do later.

ABLE Bodies Practice Session 3

Supplies

- Masking tape for creating The Straight and Narrow
- Printouts of any activities, available at www.HumanKinetics.com/ABLEBodiesBalanceTraining

Advance Preparation

Lay down the tape for The Straight and Narrow.

Active Warm-Up

None needed today.

Flexibility

- Seated Whole-Body Stretch

Posture and Core Stability

- Tall Sits
- Add Whooh, Whoohh, Whooohhh!
- Forklifts

Balance and Mobility

- The Straight and Narrow (Participants take turns doing this one.)

Strength for a Purpose

- Seated Heel Raises
- Seated Toe Raises
- Ducks and Pigeons

Overall Objectives

Continue to reinforce what they learn in class. Help them learn how to do all the exercises. Enjoy!

Venus de Milo Arms

Supplies

- Written plan
- Equipment list (supplies for activities)
  - Balloons or Slo Mo balls, one per person
  - Thera-Bands, one per person
  - Masking tape
  - Easy-listening music for WalkAbout
- Activity printouts—Printouts are available at www.HumanKinetics.com/ABLEBodiesBalanceTraining
  - WalkAbout
  - Seated Whole-Body Stretch
  - Venus de Milo Arms
  - Knee Lift, Abs In
  - When Push Comes to Shove
  - Seated Side Steps with a Thera-Band
  - Flag Salutes (seated)
  - Straight-Ahead Lat Pull-Down
  - Seated Heel Raises
  - Seated Toe Raises
  - Right Hook, Left Hook
  - Teeter-Totter Chair Stands
  - The Straight and Narrow
- Participant homework for session 4
- Rosters and name tags

Advance Preparations

- Plan to sit somewhere different this week, change rooms if possible. This way, participants will learn ABLE Bodies methods in a variety of contexts. Check that the new area is clear from any fall risks.
- Set up chairs. Provide a clear view and a safe exercise space for each participant.
- Place a Thera-Band on each chair.
- Cue up music for WalkAbout.
- Set up the obstacle course for WalkAbout. Plan to include
  - an easy figure-8 pattern
  - a narrow space through which they will need to navigate
- Put down masking tape lines for The Straight and Narrow.
- Be sure you know how to do each activity correctly; use printouts for extra confidence.

Warm-Up (Cardiorespiratory Endurance)

Today, before class starts, have some easy-listening music on and ask those that will to walk around the room on your obstacle course. This will be your active warm-up.

- They should simply walk and talk and enjoy the music.
- Cue them to walk tall, with shoulders over hips, abs in, and ribs lifted. If they have walkers, cue them to walk closer to their walkers.

- Cue them to do the bent over posture walk (hunched over with shuffling feet) and then walk tall. Do they notice many differences and which feels best?
- Do they remember Posture Affects Function and Balance and how posture affects stepping?
- Stop the activity no more than 5 minutes into class time.
- Invite everyone to be seated.

Opening

On time with a welcome! Thank them for trying the WalkAbout.

Attendance/Roll Call

Offer a pat on the back to anyone making their fourth class.

Announcements

If appropriate thank them for coming to the new location.

Review and Preview

- Review: Previously they've been exploring how good flexibility and core stability makes them feel.
- Preview: Today they'll learn how core stability can make them very difficult. Hmmm.

ABLE Bodies Components

Flexibility

- Seated Whole-Body Stretch
- Venus de Milo Arms

Posture and Core Stability

- Knee Lift, Abs In
- When Push Comes to Shove

Strength for a Purpose

Normally you'd do balance before strength, but they've been on their feet a lot already, so it's a good time to do a few seated activities with the Thera-Bands.

This is their first time using Thera-Bands. Take a few minutes to explain how to use the band. Explain how they can adjust the amount of resistance they use. Demonstrate how it may be more comfortable to wrap the bands around the palms of their hands instead of around their fingers (band can squeeze arthritic fingers). Maybe you can offer bands of different strengths and colors.

- Seated Side Steps with a Thera-Band
- Flag Salutes (seated)
- Straight-Ahead Lat Pull-Down
- Seated Heel Raises
- Seated Toe Raises
- Right Hook, Left Hook
- Teeter-Totter Chair Stands: This will be their first Chair Stands. Take time to tell the story about why we call them Teeter Totter Chair Stands.

Balance and Mobility

The Straight and Narrow. Participants take turns walking their chosen path. Emphasize visual targets (they should focus on the horizon, if they can) and good core stability.

Closing

On time with a thank you!

Take-Home Message

Chair stands get a little easier just by changing their foot position and adding a little momentum. It's all stuff they learned in kindergarten or on a playground. Venus de Milo Arms and the kind of core stability they used in When Push Comes to Shove can make their lives easier, too, by making them more stable.

Hook

Be ready for a little Change of Pace next session!

Homework and Reminders

Hand out the homework and review their new assignment. Answer any questions. Announce the practice session. Remind them to do their homework twice each week. Preach about using good posture this week.

Fun and Inspiration

Praise a few specific examples of good work on their part. End with a song, a mantra, an inspiring quote, or a funny joke and your thanks for coming along on this adventure in better living through exercise. Make notes of any difficulties you had or activities you did not get to but would like to do another time.

ABLE Bodies Practice Session 4

Supplies

- Thera-Bands, one per person
- Masking tape for warm up
- Printouts of any activities, available at www.HumanKinetics.com/ABLEBodiesBalanceTraining

Advance Preparation

- Lay down a few tandem lines, beside a handrail or other support, for the Walk-About warm-up.
- Plan WalkAbout to include a figure-8 pattern and a circle to walk around, as well as the tandem line. Plan to put yourself nearby to hold hands, as necessary.

Active Warm-Up

- WalkAbout

Flexibility

- Seated Whole-Body Stretch
- Venus de Milo Arms—just a short version

Posture and Core Stability

- Instructor's choice

Strength for a Purpose

- Teeter-Totter Chair Stands

Posture and Core Stability

- Instructor's choice

Strength for a Purpose

- Teeter-Totter Chair Stands

Have your group sit back down for these

- Flag Salutes
- Seated Side Steps With a Thera-Band
- Rows With Checkmark Feet and a Thera-Band
- Seated Leg Press With a Thera-Band
- Seated Toe Raises
- Seated Heel Raises (If group is ready, do Heel Raises standing.)

Overall Objective

Master the Teeter-Totter Chair Stand. It is one of the most functional strength exercises.

Change of Pace

Supplies

- Written plan
- Equipment list (supplies for activities)
  - Thera-Bands, 1 per participant
  - 1 or 2 sets of walking sticks
  - Magazines or .5- to 1-pound (.25- to .5-kilogram) weights, 2 per participant
- Activity printouts—Printouts are available at www.HumanKinetics.com/ABLEBodiesBalanceTraining
  - Four Corners (Part of Games in chapter 8)
  - Seated Whole-Body Stretch
  - Farmer's Stretch
  - Forklifts
  - Show Me the Money
  - Traffic School (specifically Change of Pace; Red Light, Green Light; Window Shopping; London Bridge; and Traffic Circles)
  - Opposing Circles and High Fives
  - Straight-Ahead Lat Pull-Down
  - Seated Side Steps With a Thera-Band
  - Teeter-Totter Chair Stands
  - Seated Heel Raises
  - Standing Heel Raises
- Participant homework for session 5
- Rosters and name tags

Advance Preparation

- Set up chairs for Four Corners.
- Set up chairs for class time. Provide a clear view and a safe exercise space for each participant. Place a Thera-Band on each chair.
- Be sure you know how to do each activity correctly; use printouts for any extra help you may need.

Opening

On time with a welcome!

Attendance/Roll Call

Take roll; who made it to class for the fifth time?

Announcements

Make any necessary announcements.

Review and Preview

- Review: Did anybody think about Venus de Milo arms this week while they were reaching for something? Perfect! (Reach in different directions to show increased range of motion possible with Venus de Milo arms). How about core stability? (Sit tall, exhale forcefully, and make a humph! sound as you pull your shoulder blades back and down, bracing your torso.) Have them do the same, with a humph, too! Who did their homework? Nice job! How are chair stands going? Getting a little easier? (Practice one or two with them: Lean back, lean forward, press down, stand up.)
- Preview: This week they'll be on their feet a little more, changing things up a bit.

ABLE Bodies Components

Cardiorespiratory Endurance

Four Corners

Flexibility

- Seated Whole-Body Stretch
- Farmer's Stretch; this is the first stretch we've done standing. It can replace Proud Mary in the Seated Whole-Body Stretch, for those who like it.

Posture and Core Stability

- Forklifts
- Show Me the Money

Balance and Mobility

Balance in this session is best done in two parts. The two parts are separated by time spent seated. Do Traffic School first and then let them sit so they're off their feet for awhile. During the time seated, do the seated strength training. Then they should be fresh again and ready to do the remaining balance activities, Heavy Hands and Walking Sticks.

- Traffic School
  - Change of Pace
  - Red Light, Green Light
  - Window Shopping
  - London Bridge
  - Traffic Circles
- Opposing Circles and High Fives (this one is easily added to Traffic School).

Strength for a Purpose

- Straight-Ahead Lat Pull-Down
- Seated Side Steps With a Thera-Band
- Teeter-Totter Chair Stands
- Heel Raises, Seated or Standing (their choice)

More Balance and Mobility

- Heavy Hands (This activity is done seated at first, then done while standing.)
- Walking Sticks (Have them take turns; they will learn and have fun watching others, too.)

Closing

On time with a thank you!

Take-Home Message

Speeding up, slowing down, changing directions, and even arms swings are all challenges to balance. What kinds of things help with that? (Good posture and core stability, using visual targets.)

Hook

Beginning next week, they'll never look at their belly buttons in quite the same way again. Come and see why next session!

Homework and Reminders

Hand out their homework and review their new assignment. Answer any questions. Remind them that strength is a cornerstone of better balance. Participants will see improvement sooner if they do extra work on their own. Twice each week they should do their homework.

Suggest too, that this week they practice using visual targets when they are walking about. Ask them to come back next time and tell the group if it helps. Announce when the practice session will be held and invite them to come. It's an easy way to burn a few extra calories with their friends.

Fun and Inspiration

- Praise a few specific examples of good work on their part. Has someone seen improvements or signs of change?
- End with a song, a mantra, an inspiring quote, or a funny joke and your thanks for coming. More adventures next week.

Make notes of any difficulties you had or activities you did not get to but would like to do another time.

ABLE Bodies Practice Session 5

Supplies

- Thera-Bands
- Printouts of activities, available at www.HumanKinetics.com/ABLEBodiesBalanceTraining

Advance Preparation

- Set up chairs and put out Thera-Bands
- Prepare space for Traffic School

Active Warm-Up

- Traffic School

Flexibility

- Seated Whole-Body Stretch
- Farmer's Stretch

Posture and Core Stability

- Forklifts

Strength for a Purpose

- Balloon Knee Squeezes
- Waist Whittlers
- Seated Side Steps With a Thera-Band
- Teeter-Totter Chair Stands
- Standing Heel Raises

Balance and Mobility

- No extra activities today

Overall Objectives

- Focus on various tasks done while walking.
- Practice adjusting for needed changes in speed, direction, goals, and obstacles.
- Can they walk and talk?
- Move about and enjoy the activity and each other.

Belly Button Training

Supplies

- Written plan
- Equipment list (supplies for activities)
  - Thera-Bands, 1 per person
  - Masking tape
  - Music player and some soft, slow music
  - Candy kisses or other small prizes for completing homework or accomplishments
- Activity printouts—Printouts are available at www.HumanKinetics.com/ABLEBodiesBalanceTraining
  - WalkAbout
  - Traffic School
  - Seated Whole-Body Stretch
  - Look and See Flexibility
  - Farmer's Stretch
  - Carry the Baby
  - High Rollers
  - The Up and Up
  - Knee Lift, Abs In
  - Tall Standing
  - Belly Button Training
  - Belly Stands

  - Belly Weight Shifts
  - Belly Weight Shifts to a Single-Leg Stand
  - Walk and Waddle
  - Agility Ladders
  - Overhead Lat Pull-Down
  - Teeter-Totter Chair Stands
  - Standing Heel Raises
  - Standing Toe Raises
  - Side Steps Walking
  - Push-Backs with Genie Arms
  - Pass the Duck (for practice session)
  - The Straight and Narrow (for practice session)
- Participant homework for session 6
- Rosters and name tags

Advance Preparation

- Put down tape for Walk and Waddle and Agility Ladders.
- Make sure balance support is beside Walk and Waddle and Agility Ladders.
- Put out chairs for observers of the line challenges.
- Make sure WalkAbout area is planned, safe, and ready.
- Make changes in the environment.
  - Change the chair arrangement, the side of the room, or the room itself.
  - Practice how much you will dim the lights. Not too much, just enough to get their attention.
- Set up chairs. Provide clear view and a safe exercise space for each participant.
- Be sure you know how to do each activity correctly; use printouts for any extra help you may need.

Active Warm-Up (Cardiorespiratory Endurance)

WalkAbout. Dim the lights (just enough to notice); play easy listening music. Remind participants that WalkAbouts are optional. People who are uncomfortable, unable, or simply prefer not to join in can simply sit down and get ready for class.

- Cue tall posture.
- Cue heel–toe pattern.
- Cue arm swings.
- Cue an occasional change of pace.
- Cue direction changes.

Bring lights back up and do Window Shopping (walking with head turns). Can also cue

- Opposing Circles
- High Fives
- London Bridges

Opening

On time with a welcome!

Attendance/Roll Call

Take attendance; who is present?

Announcements

Make any necessary announcements.

IceBreaker

The darkened room will probably have already gotten their attention, that's just fine. Those that came late may be wishing they'd been on time. Perfect; it may motivate them for the next session.

Review and Preview

- Review: Explain why you set the lights so low; so they will use some of their other sensory systems for balance. You can tell them it's a progression to The Ball Game, Coming to Your Senses, and Dancing With the Dragon (reviewing links prior knowledge to this activity). By reducing information from one sense, the other sensory systems are engaged and facilitated. Other than that, are they finding themselves walking taller more often? Is it helping? Who did homework? Good job! Toss or hand out small prizes to those who raise their hands.
- Preview: Today, it all centers on our Belly Buttons. And you do mean it centers on our belly button.

ABLE Bodies Components

Flexibility

Before you start, dim the lights again and play slow, nice music. Invite them to take off their shoes and rub their feet on the carpet.

- Seated Whole-Body Stretch
  - Can they feel the vibration or a little tickle in their feet from rubbing them on the floor?
  - Can they feel the firmness of the floor? Can they feel the texture of the floor?
  - Close their eyes and feel the floor again.
- Do Seated Whole-Body Stretch, but add
  - Look and See Flexibility
  - Farmer's Stretch
  - Carry the Baby

Posture and Core Stability

Pick two of these activities.

- High Rollers
- The Up and Up
- Knee Lift, Abs In
- Tall Standing: Cue soft knees and tall standing posture.

Balance and Mobility

- Belly Button Training
  - Belly Stands
  - Belly Weight Shifts
  - Belly Weight Shifts to a Single-Leg Stand

Rest break. Maybe do a seated strength exercise or stretch.

- Agility Ladders: Take turns and hold their hands.
- Walk and Waddle: Take turns and hold their hands.

Strength for a Purpose

- Overhead Lat Pull-Downs
- Teeter-Totter Chair Stands
- Standing Heel Raises (see if you can get them to do a little heel-to-toe rocking)
- Side Steps Walking

Closing

On time with a thank you!

Take-Home Message

Bellies are interesting balance aids. Participants should be thinking this week about how their belly button relates to where they feel their balance.

Hook

What's up for next session? It'll be a *reach*, that's for sure! Hope you all can come!

Homework and Reminders

Hand out the homework, review their new assignment, and answer questions. Tell participants to keep working on their strength and posture homework; it will benefit their balance and mobility activities in class. They should do their homework twice a week. Extol the virtues of using good posture this week.

Announce when the practice session will be held. They will be playing a game called Pass the Duck and doing more Belly Button Training.

Fun and Inspiration

- Praise a few specific examples of good work on their part. Share improvements you have observed. Give out the rest of the candy kisses for jobs well done.
- End with a song, a mantra, an inspiring quote, or a funny joke and your thanks for coming to Belly Button Training. Now they should go out and play with theirs!

Make notes of any difficulties you had or activities you did not get to but would like to do another time.

ABLE Bodies Practice Session 6

Supplies

- A 2-4 pound (1-2 kilogram) object for Pass the Duck
- Masking tape
- Balloons or Slo Mo balls
- Printouts of any activities, available at www.HumanKinetics.com/ABLEBodiesBalanceTraining

Advance Preparation

- Set up chairs and music for Pass the Duck
- Put down lines for Walk and Waddle or Agility Ladder

Active Warm-Up

Not this session; lots to do today.

Flexibility

- Seated Whole-Body Stretch

Posture and Core Stability

- Push-Backs with Genie Arms
- Pass the Duck

Balance and Mobility

- Belly Button Training
  - Standing
  - Belly Sways
  - Belly Weight Shifts to a Single-Leg Stand
- The Straight and Narrow
  - For gait variability, have participants walk inside, then outside, then inside, and then outside the lines.
  - Have them take turns.
  - Cue tall posture
  - Be available to hold hands.
- Agility Ladders
  - Have them do forward stepping, working on stride length.
  - Talk with participants about their belly button following their foot to each rung.

Strength for a Purpose (If Time)

- Teeter-Totter Chair Stands

Do they notice that the starting position (leaning forward and placing heels behind their knees) lines up their belly buttons over their feet? That is part of what makes it easier to get up. Then as they rise up, it will help if they think to bring their bellies up and over their feet. Try it again thinking through these concepts. Voilá, you're up easy and we're done for the day! Thanks for coming!

Overall Objective

- Focus on Belly Button Sensations. If you look, you'll find that you can use it in lots of places.

It's a Reach

Supplies

- Written plan
- Equipment list (supplies for activities)
  - Balloons, 1 per person
  - Thera-Bands, 1 per person
  - Masking tape
  - Toys or candies for It's a Reach
  - Agility discs, 6 to 12 if available
  - Half-rounds, 3 or 4 (available from equipment stores and Web sites)
- Activity printouts—Printouts are available at www.HumanKinetics.com/ABLEBodiesBalanceTraining
  - WalkAbout
  - Seated Whole-Body Stretch
  - Farmer's Stretch
  - Carry the Baby
  - The Up and Up
  - Push-Backs
  - Balloon Lifts
  - Push Up and Think Thin (with a balloon)
  - Balloon Lap Press-Down
  - Standing Heel Raises
  - It's a Reach
  - Heel Raises and Rocking on a Half-Round
  - Bows and Arrows
  - Knee Lift, Abs In
  - Marching in Place (Seated)
  - Marching in Place (Standing)
  - Clock Stepping (for practice session)
- Participant homework for session 7
- Rosters and name tags

Advance Preparation

- Set up chairs. Provide a clear view and a safe exercise space for each participant.
- Be sure you know how to do each activity correctly; use printouts for any extra help you may need.
- Plan Walkabout. Tape down a tandem line for The Straight and Narrow by a handrail and add a few agility discs to form a figure-eight pattern or turn-around. Set these beside a handrail or row of chairs for balance safety.
- Tape down agility ladder along a wall, handrail, or row of chairs.

Active Warm-Up

Play easy-listening music, if you like, while having your participants do a WalkAbout.

- Cue tall posture.
- Cue heel–toe patterns.
- Cue arm swings, head turns.
- Change up pace and stride (quick, slow, wide, narrow).
- Have them walk in a figure-eight pattern.

- Stand beside the tandem line and The Straight and Narrow so you can provide extra balance safety.
- Add a dual task: Have them recite a fun poem or sing out loud together.

Opening

On time with a welcome!

Attendance/Roll Call

Take roll; is everyone there?

Announcements

Make any necessary announcements.

Review and Preview

- Review: Have they noticed the WalkAbouts are more involved and normally practice what they've been learning? Practice helps.
- Preview: Reaching for what is just out of grasp is human nature. Who's to say they shouldn't keep reaching for the things they want? But on a practical level, there are times when overreaching causes a loss of balance. Today they'll learn how to stay safer while reaching.

ABLE Bodies Components

Flexibility

- Seated Whole-Body Stretch (Cue Venus de Milo Arms when doing upward reaching.)
- Farmer's Stretch
- Carry the Baby

Posture and Core Stability

- The Up and Up (cue Venus de Milo Arms.)
- Push-Backs
- Balloon Lifts
- Push Up and Think Thin With a Balloon
- Balloon Lap Press-Down

Balance and Mobility

- Standing Heel Raises. Have them do these holding on to their chairs. See if they can do some heel–toe rocking. If so, have them try.
  - Heel Raises and Rocking on a Half-Round
  - It's a Reach

Strength for a Purpose

- Balloon Lap Press-Down
- Bows and Arrows
- Knee Lift, Abs In
- Marching in Place (Seated)
- Marching in Place (Standing)

Closing

On time and with a thank you!

Take-Home Message

Safe reaching is often a matter of redistributing your weight. When reaching forward, push your hips backward and use Venus de Milo Arms. (Demonstrate this for them again.)

Hook

Next session, they can expect some good karma to come their way, because we'll learn an exercise called Buddha's Prayer (place your hands in the beginning position and bow your head, briefly). And we will use ABLE Bodies' core stability tricks from When Push Comes to Shove to help stand steady on balance pads. (Show them a balance pad if you have one; pass it around, even.)

Homework and Reminders

Hand out their homework and review their new assignment. Answer any questions. Encourage them do their homework twice each week.

Announce when the practice session will be held. It will be another chance to play on the half rounds.

Fun and Inspiration

- Praise something special that participants did today: Being quick learners, volunteering, taking a chance, or even just arriving early and ready.
- End with a song, a mantra, an inspiring quote, or a funny joke and your thanks for coming along on this adventure in better living with exercise.

Make notes of any difficulties you had or activities you did not get to but would like to do another time.

ABLE Bodies Practice Session 7

Supplies

- Music and music player
- Half-rounds
- Thera-Bands

Advance Preparation

- Have marching music selected and ready to play.
- Plan a safe place for working with half rounds
- Set up chairs for class

Cardiorespiratory Endurance, Core Stability, and Balance

- Active Warm-Up: Marching in Place (Seated or Standing)
  - Warm up by marching in place to music. Start seated. If it goes well, let those who want to do this standing. It's their choice. Head turns can be dizzying, so keep them in front of their chairs, with their back to a corner, or by a handrail for marching in place.
  - Add arm swings: If participant is standing just add one arm swing at first—that way, they can keep the other hand on their chair.
  - Add head turns: Turning head toward lifted knee is best.
  - Combine: Some may be able to do both arms swing and head turns, but be cautious.

Flexibility

- Seated Whole-Body Stretch
  - Cue for Venus de Milo Arms.

Balance and Mobility

- Heel–Toe Rocking and Heel Raises and Rocking on a Half-Round
- It's a Reach

Strength for a Purpose

- Bows and Arrows
- Teeter-Totter Chair Stands
- Clock Stepping

Overall Objective

The focus today is getting them to enjoy and master the half rounds.

Buddha's Prayer and Balance Pads

Supplies

- Written plan
- Equipment list (supplies for activities)
  - Thera-Bands
  - Masking tape
  - Balloons or Slo Mo balls, one for each participant
  - Agility discs, cones, or agility poles for slalom course, if available
  - Balance pads: Get a variety of densities and shapes, if possible. Try to find something for everyone. The softer the pad, the more difficult balancing will be.
- Activity printouts—Printouts are available at www.HumanKinetics.com/ABLEBodiesBalanceTraining
  - WalkAbout
  - Holiday Lines
  - Agility Ladders
  - Change of Pace
  - Slalom Turns
  - Seated Whole-Body Stretch
  - Gentlemen's Bow (Standing)
  - Farmer's Stretch
  - Farmer and the Hula
  - Carry the Baby
  - Buddha's Prayer
  - Genie Arms With a Twist
  - Figure-Eight Obstacle Course
  - Kayaking Arms (seated)
  - Heel-Touch and Roll-Up
  - Keeping You On Your Toes
  - Balance Pads
  - Overhead Lat Pull-Downs
  - A&W Chest Presses
  - Heel-Touch Forward, Toe-Touch Back
  - One-Legged Chair Stands
  - Pendulum Legs
- Participant homework for session 8
- Rosters and name tags

Advance Preparation

- Set up chairs. Provide a clear view and a safe exercise space for each participant.
- Be sure you know how to do each activity correctly; use printouts for any extra help you may need.
- Make sure WalkAbout is planned, safe, and ready.
- Prepare Holiday Lines.
- Prepare Agility Ladders—Rungs should be equally spaced. Place it by a handrail.
- Set up slalom turns course (linked figure-eight walking pattern) with cones or poles.
- If this is your first time using balance pads or balance mats, take extra time to plan for safely using them with your participants.

Active Warm-Up

- WalkAbout
- Holiday Lines—They should take turns, you should be available to hold hands
- Agility Ladders—They should sidestep through it
- Change of Pace—Call out the changes in pace
- Figure-Eight Obstacle Course

Opening

On time and with a welcome!

Attendance/Roll Call

Take roll.

Announcements

Make any necessary announcements.

Review and Preview

- Review: Each session so far has worked on core stability. Core stability helps keep our balance against jostling, when walking a tandem line, or when reaching for things. It also improves our form for most exercises.
- Preview: Today's session is more about core stability. They'll learn a great core stabilizing exercise. Then we'll use lessons from When Push Comes to Shove to play on the balance pads. Ready? Let's get started!

ABLE Bodies Components

Flexibility

- Seated Whole-Body Stretch—Teach and encourage those willing to do standing versions. Respect and encourage their decisions.
- Gentlemen's Bow (Standing)—Doing this one standing is new to them. Explain it carefully and provide plenty of balance support.
- Farmer's Stretch
- Carry the Baby

Posture and Core Stability

- Buddha's Prayer
- Genie Arms With a Twist

Balance and Mobility

Kayaking Arms—Prepare participants for this activity by having them sit tall, with hands on their chest. Then get them to stay tall and make figure-eight patterns with their trunks; first with their eyes open and then with their eyes closed. Then add Kayaking Arms (seated) and then with eyes closed.

- Heel-Touch and Roll-Up
- Keeping You On Your Toes

- Balance Pads: Be sure to review all the safety instructions in chapter 7 for getting participants safely onto balance pads. When they first get on, cue them to use the When Push Comes to Shove core stability. (As they draw shoulder blades back and down, they should exhale with a "Hummph!" and glue themselves to the ground.) Once they're comfortable, proceed with the activity. Try adding
    - Arm movements
    - Sways with arms on hips
    - Leg movement (small heel raises or squats)
    - Same movements on land (Ask if they notice how much easier they seem.)

Now everyone should sit and rest awhile.

Strength for a Purpose
- Overhead Lat Pull-Down (seated)
- A&W Chest Presses (seated)
- Heel-Touch Forward, Toe-Touch Back
- One-Legged Chair Stands
- Pendulum Legs

Closing

On time with a thank you!

Take-Home Message
When an individual is unsure of the ground under their feet, they pay more attention to the clues that come from vision or their vestibular balance system. Balance pads are effective balance tools because they activate and train our other balance systems.

Hook
Next session there'll be Words on the Wall in the Hall and a Hat Trick.

Homework and Reminders
Hand out their homework and review their new assignment. Answer any questions. Remind them to do their homework twice each week and to use good core stability and posture. Announce when the next practice session will be held.

Fun and Inspiration
- Praise something special that participants did today.
- End with a song, a mantra, an inspiring quote, or a funny joke and your thanks for coming along on this adventure in better living through exercise.

Make notes of any difficulties you had or activities you did not get to but would like to do later.

ABLE Bodies Practice Session 8

Supplies

- Thera-Bands
- Balance pads
- Masking tape
- Printouts of any activities, available at www.HumanKinetics.com/ABLEBodiesBalanceTraining

Advance Preparation

- Prepare WalkAbout
- Have a plan for dimming the lights, if you'd like to do that with your group

Active Warm-Up

Do a WalkAbout that includes walking through slalom turns and perhaps Holiday Lines. Consider dimming the lights or having participants recite poems or answer questions that you call out during the WalkAbout.

Flexibility

- Seated Whole-Body Stretch
- Farmer's Stretch
- Farmer and the Hula

Posture and Core Stability and Balance

- Buddha's Prayer
- Kayaking Arms
  - Eyes open
  - Eyes closed

Balance and Mobility

- Heel-Touch and Roll-Up
- Keeping You on Your Toes
- Balance Pads

Review safety ideas before you start. Safest way is with their back to the corner and a walker in front.

Strength for a Purpose

- Bows and Arrows
- One-Legged Chair Stands
- Clock Stepping

Overall Objective

- Get a little more comfortable with balance pads.

Hat Trick

Supplies

- Written plan
- Equipment list (supplies for activities)
  - Poem and pictures for Words on the Wall in the Hall
  - Thera-Bands, one per person
  - Masking tape
  - Agility cones, 6-12 if available
  - Hat box or facsimile
  - Balloons, one per person (They'll double as imaginary hat boxes for participants.)
- Activity printouts—Printouts are available at www.HumanKinetics.com/ABLEBodiesBalanceTraining
  - WalkAbout
  - Words on the Wall in the Hall
  - Seated Whole-Body Stretch
  - Look and See Flexibility
  - Push-Backs with Genie Arms
  - Genie Arms with a Twist
  - Drive Me Up the Wall
  - The Up and Up
  - Hat Trick
  - Rock Forward, Knee Lift
  - Rows With Check-Mark Feet and a Thera-Band
  - Right Cross, Left Cross and Right Hook, Left Hook
  - Cops and Robbers
  - Clock Stepping
  - Teeter-Totter Chair Stands (practice session)
  - Standing Heel Raises (practice session)
- Participant homework for session 9
- Rosters and name tags

Advance Preparation

- Set up chairs. Provide a clear view and a safe exercise space for each participant.
- Be sure you know how to do each activity correctly; use printouts for any extra help you may need.
- Set up WalkAbout
  - Tandem lines
  - Slalom course (weaving, figure-eight pattern) using agility cones or furniture

Active Warm-Up (Cardiorespiratory Endurance)

- WalkAbout: Cue them for tall posture, heel-to-toe action. Cue big steps, then little steps, fast and slow.
- Words on the Wall in the Hall

Opening

On time with a welcome!

Attendance/Roll Call

Take roll. Recognize consistent attendance and effort.

Announcements

Make any necessary announcements.

Review and Preview

- Review: A few weeks ago, doing Teeter-Totter Chair Stands, we learned how a rocking motion could make getting out of a chair easier. During It's a Reach, we explored how foot placement, core stability, and body position can make reaching out easier.
- Preview: The focus today is another risky, everyday activity—reaching for items that are overhead. To do this safely, they'll learn how to use smart foot placement, rocking, and core stability again. It's called the Hat Trick.

ABLE Bodies Components

Flexibility

- Seated Whole-Body Stretch
- Look and See Flexibility

Posture and Core Stability

- Push-Backs
- Genie Arms With a Twist
- Drive Me Up the Wall: This activity is useful for the Hat Trick, which they will do later in this session. Those who prefer to stay seated can do The Up and Up.

Balance and Mobility

- Rock Back, Knee Lift
- Rock Forward, Knee Lift
- Hat Trick
- Get Up and Go Relay (optional; can also be done after strength training if your participants need time to rest.)

Strength for a Purpose

- Rows with Check-Mark Feet and a Thera-Band
- Right Cross, Left Cross and Right Hook, Left Hook
- Cops and Robbers
- Clock Stepping
- Standing Heel Raises

Closing

On time with a thank you!

Take-Home Message

Whenever they reach up this week, they should remember some of the ideas they've learned in class today:

- Core stability
- Foot position
- Pulling the retrieved object toward you rather than overhead

Hook

Next session they'll glow in the dark and learn how helpful a single bright spot can be used for balance.

Homework and Reminders

Hand out their homework and review their new assignment. Answer any questions. Remind them to do their homework twice each week. Extol the virtues of good posture and core stability.

Fun and Inspiration

- Praise something special that participants did today, such as great attendance, arriving early and ready, learning quickly, volunteering, taking a chance, and so on.
- End with a song, a mantra, an inspiring quote, or a funny joke and your thanks for coming.

Make notes of any difficulties you had or activities you did not get to but would like to do later.

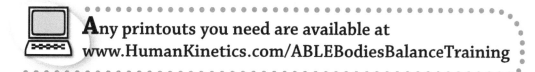

ABLE Bodies Practice Session 9

Supplies

- Masking tape
- Hat box or similarly-sized container
- Balloons

Advance Preparation

- Prepare Words on the Wall in the Hall for use in your WalkAbout
- Set up for Hat Trick

Active Warm-Up

- WalkAbout
- Words on the Wall in the Hall
- Your choice

Flexibility

- Farmer's Stretch
- Farmer and the Hula
- Seated Whole-Body Stretch

Balance and Mobility

- Rock Back, Knee Lift
- Rock Forward, Knee Lift
- Heel-Touch and Roll-Up
- Hat Trick

Strength for a Purpose

- Bows and Arrows
- Teeter-Totter Chair Stands (one-legged)
- Clock Stepping
- Hat Trick

Glow in the Dark

Supplies

- Written plan
- Equipment list (supplies for activities)
  - Music and music player
  - Thera-Bands, one for each person
  - Masking tape
  - Balance pads, 4 to 10 in a variety if possible
  - Flashlights, one per person, if possible (check that they all work)
  - Balloons, one per person (see if you can get ones that glow in the dark)
- Activity printouts—Printouts are available at www.HumanKinetics.com/ABLEBodiesBalanceTraining
  - WalkAbout
  - Seated Whole-Body Stretch
  - Lunge Stretch
  - Curl Up and Sit Tall
  - Follow the Light
  - Over and Back
  - Step-Ball-Change
  - Big Steps
  - Pendulum Legs on a Tandem Line
  - Straight-Ahead Lat Pull-Down
  - Knee Crosses
  - Side Steps with a Thera-Band
  - The Up and Up
  - Bows and Arrows
  - Seated Balloon or Beach-Ball Volleyball
  - Toe Taps and Head Nods (for practice session)
  - Some Simple Standing Moves (for practice session)
  - Ball on the Wall (for practice session)
- Participant homework for session 10
- Rosters and name tags

Advance Preparation

- Set up chairs. Provide a clear view and a safe exercise space for each participant.
- Be sure you know how to do each activity correctly; use printouts for any extra help you may need.
- Prepare for WalkAbout—Include a slalom (figure-eight) course. Place a nonskid balance pad or two in your course near where you can supervise or where there will be ample balance support, such as in a corner or between two sturdy chairs.
- Prepare for Walk the Line challenges—Tape a line 18 to 24 inches (46 to 61 centimeters) behind each chair, perpendicular to the chair back.

Active Warm-Up (Cardiorespiratory Endurance and Balance)

- WalkAbout with music
- Walking and marching steps
  - Cue big steps
  - Cue arm swings and head turns (watch them carefully)

- Ask them to try the balance pads. Plant yourself there for safety. This activity is only for those who are willing to try. They can step up and over the pad. Or they can try getting on the pad, find their balance, then lift one arm at a time or take little steps on it.

Opening

On time with a welcome!

Attendance/Roll Call

Take roll.

Announcements

Make any necessary announcements.

Review and Preview

- Review: Previously they've used visual targets to guide them down all kinds of tandem lines or to hold their balance when standing. They've learned that focusing on a visual target helps with balance.
- Preview: The focus today is also on visual targeting and on looking ahead while walking. They'll use flashlights to guide their vision. It will be fun and not too scary. Tell participants to only try what they are comfortable doing.

ABLE Bodies Components

Flexibility

- Seated Whole-Body Stretch
- Lunge Stretch

Posture and Core Stability

- Curl Up and Sit Tall

Balance and Mobility

- Follow the Light
- Do these Walk the Line activities from chapter 7
  - Over and Back
  - Step-Ball-Change
  - Big Steps
  - Pendulum Legs on a Tandem Line

Strength for a Purpose

Do these while seated for a rest break.
- Straight-Ahead Lat Pull-Down
- Knee Crosses
- Bows and Arrows
- Side Steps With a Thera-Band

Balance and Mobility (yes, again; just one more)

- Seated Balloon Volleyball with glow-in-the-dark balloons
  - Move chairs into circles of three to five participants.
  - Dim the lights just enough so the balloons will glow a bit.

Closing

On time with a thank you!

Take-Home Message

Participants should look ahead when they walk, even if it's just a little farther than normal. Their path will be more direct and their balance more natural.

Hook

Next week they'll be Puddle Jumping and having fun on the river.

Homework and Reminders

Participants will improve their balance sooner if they do a little extra work on their own. Twice each week they should do their homework. Hand out the homework, review their new assignment, and answer questions.

Announce when the practice session will be held. This time they'll learn a new balance aid called Step and Stop.

Fun and Inspiration

- Praise something special that participants did today.
- End with a song, a mantra, an inspiring quote, or a funny joke and your thanks for working hard.

Make notes of any difficulties you had or activities you did not get to but would like to do another time.

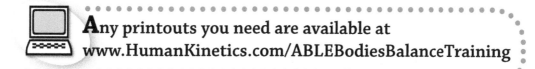
Any printouts you need are available at www.HumanKinetics.com/ABLEBodiesBalanceTraining

ABLE Bodies Practice Session 10

Supplies

- Balloons, one per person
- Masking tape
- Flashlights, one per person, if possible
- Music and music player

Advance Preparation

- Prepare lines for Walk the Line challenges and for Step and Stop
- Be sure the flashlights work
- Set up chairs
- Cue up music

Active Warm-Up

From Rhythm and Moves, practice arm swings and head turns. Consider

- Toe Taps and Head Nods
- Some Simple Standing moves

Flexibility

- Seated Whole-Body Stretch
- Lunge Stretch
- Carry the Baby
- Gentlemen's Bow (Standing)

Balance and Mobility

- Step and Stop
- Activities from Walk the Line
  - Over and Back
  - Step-Ball-Change
  - Big Steps
  - Pendulum Legs on a Tandem Line
- Follow the Light (just a quick run through)

Strength for a Purpose (if time)

- Ball on the Wall

Overall Objective

- This practice is very busy, with lots of variety. I'd guess the objective is to get through it and enjoy the variety!

Puddle Jumping

Supplies

- Written plan
- Equipment list (supplies for activities)
  - Pictures, sunglasses, and props for Walk in the Park
  - Balloons, one per person
  - Thera-Bands, one per person
  - Balance pads, 4 to 6 and in a variety of densities, if possible
  - Masking tape
  - Agility dots, 12 to 18 with nonskid surface
  - Poly beam, if available
- Activity printouts—Printouts are available at www.HumanKinetics.com/ABLEBodiesBalanceTraining
  - Walk in the Park
  - Seated Whole-Body Stretch
  - Farmer's Stretch
  - Farmer and the Hula
  - Carry the Baby
  - Gentlemen's Bow (standing)
  - Balloon Lifts
  - Tap and Catch a Balloon
  - Rows With Check-Mark Feet and a Thera-Band
  - A&W Chest Presses
  - Balloon Lap Press-Down
  - H-Lines
  - Puddle Jumping
  - Belly Steps
  - Lazy River
  - Buddha's Prayer (practice session)
- Participant homework for session 11
- Rosters and name tags

Advance Preparation

- Set up chairs. Provide a clear view and a safe exercise space for each participant.
- Be sure you know how to do each activity correctly; use printouts for any extra help you may need.
- Prepare Walk in the Park. (Put up pictures and arrange furniture in a figure-eight pattern.)
- Prepare an H-line for each participant.
- Tape down river banks for River Fun. Add at least one bridge across made of masking tape.
- If you haven't done so already, this is a great time to bring out your camera and take a few pictures.

Active Warm Up (Cardiorespiratory Endurance and Balance)

- Walk in the Park
  - Birds, bees, squirrels, sunglasses, whatever. Use slalom pathways and a London Bridge.

Opening

On time with a welcome!

Attendance/Roll Call

Take roll. Did everyone have fun?

Announcements

Make any necessary announcements.

Review and Preview

- Review: We've learned a lot so far in 10 sessions! Ask if anyone would share what has been most helpful to them. How has learning about momentum helped them? (Remember Teeter-Totter Chair Stands and Arm Swings?)
- Preview: Sometimes, though, momentum is hard to control, such as when you stop suddenly or do a too-quick weight shift. Today, Puddle Jumping will give them a chance to practice controlling momentum.

ABLE Bodies Components

Flexibility

- Seated Whole-Body Stretch
- Farmer's Stretch
- Farmer and the Hula
- Carry the Baby
- Gentlemen's Bow (standing)

Posture and Core Stability

- Balloon Lifts
- Tap and Catch a Balloon

Balance and Mobility

- H-Lines

Strength for a Purpose

- Rows With Check-Mark Feet and a Thera-Band
- A&W Chest Presses
- Balloon Lap Press-Down

Balance and Mobility

- Puddle Jumping
  - Cue them to take a Belly Step toward each next dot.

- Lazy River (from River Fun in chapter 7)
  - Be sure to put down a few bridges to cross (one can be the poly beam).
  - Teach them to use Belly Steps to cross the Lazy River at the narrower places.

Closing

On time and with a thank you!

Take-Home Message

Step and Stop and Puddle Jumping made us work to control momentum. Belly Steps helped us move in our desired direction, more easily. Belly Steps helped us get from one puddle to the next.

Now we know lots of ways to realign our wobbling balance—there's everything we did today plus ideas from other weeks, such as the glue-me-down "humph!" we learned from When Push Comes to Shove.

Hook

Next week they'll use music in a new way with Waltzing Matilda. Music will help them find a rhythm and anticipate how to move.

Homework and Reminders

Hand out their homework and review their new assignment. Answer any questions. Remind them to do their homework twice each week. Announce the next practice session.

Fun and Inspiration

- Let them know how great they're doing! Give a few examples that you have observed or enjoyed.
- End with a song, a mantra, an inspiring quote, or a funny joke and your thanks for coming along on this adventure in better living through exercise.

Make notes of any difficulties you had or activities you did not get to but would like to do another time.

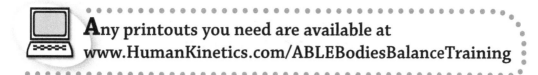
Any printouts you need are available at
www.HumanKinetics.com/ABLEBodiesBalanceTraining

ABLE Bodies Practice Session 11

Supplies

- 12 to 18 nonskid agility dots
- Masking tape
- Music and music player
- 4 to 6 balance pads

Advance Preparation

- Prepare H-Lines and Puddle Jumping

Active Warm-Up

Warm-up with marching and arm swings to music

Flexibility

- Seated Whole-Body Stretch
- Gentlemen's Bow (standing or seated)
- Carry the Baby

Posture and Core Stability / Strength for a Purpose

- Forklifts
- Buddha's Prayer

Balance and Mobility

- H-Lines
- Puddle Jumping
  - Be sure to cue them to Belly Step from dot to dot and to control their stopping with upright posture and core stability.

Strength for a Purpose

- Clock Stepping
- Teeter-Totter Chair Stands

Overall Objective

- Using Belly Steps and controlling momentum.

The Magic in Music

Supplies

- Written plan
- Equipment list (supplies for activities)
  - Music and music player
  - Thera-Bands, one per person
  - Masking tape
  - Agility dots, 6 to 12 with nonskid surface
  - Poly beam, if available
- Activity printouts—Printouts are available at www.HumanKinetics.com/ABLEBodiesBalanceTraining
  - Walk in the Park
  - Seated Whole-Body Stretch
  - Lunge Stretch
  - Farmer's Stretch
  - Sunbursts
  - Thumb Rolls
  - Knee Lift, Abs In
  - A&Ws at the YMCA
  - Some Simple Standing Moves
  - Box Step
  - Waltzing Matilda
  - Step Together, Step Turns
  - Rows With Check-Mark Feet and a Thera-Band
  - Lazy River
  - Category 3 River
  - Walk and Waddle
  - Allemande Left
- Participant homework for session 12
- Rosters and name tags

Advance Preparation

- Set up chairs. Provide a clear view and a safe exercise space for each participant.
- Be sure you know how to do each activity correctly; use printouts for any extra help you may need.
- Plan Walk in the Park
- Organize and cue music
  - For Walking and Waddle, try *New York, New York*. There are lots of good versions, including the instrumental version by Ray Anthony.
  - For Box Step, try *Blueberry Hill* by Fats Domino.
  - For Step Together, Step Turns, try *Theme From A Summer Place* by Percy Faith and his orchestra. (I find that nothing is better than waltzing music for this activity.)
  - For the strength exercise, try *YMCA* by The Village People.
- Lay down tape for Walk and Waddle
- Create the Lazy River or Class 3 River course
- This session is another great opportunity to take a few pictures of your participants.

Active Warm-Up (Cardiorespiratory Endurance)

- Walk in the Park (Play music and encourage arm swings and head turns.)

Opening

On time with a welcome!

Attendance/Roll Call

Take roll. Did everyone like the music in the park?

Announcements

Make any necessary announcements.

Review and Preview

- Review: Last session they worked on stopping momentum with Puddle Jumping.
- Preview: This week they will work at maintaining momentum using music with Rhythm and Moves.

ABLE Bodies Components

Flexibility

- Seated Whole-Body Stretch
- Lunge Stretch
- Farmer's Stretch combined with Sunbursts

Posture and Core Stability

- Thumb Rolls
- Knee Lift, Abs In (seated or standing)

Strength for a Purpose

- A&Ws at the YMCA to music (cue great core stablility)

Balance and Mobility

Rhythm and Moves

- Some Simple Standing Moves
  - Try standing or walking with big arm swings to *New York, New York*
- Box Step
  - Try activity with *Blueberry Hill*
  - Step with just half-tempo to start. Do one step at a time (like Step and Stop).
  - Do the entire song, if your group is able (make it more aerobic).
- Waltzing Matilda
  - Try activity with *Theme From A Summer Place*
  - Remember, no music the first time through, just sidestepping. They will appreciate the magic in the music more that way.
  - Start the music. When the music starts, they'll notice how their whole body dances.

- As they get comfortable, cue bigger sidesteps. Make it more like walking side lunges.
  - Enjoy the rhythm and waltzing.
- Step Together, Step Turns

Strength for a Purpose
- Rows With Check-Mark Feet and a Thera-Band

More Balance and Mobility
- River Fun—Do something between Lazy River and Category 3 River
  - Walk the shores.
  - Cross at narrowest spots using lunge steps.
  - Cross using agility dots like stepping stones.
  - Cross using masking-tape bridges.
  - Cross using poly beam.
- Walk and Waddle—Do the musical progression.
  - Try *New York, New York* by Frank Sinatra.
  - Ask them if they notice how their balance moves from one foot to the other. (It should remind them of Belly Button Training.)

Closing

On time and with a thank you!

Take-Home Message

With great music, the feet and even the whole body move better. Music helps us anticipate and maintain rhythm and coordination. It's almost magical!

Hook

More music next time!

Homework and Reminders

Hand out their homework and review their new assignment. Answer any questions. Remind them to do their homework twice each week. Announce when the practice session will be held.

Fun and Inspiration
- Praise something special that participants did today.
- End with a song, a mantra, an inspiring quote, or a funny joke and your thanks for coming along on this adventure in better living through exercise.

Make notes of any difficulties you had or activities you did not get to but would like to do later.

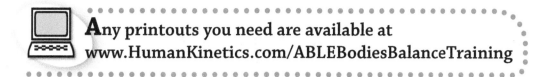

Any printouts you need are available at
www.HumanKinetics.com/ABLEBodiesBalanceTraining

ABLE Bodies Practice Session 12

Supplies
- Music and a music player

Advance Preparation
- Have music cued and ready

Active Warm-Up
- Allemande Left

Flexibility
- Seated Whole-Body Stretch
- Lunge Stretch (Standing with reaching arms)
- Carry the Baby
- Gentlemen's Bow (Standing)

Posture and Core Stability
- A&Ws at the YMCA—Do it to the music, again

Balance and Mobility
- Box Step
- Waltzing Matilda
- Step Together, Step Turns

Strength for a Purpose
- Teeter-Totter Chair Stands

Overall Objective
- Get them to believe in the magic and fun of music

Rock and Roll Heel–Toe

Supplies

- Written plan
- Equipment list (supplies for activities)
  - Music and music player: For warm-up music, try something country-western. For Rock and Walk, try *My Girl* by the Rolling Stones.
  - Thera-Bands, one per person
  - Balloons, one per person
  - Masking tape
  - Agility dots, 6 to 12 with nonskid surface
  - Poly beam, if available
- Activity printouts—Printouts are available at www.HumanKinetics.com/ABLEBodiesBalanceTraining
  - WalkAbout
  - Easy Agility Grid
  - Pivot Turns and Corners
  - Seated Whole-Body Stretch
  - Lunge Stretch
  - Farmer and the Hula
  - Waist Whittlers
  - Wall Push-Ups
  - Show Me the Money
  - Shallow Squats
  - Balloon Lifts
  - Pendulum Legs
  - Wall Push-Offs
  - Heel-Touch Forward, Toe-Touch Back
  - Country-Western Heel and Toe
  - Rock and Walk
  - Box Step
- Participant homework for session 13
- Rosters and name tags

Advance Preparation

- Set up chairs. Provide a clear view and a safe exercise space for each participant.
- Be sure you know how to do each activity correctly; use printouts for any need extra help you may need.
- Have music cued and ready.
- Prepare WalkAbout.
  - It can include puddles to jump (next to a handrail), slalom turns, Pivot Turns and Corners, and an Easy Agility Grid.
- Be ready to take lots of great pictures of your participants.

Active Warm-Up (Cardiorespiratory Endurance)

- WalkAbout
  - Cue for Change of Pace, big step, quick steps, and upright posture.
  - Put yourself by the Agility Grid to hold hands.

Opening

On time with a welcome!

Attendance/Roll Call

Take roll. Last time was really fun. It's nice to have everyone back.

Ice Breaker

Smell the Coffee (It's not that we need an icebreaker at week 13; it's just a nice start to the day!)

Announcements

Make any necessary announcements.

Review and Preview

- Review: We used music last session and it was so helpful and fun. It made our moves smooth and coordinated.
- Preview: We'll be using music again this week. We're going to Rock and Walk.

ABLE Bodies Components

Flexibility

- Seated Whole-Body Stretch
- Lunge Stretch

Posture and Core Stability

- Waist Whittlers
- Show Me the Money

Strength for a Purpose

- Shallow Squats (combine with Balloon Lifts, if appropriate)
- Pendulum Legs
- Wall Push-Offs
- Heel-Touch Forward, Toe-Touch Back

Balance and Mobility

- Country-Western Heel and Toe
- Rock and Walk

Progress from a tandem line to the poly beam, if participants are able and willing.

Closing

On time and with a thank you!

Take-Home Message

Country-Western Heel and Toe can help with foot and leg motion for gait (leg swing and heel plant). Rock and Walk explored the rhythms of walking and how they transfer their weight from one foot to the next.

Hook

Next week we'll explore some of Life's Little Hurdles—literally!

Homework and Reminders

Hand out their homework and review their new assignment. Answer any questions. Remind them to do their homework twice each week. They should also walk with tall, upright, and rib-lifted posture.

Practice Session

Announce when the practice session will be held. This session will practice class activities and review how to do the ABLE bodies exercises correctly. Mention what the session will review.

Announce the next practice session

Fun and Inspiration

- Praise something special that participants did today, such as great attendance, arriving early and ready, learning quickly, volunteering, taking a chance, and so on.
- End with a song, a mantra, an inspiring quote, or a funny joke and your thanks for their continued efforts.

Make notes of any difficulties you had or activities you did not get to but would like to do at another time.

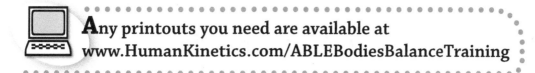
ABLE Bodies Practice Session 13

Supplies

- Music and music player
- Balloons or Slo Mo balls, one per person
- Masking tape

Advance Preparation

- Lay down tandem line for warm-up
- Organize and cue up music

Active Warm-Up

- Walking to music with big steps, arm swings, and singing along.
- Be a pied piper and lead them through turns.
- Follow a tandem line, along a handrail.

Flexibility

- Start with Farmer's Stretch; add a Sunburst
- Farmer and the Hula
- Lunge Stretch
- Seated Whole-Body Stretch

Posture and Core Stability

- Waist Whittlers
- Wall Push-Ups

Balance and Mobility

- Country-Western Heel and Toe
- Rock and Walk

Strength for a Purpose

- Teeter-Totter Chair Stands

Overall Objective

- Enjoying the music and all they can do

Life's Little Hurdles

Supplies

- Written session plan
- Equipment list (supplies for activities)
  - Prepare music for Rock and Walk and Waltzing Matilda
  - Thera-Bands, one per person
  - Masking tape
  - Soccer-type balls made out of paper, two to three per class
  - Hurdles (6-inch [15-centimeter], brightly colored, light-weight plastic ones that flip to lay flat), 6 to 12 per class
  - Poly balance beam (optional, if available)
- Activity printouts—Printouts are available at www.HumanKinetics.com/ABLEBodiesBalanceTraining
  - Seated Whole-Body Stretch
  - Rock and Walk
  - Waltzing Matilda
  - Sidestepping to Music
  - Step Together, Step Turns
  - Shake a Leg
  - Life's Little Hurdles—Sidestep over several hurdles
  - Life's Little Hurdles—Heel–toe walking over hurdles
  - Soccer Drill
  - Playground Swings—See Curl Up and Sit Tall
  - Purse Snatcher
  - Bows and Arrows
  - Side Steps With a Thera-Band (Standing or Seated)
  - Knee Lift, Abs In
- Participant homework for session 14
- Rosters and name tags

Advance Preparation

- Set up chairs. Provide a clear view and a safe exercise space for each participant.
- Be sure you know how to do each activity correctly; use the printouts for any extra help you may need.
- Organize and cue music.
  - You'll need music for the Active Warm-Up. (Find something instrumental, slow, and pretty. I like pianist Wally Clark's *Wild Mountain Thyme*, *Twelfth of Never*, and *As Time Goes By*.)
  - Suggestions for Rock and Walk and waltzing are below or use the same songs from the last session or some of your own favorites.

- Make and tape paper soccer balls
  - Paper balls work great for older participants because they don't fly as far or as fast as real balls or balloons.
  - Crumple up and densely pack newspaper into soccer-sized balls. Wrap tape around each ball, with about 4 bands of tape, so they will keep their shape.
- Prepare soccer playing field.
  - Make a goal box or two out of tape, netting, or furniture.
  - Lay down a few long tape lines about 9 feet (3 meters), to be ball guides that lead towards goal.
- Tape down lines for Rock and Walk.
  - You might be able to use lines in the soccer field
  - If appropriate, lay out poly beams.

Opening

On time and with a welcome!

Attendance/Roll Call

Take roll; is everyone there?

Announcements

Make any necessary announcements

Review and Preview

- Review: Over the past weeks, we've done a few activities to increase our step length. Some examples have been marching, big steps, and Belly Steps.
- Preview: We need good step height for everyday tasks such as climbing steps and stepping over clutter. Today we'll use hurdles to work on step height.

ABLE Bodies Components

Flexibility

Do these activities while playing relaxing, soft music. Note that we are starting with flexibility in order to warm-up for musical pieces to follow.

- Seated Whole-Body Stretch

Cardiorespiratory Endurance and Balance

- Waltzing Matilda
- Step Together, Step Turns
- Rock and Walk
  - Try doing this on tape lines or poly beams.
  - They should take turns with you there to hold hands, or pair them up.
  - Cue using tall, upright posture, visualizing targets, stabilizing their core, and following the music.
  - For music consider using *My Girl* by The Rolling Stones, *Hackensack* by Fountains of Wayne, or *Tennessee Waltz* by Patti Page.

Posture and Core Stability

- Playground Swing (see Curl Up and Sit Tall)
- Purse Snatcher

Balance and Mobility

- Shake a Leg
- Life's Little Hurdles—Sidestep over several hurdles
- Life's Little Hurdles—Heel–Toe Walking over hurdles

To ensure a safe activity, try the following:

- Have participants take turns with hurdles
- Hold their hands or forearms
- Start out with hurdles set flat
- Have participants master one hurdle before attempting a series of hurdles
- Cue previous learning
  - High knees make for bigger steps, and Belly Button Training will help them get over the hurdle better.
  - With each step, they need to move their torso over, too, not just their foot.

Strength for a Purpose

- Bows and Arrows
- Side Steps With a Thera-Band (can be done standing or seated)
- Knee Lift, Abs In (remind them that this activity improves step height and core stability)

Balance and Mobility (a little more)

- Soccer Drill
  - Show participants how to gently nudge-kick a ball, with side of their foot, down the line you've taped down.
  - Make it more fun by timing them.
  - Give everyone two tries.

Closing

On time and with a thank you!

Take-Home Message

Life's Little Hurdles is practice for stepping over everyday clutter and obstacles, such as phone books and shoe boxes. Today they used step height (high knees) and Belly Button Training to help with hurdles. They probably discovered that core control, upright posture, and visual targets all help, too. Have they noticed all the skills they're learning *and* using?

Hook

Hedgehogs are next week. What do hedgehogs have to do with balance training? Come next week and find out!

Homework and Reminders

Hand out their homework and review their new assignment. Answer any questions. Remind them to do their homework twice each week. Be sure to practice how they'll do Shake a Leg on their own. Encourage them to use tall, upright posture this week. Announce when the practice session will be held.

Fun and Inspiration

- Praise something special that participants have accomplished. Mention the awesome hurdle work they did, great attendance, arriving early and ready, learning quickly, volunteering, and taking a chance.
- End with a song, a mantra, an inspiring quote, or a funny joke and your thanks for coming along on this adventure in better living through exercise.

Make notes of any difficulties you had or activities you did not get to but would like to do another time.

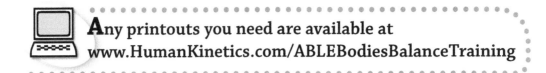
ABLE Bodies Practice Session 14

Supplies

- Music
- Thera-Bands
- Hurdles

Advance Preparation

Prepare for musical activities and hurdles.

Active Warm-Up

Perform these activities with music.

- Walking
- Marching
- Big steps
- Rock and Walk
- Waltzing

Flexibility

- Start with Farmer's Stretch.
- Add Sunbursts.

Have them compare and vote on their preferences between these stretches:

- Farmer's Stretch vs. Proud Mary vs. Lunge Stretch with reaching arms
- (Parentheticals) vs. Carry the Baby
- Gentlemen's Bow—seated vs. standing

Posture and Core Stability

- Playground Swings (see Curl Up and Sit Tall)
- Purse Snatcher

Balance and Mobility

- Shake a Leg
- Life's Little Hurdles (practice with hurdles)

Strength for a Purpose

- Side Steps With a Thera-Band

Overall Objective

- Keep on, keeping on. Progress is happening! Get them to notice their improvements.

Hail the Hedgehogs

Supplies

- Written plan
- Equipment list (supplies for activities)
    - Thera-Bands, one per person
    - Masking tape
    - Steps, one or two, risers optional
    - Agility dots, 6 to 12 with nonskid surface
    - Hedgehogs, 6 to 12
    - Poly beam
    - Music and music player, if desired
- Activity printouts—Printouts are available at www.HumanKinetics.com/ABLEBodiesBalanceTraining
    - WalkAbout
    - Traffic School
    - Seated Whole-Body Stretch
    - Playground Swings (see Curl Up and Sit Tall)
    - Balloon Lifts
    - One-Arm Bandits
    - Push-Backs
    - Push-Backs with Genie Arms
    - Balloon Knee Squeezes
    - Balloon Lap Press-Down
    - Flag Salutes
    - Seated Side Steps With Thera-Band
    - Front Step-Ups
    - Belly Lunges
    - Belly Up
    - The Straight and Narrow
    - Walk and Waddle
    - Tight Tandem Walking on a Line or Beam
    - Put Your Best Foot Up and Get Off Easy
    - Bop the Hedgehogs
    - River Fun
- Participant homework for session 15
- Rosters and name tags

Advance Preparation

- Set up chairs. Provide a clear view and a safe exercise space for each participant.
- Be sure you know how to do each activity correctly; use printouts for any need extra help you may need.
- Organize and cue music.
- Make sure first WalkAbout area is ready and safe.
- Prepare second WalkAbout area, in another room if available.
    - Changing environments will help their learning process
- Lay down tape for Holiday Lines, Lazy River (V-shaped), Walk and Waddle, or The Straight and Narrow (or just plain tandem lines) beside handrail.
- Set out dots for Puddle Jumping.
- Place poly beam beside a handrail.
- This session is a great opportunity to take photos of your participants.

Active Warm-Up (Cardiorespiratory Endurance)

- First WalkAbout
  - Cue for Traffic School challenges: slow, fast, big, small, change direction, curved paths, London Bridges, and window shopping.
  - Do some high fives and opposing circles.
  - March with arm swings.
  - Sing, spell, or do math out loud.

Opening

On time and with a welcome!

Attendance/Roll Call

Take roll. Just two more sessions left.

Announcements

Make any necessary announcements.

Review and Preview

- Review: Well guys, just two sessions left and this is one of them. So far we've learned a lot about keeping our balance under challenging situations. And you have done great! You are stronger, more flexible, and better balanced than you were 3 months ago. And you know how to use posture and core stability to your advantage.
- Preview: Today you will be doing two Walkabouts. You just finished the first. The second will be trickier, with lots of activities to choose from. Choose the ones you like the best or find the most challenging. Ask for help if you need it. Do only what you are 90 percent sure that you can do safely. When you are done with that playground, you'll be off to conquer the new challenge for today, hedgehogs. (Be sure to show them the hedgehogs.) Ready? Let's get going!

ABLE Bodies Components

Flexibility

- Seated Whole-Body Stretch

Invite those who are able to do standing versions of stretches: Proud Mary (or Lunge Stretch), (Parentheticals) (or Carry the Baby), Gentlemen's Bow (seated or standing).

Posture and Core Stability

- Playground Swings (see Curl Up and Sit Tall)
- Balloon Lifts

Balance and Mobility

- Second WalkAbout—It's like a big playground

There's a lot to choose from on this playground. You'd like them to walk about normally first, and check out all the equipment. Then, when they're ready they should choose three things that they want to try. The rules are simple. First, they should ask for help, even if they just think that they may need it. Second, they should only do what they're

90 percent confident that they can do well. (Place yourself between Puddle Jumping and River Fun; the rest of the challenges should have been placed beside handrails. They can choose three of the following choices.

- Belly Lunges across the V-shaped River. They keep crossing it until they can't anymore.
- Puddle Jumping
- The Straight and Narrow—inside the lines, on the line, or keep switching for variability.
- Walk and Waddle—wide-set agility dots provide for wide, lumbering steps
- Tight Tandem Walking on a Line or Beam—Tight tandem means the heel of one foot lands touching the toe of the one behind it. (These challenges need to be done by you or a handrail.)
- Holiday Lines—Look ahead to the next turn.

Strength for a Purpose
- One-Armed Bandits
- Front Step-Ups

Balance and Mobility (yet again)
- Put Your Best Foot Up and Get Off Easy
- Belly Up—climbing stairs
- Bop the Hedgehogs (You can start with agility dots as hedgehogs.)

Closing

On time and with a thank you!

Take-Home Message

Wow! What a group of skills they now have for everyday living and better balance. Getting out of chairs, reaching with Venus de Milo Arms, climbing stairs, and avoiding obstacles are all a little easier. They've been on balance pads, balance beams, and hedgehogs. They've walked the line—tandem lines, wide lines, and squiggly lines. Together they've danced, crossed rivers, and played soccer and volleyball. Tell participants good job, one and all! They're awesome. Do they feel better? Are they moving better? Are they stronger? Are they more flexible? Encourage them to keep up the practice and find ways to make their sessions more enjoyable for them.

Hook

There's just one class to go. It will be a culmination of their many new skills and a fun celebration of their progress. It's game day!

Homework and Reminders

Hand out their homework and review their new assignment. This is the last homework assignment! Wow, that went fast. Answer any questions. Remind them to do their homework twice a week. If you are planning to re-test them, then tell them when. Encourage them to continue doing their homework. Announce when the last practice session will be held.

Fun and Inspiration

- Are they ready to graduate? (The next session is graduation, unless you want to wait until after the testing.) What a great job they've done.
- End with a song, a mantra, an inspiring quote, or a funny joke and your thanks.

Make notes of any difficulties you had or activities you did not get to but would like to do another time. If you've taken photographs of your participants, now is the time to get them ready. see if you have a good one of everyone who will receive a certificate. Consider adding the photo to their certificate.

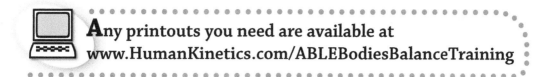
ABLE Bodies Practice Session 15

Supplies

- Balloons, one per person
- Thera-Bands, one per person
- Masking tape
- Agility discs, 6 to 12
- Hedgehogs, 6 to 12
- Poly beam, if available
- Steps, one to two, risers are optional

Advance Preparation

Prepare River of Fun with tape, balance beams, agility dots, and hedgehogs acting as crossing aids. Make easy ways to cross and more challenging ways.

Warm-Up

- WalkAbout
    - Cue slow, fast, big steps, small steps, changes in direction, slalom course, arm swings, window shopping.
- Put Your Best Foot Up and Get Off Easy
    - Work with them individually at the step to practice getting up on it and back down safely.

Flexibility

- Seated and standing versions of Whole-Body Stretch

Posture and Core Stability

- Balloon Lifts
- Balloon Lap Press-Down
- Push-Backs with Genie Arms

Balance and Mobility

- Bop the Hedgehogs
- River Fun
    - Help participants cross the river using beams, agility dots, balance mats, and maybe hedgehogs.

Strength for a Purpose

- Flag Salutes
- Balloon Knee Squeezes with arms reaching
- Put Your Best Foot Up and Get Off Easy
- Seated Side Steps With a Thera-Band

Overall Objective

- Being playful, but persistent about training for better balance

Game Day

Supplies

- Written plan
- Equipment list (supplies for activities)
  - Music and music player
  - Sunglasses, 6 pairs
  - Heads-up glasses, 3 pair if available
  - Soccer balls made of crumpled newspaper and tape, 2 per class
  - Prizes to hide in the park and candy to reach for
  - Masking tape
  - Step (risers are optional)
  - Hedgehogs, 6 to 12
  - Agility dots, 6 to 12 with nonskid surface
  - Poly beam (optional)
  - Certificate of class completion
  - Collection of all your class plans and activity printouts
  - Photographs (if you've taken any, bring them to class)
  - Balance pad (optional, for Bop the Hedgehog)
- Activity printouts—Printouts are available at www.HumanKinetics.com/ABLEBodiesBalanceTraining
  - Walk in the Park
  - Seated Whole-Body Stretch
  - Pass the Duck
  - Bop the Hedgehog
  - It's a Reach
  - Moderate Grids
  - Chain Gang
  - Relays: Get Up and Go Team Relay
  - River Fun: Alligator Pit
- Roster
- Name tags—since you may have extra guests

Advance Preparations

- Prepare and print certificates of completion (see appendix C).
- Arrange for extra staff to help.
- Develop a plan and communicate to your extra staff what you expect.
- Set up chairs. Provide a clear view and a safe exercise space for each participant.
- Be sure you know how to do each activity correctly; use printouts for any extra help you may need.

- Have Walk in the Park area planned, safe, and ready.
- Organize and cue music.
- Set up the games as if they were at a carnival.
- Put down tape for River Fun or Alligator Pit with toys and prizes inside the river.

Active Warm-Up (Cardiorespiratory Endurance)

- Walk in the Park

Play some happy music (*Oh, What a Beautiful Morning*, from Oklahoma or a version by Ray Charles). Give some of them sunglasses; others can use the heads-up glasses. Give others a large-print article to read and walk with. Others can walk with an imaginary (or real) camera, snapping pictures. Maybe a few could kick those paper soccer balls. Cue them to walk, talk, and use arm swings. Cue head turns to look at the images you've put on the walls. Pretend a big wind comes up, a lion chases them, there are puddles to step over, and friends to meet and shake hands with. Be creative. Keep your eye on them for safety. Enjoy. Maybe take pictures yourself.

Opening

On time and with a welcome!

Attendance/Roll Call

Take roll. This is our last session. Many thanks to all.

Announcements

Make any necessary announcements.

Review and Preview

- Review: Look at all we've done. Show them all of your class plans and all those printouts of activities! They will be amazed. Leave them out to look at later. If you've taken pictures through the weeks, share them now. Our cornerstones are all things that they can continue to improve, going forward—Be active, take walks, be social, do your homework, come to classes. Remember the ABLE Bodies components: Flexibility, Posture and Core Stability, Strength, and Balance. What's the best exercise? It's the one you'll do.
- Preview: Every good journey should end with a celebration. Thank them all for taking this journey with you. Today is for fun and being happy and proud of all they've accomplished. There is no goal other than to celebrate and enjoy their accomplishments.

ABLE Bodies Components

Flexibility

- Seated Whole-Body Stretch (they'll spend plenty of time on their feet)

Posture and Core Stability

- Pass the Duck

Balance and Mobility

- Bop the Hedgehogs (place a volunteer here)

- It's a Reach—for candy (place a volunteer here)
- Moderate Grids (make an agility grid)—a it's version of hop scotch (needs a volunteer or you)
- Chain Gang (man this one yourself)
- Get Up and Go Team Relay (suggested in chapter 8)
  - Its format is like the Rikli and Jones Get Up and Go test (Rikli and Jones, 2001), but way more fun! (I think the participants move much faster in a game than in a test.)
  - Form relay teams of four. Each team must send all four players around an agility cone and back.
  - The team with the fastest time wins and can challenge another team. Or you can handicap the winning team with a balance beam or tandem line or make everyone use a walker.
- From River Fun, do the Alligator Pit suggestions

Closing

On time and with a thank you!

Take-Home Message

Here the journey ends.

- How many can stand up from a chair more easily?
- Who feels a little more balance confidence?
- Has anyone become more active than in the past?
- Are some tasks easier?
- I thought so! Nice work! Those are the real rewards you'll take home for all your efforts.

Hook

Being stronger and more able will help you maintain your independence longer and keep you connected to your community and doing the things you love longer. Award them their certificates; maybe individually with special remembrances, such as a story about their progress or a photo of them in class.

Fun and Inspiration

- Ask, what's the best way to stay active? The answer is to stay active.
- Ask, what's the best exercise? The answer is the one you'll do!
- Encourage them to stay active and playful. Tell them you hope they've enjoyed the class as much as you've enjoyed teaching it.
- Thank your volunteers. You couldn't have done this day without them.
- Thank all of your participants again for coming along on this adventure and journey with you.

Note that there is no homework nor a practice session this week.

• •

Template for ABLE Bodies Balance Training Sessions

Are you ready to create your own sessions of ABLE Bodies training? Great! Here's a template you can use to ensure you're covering all of the components and creating an effective session for your clients.

Supplies

- Written plan
- Equipment list (supplies for activities)
- Activity printouts (cheat sheets or any notes you may need)
- Participant homework, printed and ready to hand out
- Roster of names and name tags

Advance Preparation

- Set up chairs. Provide a clear view and a safe exercise space for each participant.
- Be sure you know how to do each activity correctly; use printouts for any extra help you may need.
-
-
-

Warm-Up (Cardiorespiratory Endurance)

-
-

Opening

- Welcome
- Attendance/Roll Call
- Icebreaker (optional; may not be needed for every class)
- Set expectations (optional; may only be needed in first class session)
- Announcements
- Review and preview

Flexibility

-
-

Posture and Core Stability

-
-

Strength for a Purpose

-
-

Balance and Mobility

-
-

Cardiorespiratory Endurance (If not done as warm-up)

-
-

Closing

- Take-home message
- Hook
- Homework and reminders
- Fun and inspiration

Certificate of Completion

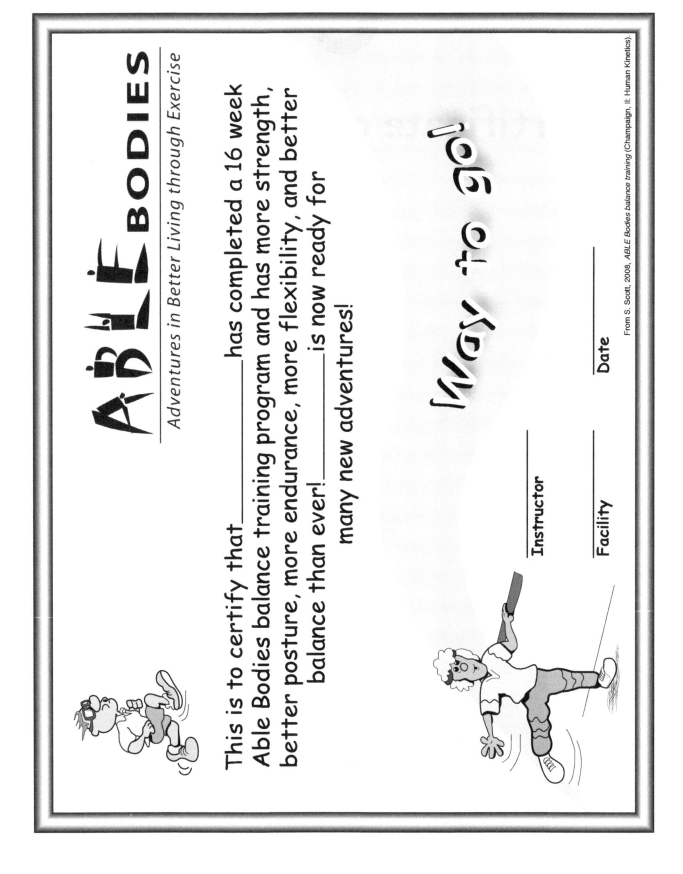

ABLE BODIES

Adventures in Better Living through Exercise

This is to certify that _____ has completed a 16 week Able Bodies balance training program and has more strength, better posture, more endurance, more flexibility, and better balance than ever! _____ is now ready for many new adventures!

Way to go!

Instructor _____

Date _____

Facility _____

Position Glossary

This handy reference tool helps you quickly locate basic positions and modifications, safety positions, and instructor techniques.

BASIC POSITIONS AND MODIFICATIONS

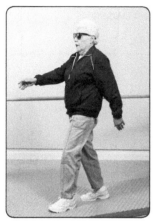

Adding impairments to standing and walking

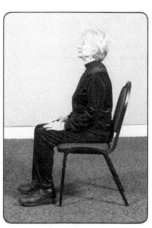

Seated at back of chair with hips touching

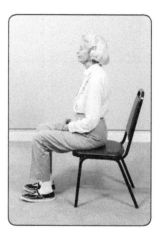

Seated at front of chair (tall sit)

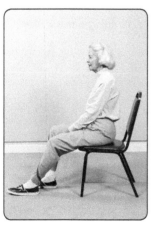

Seated with feet tandem

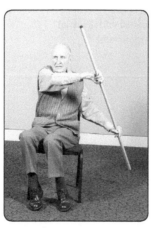

Seated with arm movements

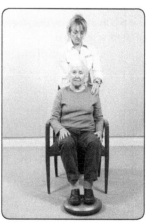

Seated with feet on a balance disc

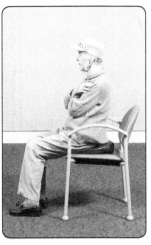

Seated on a balance disc

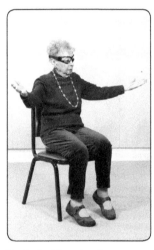

Seated on a balance disc with arms lifted

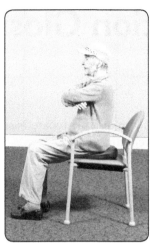

Seated on a balance disc with feet tandem

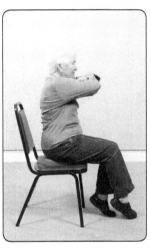

Seated on a balance disc, feet tandem, arms lifted

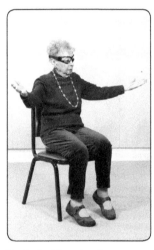

Seated with a visual impairment

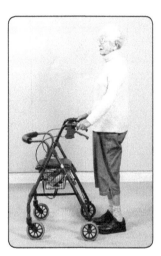

Tall standing with a walker

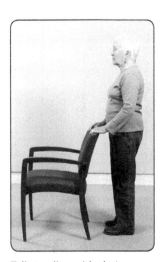

Tall standing with chair support

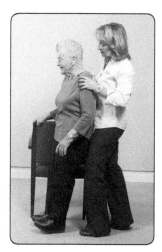

Catching a backward fall

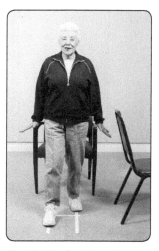

Chair behind and another beside

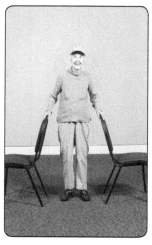

Double-chair support (standing between two chairs)

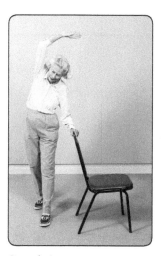

One-chair support

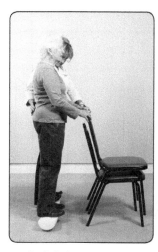

Stacked chair support

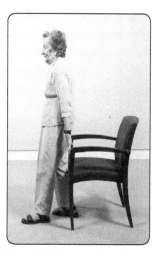

Stand with legs and hand touching front of chair

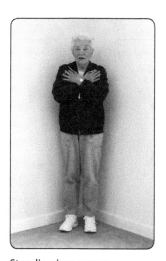

Standing in a corner

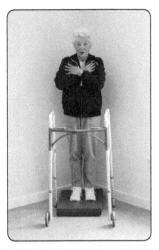

Standing in corner with walker on balance pad

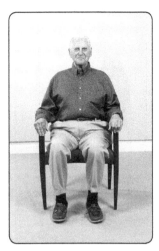

Using a chair for additional back support

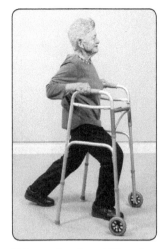

Using walker for additional support

INSTRUCTOR TECHNIQUES

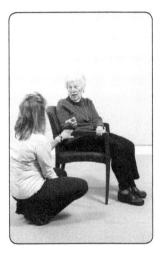

Active listening

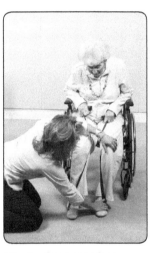

Aligning knee over foot

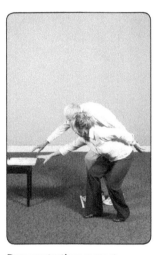

Demonstrating correct technique

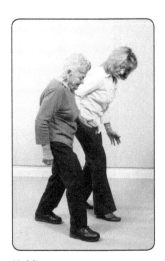

Holding one arm

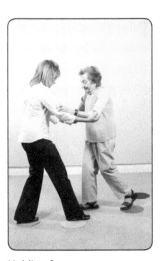

Holding forearms

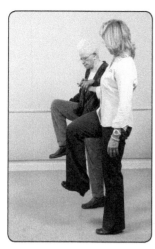

Holding hand while walking along handrail

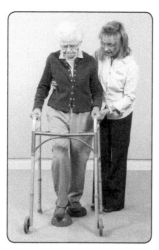

Holding torso while participant uses a walker

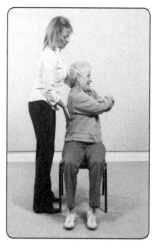

Using light touches to help find correct position

References

Alexander, N.B., M.M. Gross, J.L. Medell, M.R. Hofmeyer. 2001. Effects of functional ability and training on chair-rise biomechanics in older adults. *Journal of Gerontology Series A: Biological Sciences and Medical Sciences* 56(9): M538-547.

American Geriatrics Society, British Geriatrics Society, and American Academy of Orthopedic Surgeons Panel on Falls Prevention. 2001. Guideline for the prevention of falls in older persons. *Journal of the American Geriatrics Society* 49(5): 664-672.

Argue, J. 2000. *Parkinson's disease and the art of moving.* Oakland, CA: New Harbinger Publications, Inc.

Barnett, A., B. Smith, S. Lord, M. Williams, and A. Baumand. 2003. Community-based group exercise improves balance and reduces falls in at-risk older people: A randomized controlled trial. *Age and Aging* 32(4): 407-414.

Berg, K.O., and D. Kairy. 2002. Balance interventions to prevent falls. *Generations* 26(4): 75-81.

Campbell, A., M.J. Borrie, and G.F. Spears. 1989. Risk factors for falls in a community-based prospective study of people 70 years and older. *Journal of Gerontology* 44: 112-117.

Campbell, J.A., M.C. Robertson, M.M. Gardner, R.N. Norton, and D.M. Buchner. 1999. Fall prevention over 2 years: A randomized controlled trial in women 80 years and older. *Age and Aging* 28(6): 513-518.

Chandler, J.M., P.W. Duncan, G. Kochersberger, and S. Studenski. 1998. Is lower extremity strength gain associated with improvement in physical performance and disability in frail, community-dwelling elders? *Archives of Physical Medicine and Rehabilitation* 79(1): 24-30.

Chang, J.T., S.C. Morton, L.Z. Rubenstein, W.A. Mojica, M. Maglione, M.J. Suttrop, E.A. Roth, and P.G. Shekelle. 2004. Interventions for the prevention of falls in older adults: Systematic review and meta-analysis of randomized clinical trials. *British Medical Journal* 328(7441): 680-687.

Day, L., B. Fildes, I. Gordon, M. Fitzharris, H. Flamer, and S. Lord. 2002. Randomized factorial trial of falls prevention among older people living in their own homes. *British Medical Journal* 325(7356): 128-133.

Dunn, K. 2007. This is Your Brain on Music. *The Oregonian*, page 10.

Eng, J.J., K.S. Chu, C.M. Kim, A.S. Dawson, A. Carswell, and K.E. Hepburn. 2003. A community-based exercise program for persons with chronic stroke. *Medicine & Science in Sports & Exercise* 35(8): 1271-1278.

Gladwell, M. 2000. *The tipping point: How little things can make a big difference.* Boston: Little Brown.

Harmon, N.M., and L. Kravitz. 2007. The beat goes on: The effects of music on exercise. *IDEA Fitness Journal* 4(8): 72.

Horak, F.B., A. Mirka, and C.L. Shupert. 1989. The role of peripheral vestibular disorders in postural dyscontrol in the elderly. In *The development of posture and gait across the lifespan,* ed. M. Woollacott and A. Shumway-Cook, 253-279. Columbia, SC: University of South Carolina Press.

Hoyert, D.L., D.K. Kochanek, and S.L. Murphy. 1999. *National Vital Statistic Report* June 30; 47(19): 1-104.

Kochanek, K.C., and B.L. Smith. 2004. Deaths: Preliminary data for 2002. *National Vital Statistics Report* 52(13): 1-47.

Liu-Ambrose, T., K.M. Khan, J.J. Eng, P.A. Janssen, S.R. Lord, H.A. McKay. 2004. *Resistance and agility training reduce fall risk in women aged 75 to 85 with low bone mass: A 6-month randomized, controlled trial.* Journal of the American Geriatrics Society 52(5): 657-665.

Lord, S.R., S. Castell, J. Corcoran, et al. 2003. The effect of group exercises on physical functioning and falls in frail older people living in retirement villages: A randomized, controlled trial. *Journal of the American Geriatrics Society* 51(12): 1685-1692.

Mazzeo, R.S., P. Cavanagh, W.J. Evans, M. Fiatarone, J. Hagberg, E. McAuley, and J. Startzell. 1998. ACSM position stand: Exercise and physical activity for older adults. *Medicine & Science in Sports & Exercise* 30(6): 992-1008. Philadelphia: Lippincott, Williams, & Wilkins.

McGill, S. 2007. *Low back disorders.* Champaign, IL: Human Kinetics.

Nelson, M., W. Rejeski, S. Blair, et al. 2007. Physical Activity and Public Health in Older adults: Recommendation from the American College of Sports Medicine and the American Heart Association. *Medicine and Science in Sports and Exercise* 39(8): 1435-1445.

O'Loughlin, J.L., Y. Robitaille, J.F. Boivin, and S. Suissa. 1993. Incidence of and risk factors for falls and injurious falls among the community-dwelling elderly. *American Journal Epidemiology* 137(3): 342-354.

Province, M.A., E.C. Hadley, M.C. Hornbrook, et al. 1995. The effects of exercise on falls in elderly patients: A preplanned meta-analysis of the FICSIT trials. *Journal of the American Medical Association* 273(17): 1341-1347.

Rikli, R.E., and C.J. Jones. 2001. *Senior fitness test manual*. Champaign, IL: Human Kinetics.

Rose, D.J. 2003. *FallProof! A comprehensive balance and mobility training program*. Champaign, IL: Human Kinetics.

Rose, D.J., and S. Clark. 2000. Can the control of bodily orientation be significantly improved in a group of older adults with a history of falls? *Journal of the American Geriatrics Society* 48(3): 275-282.

Rubenstein, L.Z., and K.R. Josephson. 2002. The epidemiology of falls and syncope. *Clinics in Geriatric Medicine* 18(2):141-158.

Sacks, O. 2007. *Musicophilia: Tales of music and the brain*. New York: Knopf.

Scott, S.M., and R.I. Rosenberg. 2005. Methods to improve and maintain balance, mobility, flexibility and balance confidence in older adults. *Medicine and Science in Sports and Exercise* 37(5)(Suppl): S256.

Shumway-Cook, A., and M.H. Woollacott. 2001. *Motor control, theory and practical applications*. Baltimore: Williams and Wilkins.

Takeshima, N., N.L. Rogers, M.E. Rogers, M.M. Islam, D. Koizumi, and S. Lee. 2007. Functional Fitness Gain varies in older adults depending on exercise mode. *Medicine and Science in Sports and Exercise* 39(11): 2036-2043.

Tinetti, M.E., M. Speechly, and S.P. Ginter. 1988. Risk factors for falls among elderly persons living in the community. *New England Journal of Medicine* 319(26):1701-1707.

Wagenaar, R.C., K. Holt, M. Dubo, and C. Ho. 2003. Gait risk factors for falls in older adults: A dynamic perspective. *Journal of the American Society on Aging* 26(4): 15-21.

Wood, R.H., R. Reyes, M.A. Welsch, J. Favaloro-Sabatier, M. Sabatier, C. Matthew Lee, L.G. Johnson, and P.F. Hooper. 2001. *Medicine & Science in Sports & Exercise* 33(10): 1751-1758.

Index

Note: The italicized t or f following a page number denotes a table or figure, respectively.

About the Author

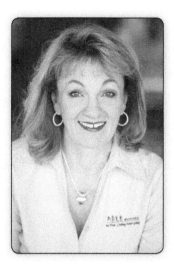

Sue Scott, MS, is an exercise consultant, balance specialist, and active living consultant. In her work with older adults and through her fitness company, Renewable Fitness, Scott focuses on bettering the health and well-being of seniors, particularly frail older adults.

Scott has over 10 years of experience working exclusively with seniors and fitness. She has worked in fitness as an educator, researcher, consultant, and personal trainer since 1986. She is certified as an American College of Sports Medicine (ACSM) health and fitness instructor and an International Dance Exercise Association (IDEA) master trainer.

Scott is the creator of the Adventures in Better Living through Exercise (ABLE) Bodies Balance Improvement Protocols. A National Blueprint on Active Aging grant in 2003 enabled Scott to research the effectiveness of the ABLE Bodies balance techniques in a randomized, controlled trial. In 2005, Scott presented her findings at the American College of Sports Medicine (ACSM) conference in Nashville as well as the International Association of Homes and Services for the Ageing (IAHSA) conference in Norway and the American Public Health Association (APHA) conference in Philadelphia.

In addition to teaching group fitness classes and personal training for seniors, Scott is collaborating with Fay Horak, PhD, John Nutt, MD, and others at Oregon Health and Science University (OHSU) to develop an at-home exercise program to delay mobility losses in Parkinson's patients. She is also working with OHSU biomedical engineers Misha Pavel and Holly Jimmison, PhD, to develop interactive exercise videos for frail seniors and for those with Alzheimer's.

In her free time, Scott enjoys skiing, mountain biking, gardening, and vacationing with her family. She and her husband, Rick, and their two children reside in Happy Valley, Oregon.

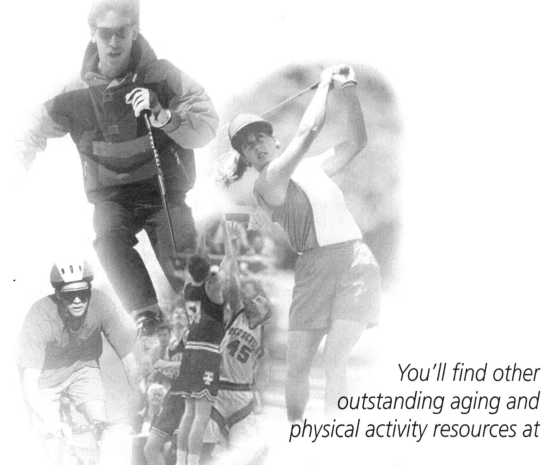